# THE COMPLETE BOOK OF
# food
## combining

## Also by Kathryn Marsden

*The Food Combining Diet*

*Food Combining in 30 Days*

*The Food Combiner's Meal Planner*

*Food Combining Two-day Detox*

*All Day Energy*

*The All Day Energy Diet*

*Superskin*

*Hotline to Health*

*Evening Primrose*

*Reader's Digest Mind & Mood Foods*
(co-author with Hazel Courteney)

*Reader's Digest Body & Beauty Foods*
(co-author with Hazel Courteney)

*Good Gut Healing*

# KATHRYN MARSDEN

## THE COMPLETE BOOK OF

# food
# combining

A new, easy-to-use guide to the
most successful diet ever

piatkus

PIATKUS

First published in Great Britain in 2000 by Piatkus
Reprinted 2005, 2006, 2008, 2009 (twice)

A CIP catalogue record for this book
is available from the British Library

ISBN 978-0-7499-2586-4

Typeset by Paul Saunders
Printed and bound in Great Britain by
MPG Books Ltd, Bodmin, Cornwall

Papers used by Piatkus are natural, renewable and recyclable
products sourced from well-managed forests and certified
in accordance with the rules of the Forest Stewardship Council.

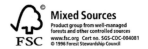

**Mixed Sources**
Product group from well-managed
forests and other controlled sources
www.fsc.org  Cert no. SGS-COC-004081
© 1996 Forest Stewardship Council
FSC

Piatkus
An imprint of
Little, Brown Book Group
100 Victoria Embankment
London EC4Y 0DY

An Hachette UK Company
www.hachette.co.uk

www.piatkus.co.uk

*For Gill and for Sarah, dear and precious friends*

. . . may a slow wind work these words of love
around you an invisible cloak to mind your life

*Anam Cara – Spiritual Wisdom from the Celtic World,*
John O'Donohue (Bantam Books)

## Note on previous printer's error

When *The Complete Book of Food Combining* first came out in hardback and also in large format softback, page 21 unfortunately contained a printer's error which listed Butter as a protein! Whoops! My apologies. The mistake has been corrected for this new paperback edition. Butter is, of course, a fat and, for the purposes of food combining, will combine successfully with proteins or starches. See page 434 for detailed information on fats and oils.

Kathryn Marsden

# Contents

## PART TWO  Food Combining to Improve Your Health

## PART THREE Over 50 Fabulous Food Combining Recipes

Kathryn regrets that, due to the cost and time involved in dealing with her already overloaded mailbag, she can no longer reply individually to letters nor is she able to comment on or advise on specific case histories. She is, however, always delighted to hear from readers and promises to read every letter.

# *Spiral*

The wild vortex that whirls cabbages into
Labyrinths of crunchy green
Shapes the horns of a ram
Coils the timeless serpent and
Etches curves into sea shells so smooth
You hardly dare to touch them

Spiral energy
The symbol of creative power
Turns the seasons
Weaves DNA
Rolls thunder
Spins the sun and the moon
Balances the earth's rotation
Encourages health and healing
And links friends in love, thought and deed

Spiral energy
May it bless you and
As a drop of water touches the stillness of the pool
May healing spin from the centre of your being and
Completely and safely
Bring harmony to your life and
Keep you well.

This glorious poem was sent to me some years ago in a Christmas card. I have no idea who wrote it and so am unable to credit the author but would be happy to do so if someone can identify his or her work. In the meantime, I hope he or she will not mind my sharing it with you.

# Acknowledgements

Armfuls of gratitude and appreciation to:

Gillian Hamer, Rhaya Jordan and Jamie Gisby for their practitioner expertise, to Barbara Griggs for her Foreword, to Alan Simpson for helping with early edits, and to my very special agent Michael Alcock for his friendship and guidance.

Thanks also to Alice Booth, Lynne Booth, Jean Cooper, Muriel Dubourdieu, Vera Garschagen, Patricia Hubbard, Alan Johnson, Mary King, Carol Newton, Jan Robinson, Rose Rosney and to my mother for their recipe contributions.

To Judy Piatkus, Rachel Winning and Katie Andrews for their warm welcome and to Anne Lawrance for her sensible and gifted editing. And to Paul Saunders for his creative design and layout.

And finally and most especially to my dear and delightful husband Richard who, for the year that it has taken to get this work on to the word processor, kept the ship afloat and did everything domestic, including the ironing! Somehow, he stayed sane throughout, and still found time to soothe my furrowed brow, cricked neck and stiff shoulders, and above all to make me laugh. I will love you for the rest of my life.

# Foreword

first came across food combining 15 years ago, when I was asked to write about it for a glossy magazine. I studied the available texts with astonishment. Don't mix foods that fight? Don't mix starch and protein? Don't eat fish and chips? No more bread and cheese – of which J C Squire once wrote, 'What God hath joined together, let no man put asunder.'

Baffled, I sought out a knowledgeable friend – Lilian Schofield, Director of London's pioneering healthfood shop, Wholefood. 'Does it really work?' I asked her.

'Oh yes,' she told me. 'And you'll find you have a mind as clear as a bell, too.'

I tried it out for a week: it wasn't all that complicated. At the end of those seven days, I had mysteriously shed two or three surplus pounds, though I certainly hadn't been consciously dieting. Digestive problems of which I had hardly been aware had eased off, leaving me with a digestive peace that was a whole new experience. And yes, my mental functioning seemed to have shifted up a gear.

I cannot pretend that I have been a faithful food combiner ever since. But at times when my vital energies seemed in decline, my mental processes were fuzzy, or when my digestive system intruded on my notice, I have found it a marvellous tool for restoring all three.

However, thousands of people have probably tried food combining and then given up on it for good because different experts seemed to offer such totally different sets of rules. Are nuts protein or neutral? Are tomatoes fruits or vegetables? And why can't you eat beans – or drink a glass of wine with a plate of pasta?

Or they've given up because there were too many rules: not only did they have to remember which foods were starch and which were protein – but which were acid and which were alkaline too.

Or they've given up because they found it hard to stick to it for three meals a day, seven days a week.

It is this confusion and inflexibility, too, which has made food combining such an easy target for doctors or dieticians, who dismiss it out of hand on the basis that mixing starch and protein is 'normal'.

*The Complete Book of Food Combining* cuts through this confusion to give us a clear, fresh, simple and highly persuasive account of the system. It takes note of a number of vital new findings in the ever-expanding field of nutritional research, as well as presenting both the history and the science of food combining in an easy, readable style.

Kathryn has been food combining herself for over 17 years: she has also been prescribing it to thousands of patients who come to her nutritional consultancy with a wide spectrum of ailments. So her book is based on long practical experience – and a supremely practical user-friendly book it is, too. Kathryn puts food combining back into the normal world in which we all live – and eat and drink with friends, go out for a *pizza margarita* and a glass of wine and occasionally overdose on our favourite foods.

Much more than just another book on food combining, this is a treasury of wisdom, useful tips and delicious recipes, brimming with helpful advice about how to put the system into practice without getting bogged down by the detail.

I defy anyone to read through this book, or even just dip into it, and not be encouraged to get a grip at last on their eating habits, and work towards that digestive health which is the foundation of all well-being.

Barbara Griggs
July 2000

# Introduction

'Don't just live the length of your life, live the width
and breadth of it as well.'

Kathryn Marsden

During the research for this book, I came across a document entitled *Rules for the Preservation of Health* in which readers are advised to observe 'moderation in eating and drinking, regularity in exercise, recreation and rest, cleanliness, short hours of labour and study, equanimity of temper and equality of temperature'.

Good advice, you might say. If we were all able to follow it, we might all be a great deal healthier as a result. The surprise is that these recommendations were made nearly a century ago, before World War I. But would it have made any difference if we had listened to that advice? Since then, vast improvements in living standards, the provision of indoor plumbing and sanitation, and the advent of antibiotics and vaccinations, have certainly played their part in eradicating the infectious diseases, such as diphtheria, smallpox and typhus, that took the lives of hundreds and thousands of victims at a time.

So what has happened since? Haven't we simply swapped one set of diseases for another? Today we are troubled by different plagues – insidious and debilitating disorders that kill us slowly rather than quickly: heart and circulatory disorders, diabetes, stroke, osteoporosis (brittle bone disease) and cancer. Asthma, allergies, ulcers, irritable bowel syndrome and Chronic Fatigue Syndrome all appear to be on the increase. Obesity has reached epidemic proportions. The menopause has become an illness. Everyone you know has 'got cholesterol'. Depression and stress are two of the most common reasons for visiting the doctor. Not-so-good health, it seems, invades the quality of almost everyone's life.

With lemming-like determination, we continue to short-change our bodies: we eat and drink too much, work too long, rest too little, invite and put up with stress, ignore exercise, allow unimportant irritations to gnaw away at us, and bottle up our feelings. In an almost competitive race to see who can get sickest quickest, we take our health pretty much for granted – until it fails us. When the realisation dawns that we are not immortal and our bodies become too exhausted to fight off the latest bout of illness, panic may drive us to take stock and seek help.

Our first port of call is likely to be our doctor. No one could doubt the value of early diagnosis and of modern medical and surgical technology but it is slowly becoming clear that, if we are to make any impact on current statistics, we have to turn our attention to *preventing disease rather than waiting for it to happen before we take action.*

Improving the quality of our diet as a way of reducing the risk of degenerative illness is gaining far wider acceptance, both medically and scientifically. If it's heart disease we're trying to prevent, experts tell us that we could help matters considerably by eating less fat. If we want stronger bones, calcium-rich foods are the thing. And one of the ways we might reduce cancer risk, say researchers, is to go for foods rich in antioxidants.

We know this stuff, don't we? So why are so many of us still not eating as healthily as we could? One reason could be confusion. It's easy to get the idea that each illness needs a different diet – so how can we possibly follow all of them? Do we need to?

The good news is, in fact, that major health agencies are beginning to spread the message that one simple eating plan could lower the risk of a whole range of chronic diseases, including cancer, heart disease, stroke, diabetes and osteoporosis.

*The Complete Book of Food Combining* is a brand new, holistic approach that incorporates all of the latest health guidelines for disease prevention, together with plenty of seriously useful tips for a healthier lifestyle. As well as all that, you'll find an innovative and exciting perspective on food combining and learn why it can be such a valuable part of any successful health programme.

In this new book, you'll discover that my original simplified food combining system has been completely revised and updated. It follows the same philosophy that I have always encouraged in my nutrition practice, offering a whole health package that works closely with other important aspects of a healthy lifestyle, such as exercise, stress management and weight control. No hard regimes, no hassle. It is especially easy to follow, needs no specialist knowledge and uses everyday foods that are familiar to all of us.

Get healthy.
Get food combining.

## But Why Choose Food Combining?

'Nutritional research, like a modern star of Bethlehem, brings hope that sickness need not be a part of life.'

Adelle Davis (1904–74), US nutritionist and writer,
*The New York Times Magazine*, 20 May 1973

Food combining could probably be described as one of the most successful diets of all time, some might say the most successful. When I was asked to write my first book, *The Food Combining Diet*, in 1993, I had no idea at the time that it would be so popular and attract such an immense following. A familiar title in the bestseller lists, the book has sold hundreds of thousands of copies and, to date, has been reprinted 17 times.

So why write another food combining book?

In the decade that has passed since I began working on that first manuscript, lots of new and fascinating information has come to light that is now incorporated into *The Complete Book of Food Combining*. I really want to share that with you.

Food combining follows the simple idea that foods such as eggs, cheese, fish, meat and soya don't mix well with potatoes, rice, pasta, bread and cereals. If you've heard or read about this system before, you may have associated it with something called the Hay diet. You may even have been put off because it all sounded too troublesome to follow. (For more information on Dr Hay and the history of food combining see pages 95–8.)

Well, I agree with you.

I've always been convinced that, for some people (me included), some aspects of the diet promoted by Dr Hay are a little too rigid and too complicated – essentially not suited to our modern lifestyle.

In fact, Dr Hay's more complex methods differ in several very basic ways from the easy-to-follow style I have developed.

For almost a decade, I had used my own interpretation of food combining in my own clinic.

And my patients loved it.

It was super-simple to follow and, I felt, well suited to the mad, frenetic, no-time-to-spare lifestyle that most of us lead.

No long lists of foods to commit to memory.

No unrealistic rules and regulations.

Again, no hassle.

When a number of patients bemoaned that they'd already tried the original Hay system but found it was too hidebound by rules, regulations and endless things to remember, I decided to disentangle it a bit.

Well, quite a lot, in fact.

The more I delved, the more I realised that food combining was definitely not the crank regime it is occasionally accused of being. It was supported by plenty of sound science and a generous dollop of common sense. But it wasn't the easiest of systems to get a handle on. Someone who is already struggling with a long-term weight problem, or who hasn't been well for a while, may not feel that they can cope with a diet that takes too much time and lots of effort. The whole package needs to be clear, workable, stress-free and, above all, UNCOMPLICATED.

So that's what I did. Unravelled it, kicked out the stuff that wasn't important, added some fresh new ideas, and put it into plain, understandable language. The results were nothing short of amazing and, I have to say, in most cases, unexpected. It certainly proved to me that food combining can be just as effective, and probably much more enjoyable, when it is streamlined and simplified.

Although I felt sure that I'd see some good results, I didn't expect to see such significant changes. What actually happened was that a considerable majority of patients reported remarkable improvements and, in many cases, complete recovery from a long list of different ailments. I claim no credit for any of this, nor would I want or expect any. I did nothing more than give people an empathetic ear, moral support and the benefit of my own training. They did the work and achieved the results by putting the food combining and other health recommendations into practice.

And not just my own patients. It is wonderful to hear how those I've never met have also benefited. When people take the trouble to write to me – some have gone to endless lengths to track me down just to say how much a book or an article or a broadcast has helped them overcome a particular health problem that had plagued them for years – then I know my faith in food combining as part of a healthy lifestyle is completely justified. I still receive letters from readers and from former patients who keep me in touch with their progress and who are still convinced that the dietary changes I recommended have changed their lives for the better.

And it's not just in the UK that this happens. On business trips to the Far East, the US and Australia, I have found fit and healthy food combiners who wouldn't eat any other way. In Singapore, an ambassador's wife told me that when she started food combining everyone thought she was 'a little bit crazy' but when they saw how much her health had improved, they all followed her lead. 'Now it's a food combining embassy,' she told me.

▶ I've used my particular kind of food combining to treat all kinds of digestive disorders, and to relieve bloating and irritable bowel.

▶ It's particularly good at dealing with food allergies and also seems to strengthen resistance to hay fever.

▶ It's also one of *the* best diets for improving energy levels.

▶ Because food combining sustains and nourishes, it helps to support the body against the damaging effects of stress.

▶ And surprisingly, perhaps, food combining has proved itself a winner in the weight-loss stakes, helping to achieve steady weight loss without the need to account for every kilojoule or calorie, **and succeeding where so many other weight-loss programmes have failed.**

## So is Food Combining for You?

Well, it's important to bear in mind that nothing is a panacea for all ills. There are no magic bullets. But there is a great deal of common sense healthy eating and lifestyle advice here that can help to relieve symptoms, regulate imbalances, encourage healing and enhance well-being. Food combining is a gentle, simple, harmless system that clearly has helped a considerable number of people regain their health.

All I can say is try it.

If you've tried it before and given up, *please* give it another go. If you are an experienced food combiner but want more information, there's plenty here. If you've been struggling for years to get into shape, this could be your chance to shed those unwanted kilos for good. And if your health isn't so great and you need a lift, food combining could be the answer. I wish you the very best of good health.

## How to Use this Book

▶ Part One shows you the essential basics. And it lets you into the diet side of things straight away. In addition to the simplest and best food combining you've ever come across, you'll find plenty of short cuts, tips and easy-to-follow food charts. At the end of Part One you'll find a chapter on the history of food combining too.

▶ Once you're up and running, you can turn to specific sections in Part Two that are of special interest. In this section you'll find out how food combining can contribute so much to general well-being. It kicks off with a supersection on **healthy weight loss** (pages 112–55) which gives you all the latest on how to deal safely and effectively with weight problems – and some encouraging facts you might not have heard about before. You'll also find really practical advice on conditions that can be a problem in their own right but that can seriously hinder all your attempts to get your weight back to normal. Look up the low-down on **fluid retention** (pages 156–66), **food allergies** (pages 202–18), **good digestion** (pages 167–201), **eating disorders** (pages 273–99), **low blood sugar** (pages 300–28) and **stress** (pages 329–47). My simple **detox diet** and **skin cleansing programme** begins on page 219. And check out the importance of **proper breathing** (pages 262–72).

▶ Part Three has more than 50 fabulous recipes to get you started. These meals are all about maximum nourishment with minimum preparation. They'll help you to eat more healthily however busy you are. Either follow them exactly or, using the guidelines on pages 348 and 418, adapt them to suit your own tastes and menu preferences.

At the back of the book, there's an extensive **resources** section (pages 438–47) that gives suggestions on where to find further help if you need it and how to locate any products and services mentioned throughout the book. There's also some information on the more technical aspects of **food combining chemistry** (pages 420–37), for those who are interested.

Read on; I'm sure you'll enjoy the experience.

Kathryn Marsden
Gloucestershire, England

*Kathryn*

# PART ONE

# The Basics of Food Combining

# CHAPTER 1

# Keep it Simple

'In all your striving, let love be your guide for it is the greatest power in the universe.'

Alfred Vogel, nutrition expert and pioneer in natural medicine, 1902–96

## The Week Before...

Before you begin to food combine, do you think you could introduce some very basic healthy changes to your existing diet and shopping habits?

OK, for one week before you make any moves towards food combining, try to cut back on the following items:

▶ Alcohol

▶ Artificial sweeteners and foods that contain them

▶ Beef and pork products

▶ Coffee

▶ Cola drinks

▶ Cow's milk

▶ Cow's milk cheese

▶ Fizzy drinks

▶ Margarine-type spreads

▶ Salt

▶ Sugar

▶ Sugary foods

▶ Tea

▶ Bread and other wheat-based products such as pastry, cakes, biscuits and breakfast cereals (check labels to be sure)

Reduce your intake of tea to two cups per day and work your way towards cutting right back on coffee by the end of the week. First make it weaker and then start reducing by one cup every two days. One cup per day is a good goal to work towards. Giving up coffee overnight, especially if you are used to drinking it strong or in quantity, can cause withdrawal headaches, anxiety, restless limbs and nervous twitches. Each time you give up a coffee, substitute a cup of herbal or fruit tea, green tea, a glass of apple or carrot juice, or drink a glass of filtered water. Eventually, you might decide to give up coffee altogether. If you really can't cope without your caffeine, limit yourself to one cup of coffee and one cup of tea per day.

Also this week, re-think your shopping list. Introduce an extra fresh vegetable every day, add a small green salad as a starter to your main meal each day, and try to increase your intake of fresh fruit.

**Eating for Better Health** (pages 60–81) also has lots of useful info on how to make the best of your diet. And, for quick reference, check out my **Swap Sheet** (pages 80–1) for ideas on how to replace some not-so-healthy items in your shopping trolley with some really healthy alternatives.

Don't worry about food combinations at this point. We'll be introducing these later on.

During this first preparation week, continue reading *The Complete Book of Food Combining*. The chapters that follow not only explain food combining in more detail, but also contain lots of good health and lifestyle advice on healthy weight loss, fluid retention, food allergies, detoxification, stress, balancing blood sugar, enjoyable exercise, and much more.

## The Only Two Rules You Need to Follow

The secret behind the success of my kind of food combining is its absolute simplicity. Take some time now to familiarise yourself with the only two guidelines you will ever need to remember:

> ## ! ESSENTIAL
>
> **1. THE FIRST RULE**
> Eat fruit on an empty stomach.
>
> **2. THE SECOND RULE**
> Don't combine *concentrated* proteins with *concentrated* starches at the same meal.
>
> You can use the chart on page 15 as an initial guide.
> But don't go there just yet.
>
> Before you introduce rule 2, follow rule 1 (the fruit rule) for a full week.

## Eat Fruit on an Empty Stomach

On page 10, I've suggested that you cut out a few of the not-so-helpful foods from your regular shopping list. During your week of preparation, it's also a good idea to begin eating fruit and drinking fruit juices separately from other foods. **Remember: don't make any effort to food combine until you have followed the guidelines on pages 10–11 and, at the same time, completed one full week of just separating your fruit intake from other foods.**

**There are lots of ways to get more fruit into your diet. For example, do you think you could:**

▶ Drink a glass of fresh juice first thing in the morning – as soon as you get up. Then have breakfast after you've washed and dressed.
*Or*

▶ Eat two or three pieces of fresh fruit as a refreshing light breakfast instead of your usual breakfast once or twice a week?
*Or*

▶ Have an apple, a pear or a couple of bananas as a mid-morning snack instead of coffee and biscuits?
*Or*

▶ If you need a lift in the middle of the afternoon, enjoy a glass of fresh fruit juice instead of tea.
*Or*

▶ Instead of eating fruit as a dessert after your evening meal, why not have melon, grapes or a fresh fruit salad as a starter?

Try to leave about 15 minutes between your fruit starter and your main course. By eating fruit on an empty stomach, you'll be helping your digestion to work more efficiently. You will also probably notice that you are eating more fruit than before.

Always dilute pure fruit juice with about 30 per cent water.

**Remember**

It's fine to eat fruit or drink juices:
- first thing in the morning
- between meals
- as a starter or aperitif

*but don't* eat fruit or drink juices:
- *with other foods*
- *in the middle of a meal*
- *as a dessert*

After you have followed the first rule for a week, introduce
**the second rule**.

## Don't Combine Proteins and Starches at the Same Meal

At the outset, this can seem a daunting prospect. Isn't it going to be
difficult to face a diet that says no more bread and cheese, fish and
chips, burger and fries or meat and potatoes?

There is no need to avoid these familiar combinations forever. If you
have a real craving for a particular protein/starch dish, then enjoy it –
say – once or twice a week. I'm not asking you to food combine every
day. Nothing terrible is going to happen to you if you have days off!

Remember that *The Complete Book of Food Combining* encourages
flexibility. If you're at a restaurant, out with friends or at a business
lunch and you find it isn't easy to food combine, then don't bother
about it, although food combining outside the home isn't as difficult
as you might imagine. I'll be covering this aspect later on – but, in the
meantime, just concentrate on food combining when you are at home.

## Start Slowly

To begin with, I'm suggesting that you food combine for only **one
meal** on **one day** each week. You might choose Wednesday lunchtime,
Thursday supper or Sunday breakfast. Whenever suits you.

Then, once you feel confident, increase this so that you are food
combining **one meal only (lunch *or* dinner)** for two days each week,
then lunch or dinner on three days, then four, then five.

Let's look at that again: all you have to do is introduce one food combined meal on just one day per week to begin with. If, eventually, you're
combining carefully for around **five days out of every seven** or for
**two meals out of three**, you should gain considerable benefit.

## HERE'S A RECAP

To begin to food combine successfully, there a'
need to remember:

### 1. THE FIRST RULE

Eat fruit on its own, before or between meals.

### 2. THE SECOND RULE

Don't mix concentrated, high-quality proteins with very starchy foods
at the same meal.

Use this list as an initial guide: don't mix anything in the left-hand
column with any foods from the other two columns.

| Proteins | Starches | |
|---|---|---|
| Beef | Barley | Pasta |
| Canned fish (such as | Basmati rice | Pastry |
| salmon, sardines, | Biscuits | Pitta bread |
| mackerel and tuna) | Bread | Porridge |
| Cheese | Brown rice | Potatoes |
| Chicken | Bulgur | Pulses (all kinds *except* |
| Eggs | Buns | soya) |
| Fish | Ciabatta | Pumpernickel (black rye) |
| Game | Corn (maize) | Rice |
| Lamb | Couscous | Rice cakes |
| Lamb's liver | Crackers | Rye |
| Pork | Durum semolina | Rye bread |
| Quorn | (most dried pasta) | Rye crackers |
| Shellfish | Flour (all kinds) | Scones |
| Soya beans | Kamut (pasta) | Soda bread |
| Soya milk | Kasha (buckwheat) | Spelt (pasta) |
| TVP (textured vegetable | Matzos | Sweet potatoes |
| protein) | Millet | Tortillas (wraps) |
| Tofu/beancurd | Muesli | Yams |
| Turkey | Oats | |
| Oat biscuits | | |

Choose organic meat,
milk, cheese, eggs and
poultry whenever possible
and non-GM organic soya.

these basic food combining principles as stepping stones to ving energy and digestive function. As you progress towards e food combined meals, you should notice that you feel lighter, ghter and fitter. Accept that it's necessary to compromise and don't worry if you don't get it right every day. We live in a stressful world where it is hardly ever possible to eat the perfect diet. Be flexible; do the best you can.

That's all there is to it.

Honestly.

These two guidelines are the only ones you need to follow. Forget everything you have been told about food combining or might have read about it elsewhere.

Just eat fruit separately and don't mix the major proteins and starches and

**You've got it!**

# Going into Detail

'Nature never produced a sandwich.'

Dr Herbert M Shelton, food combining guru 1895–1985

As we've already established, food combining is based on the simple idea that proteins and starches should not be combined at the same meal. At the outset, this can seem complicated or even daunting but is, in fact, simplicity itself.

If you've read about food combining in the past and were intimidated by too many rules, don't be put off. Forget everything you have ever heard or seen anywhere else and follow the basics set out in *The Complete Book of Food Combining*. You'll soon be completely confident about which foods combine well together.

Like me, you may have wondered why the word 'combining' was chosen in the first place. After all, it suggests mixing things together, rather than keeping them apart, doesn't it? I've always thought it would be better named '*food separation*' – although I suppose even that could leave you thinking you have to eat everything separately, which is definitely not the case.

In practical terms, food combining means nothing more than keeping concentrated starches such as rice, pasta and potatoes away from concentrated proteins like meat, eggs, cheese, and fish. There's no nonsense about having to give up long lists of 'forbidden' foods and no need to buy any kind of special diet foods either.

## So Why Don't Proteins Go with Starches?

Food combining law says that proteins are not digested well if they're combined with starchy foods. Similarly, starch isn't broken down properly if it's mixed with protein. The main reason why they seem to be mismatched is because they need different conditions in order to be properly digested. Protein foods must have an acidic stomach, whereas carbohydrates (starches) need just the opposite. For those who are interested, I've explained this incompatibility in a bit more detail on pages 175–9. In the meantime, please don't think that you have to eat everything individually. While some foods don't mix well together, others are extremely compatible. One of the great things about food combining is that it actually *increases* variety and nourishment and makes mealtimes much more interesting.

For the purposes of food combining, foods fall into three basic sections: **proteins**, **starches**, and a third group that I have called '**versatile**', all-rounders that combine happily with either proteins or starches, such as vegetables or salads.

### HERE'S A RECAP

▶ Proteins go well with versatile vegetables or salads.

▶ Starches go well with versatile vegetables or salads.

▶ But proteins and starches are not compatible.

**You can get an instant view of how this works by checking out the quick reference chart on pages 46–7.**

Now we've covered the basics, let's have a look at each of the different food combining categories.

# Proteins and Starches

When we talk in food combining terms about **proteins**, we refer specifically to the concentrated, high-class (sometimes called first-class) proteins which include meat, poultry, eggs, cheese, fish and soya.

When we refer to **starches**, we mean any kind of carbohydrate, including oats, rice, rye, couscous, pasta, bread, buns, scones, cakes, biscuits and pastry. Potatoes, sweet potatoes and corn (cobs and kernels) are also included under the starch heading.

## Almost All Foods Contain Some Protein and Some Starch, Don't They?

Yes, that's true. But it's the *quantity* of starch or protein in any particular food that decides its food combining category. As a general rule, I look at how much starch (carbohydrate) or protein there is in 100 grams of food. I draw an imaginary line at 10 per cent (in other words, 10 grams per 100 grams). Anything that contains 10 or more grams of protein per 100 grams is classed as a protein. And anything containing 10 or more grams of starch is considered a starch.

For the purposes of my kind of food combining, anything that has less than 10 per cent of starch or protein is much less likely to interfere with digestion.

**!** **TECHNICAL STUFF**

**Food combining starches**

Here are a few examples of starch content:

▶ Cooked brown rice has around 30 grams of starch but only a couple of grams of protein – so it's pretty obviously going to be classed as starch.

▶ Brown bread is one of the starchiest foods of all, at around 40 grams of carbohydrate but only 8 grams of protein.

▶ Spaghetti has about 22 grams of carbohydrate and 4 grams of protein.

▶ Potatoes are definitely starchy enough to be eaten separately from proteins, having between 15 and 17 grams of carbohydrate if they're boiled and 30 grams if they are baked in their skins. If you've read somewhere, as I did in one fairly recent health book, that potatoes are a whopping 90 per cent carbohydrate, that's either a miscalculation or a misprint because a cooked spud contains at least 60 per cent water!

See how easy it is to get confused? If you want a reliable way to check out the starch and protein portions of any kind of food, look them up in *McCance & Widdowson's Composition of Foods*, issued by the Royal Society of Chemistry and available through most libraries.

### Food combining proteins

The same method of calculating applies to proteins. Here are some examples:

▶ Most hard cheese has at least 25 grams of protein to every 100 grams but only a trace of starch.

▶ Eggs have 12 grams of protein.

▶ Most fish have around 15–20 grams and no starch.

▶ Lamb has around 20 grams of protein and no starch at all.

▶ Lean steak and roast turkey both have approximately 28 grams of protein and again, no starch.

### Yoghurt and milk

Yoghurt really deserves a special category of its own and milk is a bit of an oddball when it comes to protein classification. I'll be looking at these two foods in more detail later on in *The Complete Book of Food Combining*.

At the end of the day, you really don't need to remember any of these figures. *The Complete Book of Food Combining* has some very easy-to-use charts (pages 46–7) that give you an instant guide to the different categories without having to commit anything to memory. I'm just giving you a few examples so that you can see the reasoning behind the theory.

---

**Here's a quick reminder of how the major proteins and starches fit into food combining:**

### PROTEINS

▶ OK with salad foods

▶ OK with vegetables (but not potatoes, yams and corn)

▶ OK with oils, spreading fats, nuts, seeds and dressings

**Not OK** with starches or fruit

### Major proteins include:

| | | |
|---|---|---|
| Beef | Game | Soya products |
| Cheese | Lamb | TVP (textured vegetable protein) |
| Chicken | Pork | Tofu/beancurd |
| Eggs | Quorn | Turkey |
| Fish | Soya milk | |

### STARCHES

▶ OK with salad foods

▶ OK with vegetables

▶ OK with potatoes, yams and corn

▶ OK with oils, spreading fats, nuts, seeds and dressings

**Not OK** with proteins or fruit

## Major starchy foods include:

**All kinds of grains**
Barley
Buckwheat (kasha)
Bulgur
Couscous
Millet
Oats
Quinoa
Rice
Rye
Semolina
Wheat
Wild rice

All types of lentils, peas and beans *except soya*

**All kinds of pasta**
Buckwheat pasta
Durum semolina
Kamut
Spelt

Corn
Potatoes
Sweet potatoes
Yams

Sweet biscuits
Cakes

Cereals
Porridge
Muesli

**All kinds of bread**
Ciabatta
Crackers
Matzos
Oat biscuits
Pitta bread
Pumpernickel
Rice cakes
Rolls
Rye bread
Rye crackers
Soda bread
Wraps (tortillas)

All types of flour

# Fruit

'Fruit is, without doubt, the most beneficial, energy-giving,
life-enhancing food you can eat – if it is correctly consumed.'

Harvey and Marilyn Diamond, *Fit for Life*, 1985

Nutritious and delicious fresh fruit is a vital component of any healthy eating programme. It is an especially important part of *The Complete Book of Food Combining*. Fresh fruit is a rich store of antioxidants, nutrients that are believed to help protect us against many of the health problems associated with ageing. Antioxidants are capable of extinguishing *free radicals*, rogue molecules that trigger degeneration and disturb the immune system by mutating genetic material and impairing the function of essential enzymes. Research suggests that cataracts, cancer, cardiovascular disease and Alzheimer's disease may all be linked to free radical damage and low intake of antioxidants. Some of the most exciting research proposes that people who eat fresh fruit every day could have a 24 per cent reduction in fatal heart disease and a 32 per cent lower risk of stroke.

Fruit has another talent too. Apart from providing some useful dietary fibre, its high water content hydrates the body with nourishing fluid which helps to stir up and flush out toxins. As such, fresh fruit and fresh fruit juices are a vital part of the healthy detox programme which begins on page 219.

## So Where Does All This Fit into the Food Combining Scheme of Things?

Unfortunately, there are some aspects of food combining that have been consistently and incorrectly handed down, resulting in a number of writers crediting Dr Hay with concepts and conclusions that were never his. The fruit rule is one of them. In a nutrition book published as recently as 1997, a section on food combining states: 'Dr Hay's advice to eat fruit separately makes a lot of sense.' Eating fruit separately *does* make a lot of sense but it wasn't Dr Hay's idea and he never recommended it. Although goodness knows why not.

Dr Hay's ideas about fruit were entirely his own and at odds with all other experts. He agreed that it was essential to a healthy diet but had hard and fast rules about *when* it could be included. He put forward the idea that acid fruits should be eaten with proteins and that very sweet, ripe or starchy fruits would mix with bread and other starchy foods. This rationale is embedded into the Hay system. It has been sustained by Doris Grant, a dedicated follower of Dr Hay, and much copied in subsequent books. If you're prepared to remember which category each fruit falls in to, and it works for you, then I don't see any reason to discontinue doing it.

## Nothing Should be Written in Stone

Rightly or wrongly, I'm not into hard and fast rules. I have learnt so many new and fascinating things about health and healing, and food combining since I began working in the field of nutrition; one of the most important things to remember is that *flexibility* often achieves better results than *rigidity*. In any event, we are all so individual and what suits one person doesn't always suit another. And, I'm convinced, human nature is such that we are much less likely to have a go at something new if it seems to be too rigorous, exacting or time-consuming – and much more likely to try it out if it's easy.

I have to say that I have always found Dr Hay's rules about fruit a complicated system that doesn't sit well with my understanding of how the digestive system works. And it seems to be an area of food combining that foxes many people.

## A Change of Direction

I was the first food combining author in the UK to recommend that fruit should be eaten separately from most other foods – especially concentrated proteins and starches – having adopted this approach for many years in my own nutrition practice. I have to say that, at the time, this was done simply because it seemed to provide the best results.

For the most part, it still applies. However, in a world of nothing-is-ever-simple, there are the inevitable exceptions. In practice, I've found that some people seem to have no problem digesting fruit when they eat it with, say, cheese or yoghurt, but suffer indescribable discomfort if they consume fruit too close to other proteins such as chicken or fish. One of the most likely causes of a grumbly, gripey stomach is the combination of acidic fruit with starch. An apple eaten after a sandwich or fruit in a pastry tart are just two examples.

Apart from those writers who are faithful to the specific rules set by Dr Hay, all other leading food combining experts appear to follow the lead set by American doctor, Herbert Shelton (see page 98), and agree that fruit is best consumed on an empty stomach. This is the route that seems especially beneficial to people who suffer from any kind of digestive or bowel disorder such as heartburn, bloating, flatulence, irritable bowel, malabsorption syndrome or overweight.

## Delay Can Mean Indigestion

Dr Shelton wrote that when fruit is delayed in the stomach because it has accompanied other food, not only is much of the goodness lost but the rest of the meal also spoils. Things go off and get smelly! Bacteria get to work. Proteins decompose and starches ferment, causing acidity, bloating, burning and gas.

This was certainly my own experience as a practitioner. I have met many people who, because they believed that it was healthier to eat fruit after a meal than, say, a calorie-laden dessert, chose an apple or a bowl of fruit salad instead of a piece of pie or a chocolate mousse. When they suffered severe indigestion, they would analyse their meal in detail and blame almost any part of it other than the fruit. A natural enough thing to do. Fruit is good for you; it couldn't be that. However, following detailed observations of feeding patterns and habits, the troublemaker has often been found to be the fruit.

Many of the patients I've seen over the years have been referred to me with digestive disorders. Almost without exception, by extracting fruit from their main diet and eating it separately from other foods, many a case of heartburn and flatulence has been avoided.

## How Fruit is Digested

### On its own = effortless digestion

Fruit undergoes very little digestion in the mouth and none in the stomach. Unlike the breakdown of proteins and starches, which seize huge amounts of energy from the body while they are going through the process of digestion, fruit requires very little energy indeed. When eaten on its own, it's able to pass quickly and efficiently to the next stage of the digestive process – the small intestine.

### With other food = not so smooth

Fruit acids inhibit protein digestion because they restrict the production of stomach acids as well as destroying the protein-splitting enzyme, pepsin. Herbert Shelton stated that all fruit acids, including those in apples, cherries, grapes, grapefruit, lemons, peaches and oranges are a '*severe check to hydrochloric acid secretion and thus interfere with protein digestion*'. And when it comes to starches, all acids – fruit acid being no exception – put a stop to starch digestion because they disturb the alkaline medium needed by the starch-digesting enzymes. This doesn't make fruit a bad food. On the contrary. Fruit belongs to the 'superfood' category. But much of its goodness is likely to be wasted if it's eaten either during or immediately after a meal.

### Fast transit

Another important factor is that different foods require different journey times to navigate their way through the digestive system. Most proteins, for example, chug along on the slow train, taking several hours to make the trip. By comparison, fruit jumps aboard the Rapid Transit enabling a free and clear run through the stomach. Once in the small intestine, the concentrated natural sugars, vitamins and minerals are quickly absorbed.

Authors Harvey and Marilyn Diamond, who have also followed much of Dr Shelton's work, suggest that eating fruit or drinking fruit juice with, or directly after a meal will deprive the body of the cleansing benefits of fruit taken alone. Unless you have totally numbed your system after years of dietary abuse, they say, you will probably experience discomfort and indigestion as the fruit ferments in your stomach. If you're lucky enough to get away with it – in other words you don't burp, belch, bloat, fart or feel nauseous – it doesn't necessarily mean you digested well, only that the body is, yet again, proving itself incredibly tolerant and compliant.

---

**Author's note**

I remember one senior university lecturer once warning television viewers that food combining was bad because it recommended avoiding fruit. Comments such as these are way off the mark and a classic example of an alleged expert, who knows nothing about the subject, putting their mouth into gear before their brain is engaged. On further questioning, it transpired that this person had never read any of the leading books on the subject and had confused the instruction to eat fruit separately as advice to eat no fruit at all. Of the many food combining books available, I cannot find one that tells us we shouldn't eat fruit. Food combining actually encourages us to eat more of this delicious nutritious food.

---

**!** **ESSENTIAL**

**Here is the fruit rule:**

▶ Eat plenty of fruit – two or three pieces a day is an ideal amount.

▶ Eat fruit on an empty stomach. Either between meals or at the beginning of a meal, not with it, in the middle of it or immediately afterwards.

▶ If you eat fruit with yoghurt or occasionally with cheese, enjoy them as separate snacks.

'On an empty stomach' means either first thing in the morning or as a between-meal snack – or as a starter to a main course.

### First fruit serving

First thing in the morning, as soon as you get up. Eat any kind of fresh fruit such as grapes, grapefruit, apples, kiwi or pineapple. Or make a fresh juice. For ideas, see pages 244–5.

### Second fruit serving

Enjoy your second fruit of the day as a mid-morning snack, instead of coffee and biscuits.

### Third fruit serving

While you are preparing or waiting for your evening meal. If you are eating out in a restaurant, ask for a glass of fresh juice as an aperitif.

## How Long Between Fruit and the Main Course?

If you're eating fruit as a starter, experts say that the ideal space between your fruit and the rest of your meal is 15 minutes. That works well in the morning if you eat fruit on rising and have breakfast after you've washed and dressed. For a mid-morning snack you'll be eating fruit on its own so the question doesn't apply. In the evening it's likely that meal preparation will take long enough to allow the fruit or the juice to be properly assimilated.

### But what if you're really pushed?

Do what you can to leave a gap but if your main course comes along and you've only just taken the last mouthful of fruit or juice, don't worry about it. I have conducted a number of experiments by introducing fruit at different stages throughout a meal and then assessing levels of discomfort, pressure, gas, burping and bloating. Results are fairly consistent that fruit either on a completely empty stomach or with a gap of 10 to 15 minutes between fruit and main course are the best options. However, it is also the case that fruit as a first course, even if the main course is served straight away, seems to cause far less disruption to digestion than fruit as a dessert.

**Thirty delicious fruits to get your teeth into:**

| | | |
|---|---|---|
| Apples | Fig | Nectarines |
| Apricots | Grapefruit | Oranges |
| Bananas | Grapes | Papaya |
| Blackberries | Guava | Peaches |
| Blackcurrants | Hunza apricots | Pears |
| Blueberries | Kiwi fruit | Pineapple |
| Cherries | Lychees | Pomegranates |
| Clementines | Mandarines | Raspberries |
| Dates | Mango | Satsumas |
| Durian | Melon | Tangerines |

## What About Stewed or Baked Fruit?

Cooking is believed by some nutrition experts to change the structure of fruit, destroying nutrients and making it more acidic. If you enjoy stewed prunes, rhubarb or baked apple, don't deny yourself the treat but do be aware that cooked fruit does not appear to be digested as efficiently as raw fruit. If you have any kind of digestive problem, you may find cooked fruit aggravates the symptoms. And remember that any kind of fruit is much more inclined to upset the digestion if it's mixed with starchy pastry or crumble.

## Dried Fruit

Once dried, the sugar in fruit becomes much more concentrated and the fruit generally less acidic. Currants, raisins and sultanas, for example, have an entirely different taste and 'mouth feel' to a fresh grape. The same applies to dried apple versus fresh apple or dried apricot against fresh apricot. As a result of the drying process, they seem to combine much more comfortably with other foods than do fresh fruits. One reason may be that we tend to eat them in only relatively small amounts, compared to their fresh equivalents. My experience over the years has been that dried fruits can be added in small amounts to almost anything from curries to cereals. Don't store dried fruit for long periods, however. Buy small packs as needed and use it up well within date. Organic dried fruit is nearly always available in good health stores and also in some supermarkets and delis.

---

**About prunes**

Some people rely on prunes as an aid to efficient bowel movements. Others say that they avoid prunes because they're hard on the digestion. It's worth knowing that dried figs, apart from being packed with nourishment, can be far more gentle in their action than prunes but are still extremely effective.

---

## Exceptions to the Fruit Rule

My own researches into food combining have turned up two interesting anomalies to the fruit rule:

**1.** Cheese, which often accompanies fruit as a dessert, does not appear to putrefy as quickly as meat, fish or eggs. It's a phenomenon that was touched on over 50 years ago by Dr Shelton. No one has yet been able to ascertain any physiological reason for this difference. Although fruit and cheese are still not an ideal combination after a meal, they do seem to be less disruptive than other protein/fruit mixtures. I still wouldn't recommend eating fruit at the end of a meal, even with cheese, but a piece of sheep's or goat's cheese with, say, an apple or some grapes, could make an enjoyable and occasional snack or light meal on its own.

**2.** The other 'exception' is yoghurt. Peach, banana, grape, kiwi – any kind of fruit combines well with yoghurt. Again, it is only from experience that we find that yoghurt and fruit mixtures are digested well. No one really knows why. However, it is the case that yoghurt is already partially digested during its manufacture and so requires less work to be broken down inside the body. Although it is classed, officially, as a protein food, whole yoghurt is actually much lower in protein (around 3 or 5½ grams per 100 grams of yoghurt), than other high-class proteins, which means it does not require anything like the same amount of stomach acid or digestion time as, say, meat or poultry. For the purposes of food combining, yoghurt is **versatile**.

**3.** Banana seems to combine quite comfortably with breakfast cereals and porridge, especially if you use a rice milk or oat milk or a little cream (page 52) instead of cow's milk.

## What About Fruit Juices?

I've talked about fruit juices elsewhere in this book but, just to recap, it's worth remembering that many commercially produced cartoned or bottled juices that give the impression of being *Fresh! Real! Pure!* and unadulterated may, in fact, be reconstituted and have extra acids, sweeteners, sugar or other 'enhancers' added to them. Labelling laws are such that not all ingredients are always declared and pack information can also be very confusing. For example, it can be difficult to sus out whether or not any flavourings are real or artificial. Did you know, for example, that 'blackcurrant flavour' indicates artificial flavouring but that 'blackcurrant flavoured' means it contains the real thing!

### Juice your own

The best way to get the most nourishing juice is to make your own by putting fresh fruit through a juicing machine. There are a number of different types of machine available and, because I've been asked so many times about which machines are best and where to find them, here are a few thoughts:

▶ Before you buy, ask to see the machine dismantled and reassembled. Don't take anybody's word that the thing is easy to clean or simple to take apart or put together. Some are – but others have lots of connections and attachments that can be a fiddle to fix and difficult to clean really thoroughly.

▶ Find out what you are getting for your money, including accessories. Just because it's pictured in the brochure doesn't mean it comes as standard.

▶ Make sure you know which of the attachments are dishwasher proof and which should not be immersed in water.

▶ Most of the better-quality blenders and processors have attachments for the effortless squeezing of citrus fruit. Braun and Kenwood both make dedicated machines for juicing all kinds of fruit. Moulinex and Bosch sell processors with juicing attachments. The Magimix Le Duo is, as the name suggests, a dual- purpose machine that does citrus as well as all other kinds of fruits and vegetables. The Magimix 4100 food processor comes with two separate attachments for juicing everything from oranges and grapefruit to kiwi, apples, mango and all kinds of vegetables too. Of the makes of machine that I've tried, Magimix Le Duo and 4100 get my number one vote for simplicity, robustness and ease of cleaning. See page 440 for stockist details.

▶ Always clean juicing machines immediately after use, otherwise the fruit pulp dries on and sticks. Actually, you'll only leave it on once!

## Don't have a juicer or blender?

The next best option to having a juicer is to choose organic non-carbonated juices or at least go for those that are labelled free of artificial additives. Check the actual ingredients' tag as well. Some packs will tell you that a product is 'free' of something, for example 'sucrose free', giving the impression that there is no sugar at all, only to sneakily add other sugars such as glucose, maltose or dextrose – or artificial sweeteners – instead. Whatever type of juice you buy, dilute it with one third water. Not only does this make the juice go further, it reduces the risk of acidity to sensitive stomachs.

You'll find more on juices in the **Food Combining Detox** chapter, pages 244–5.

**IMPORTANT NOTE**

Drink home-made juices as soon as they are made so that you get the optimum nourishment from them. If juice is allowed to sit, it oxidises, changing from an alkaline-forming food to an acid-forming one that is no longer able to hold on to its store of vitamins and minerals (for more information on alkaline- and acid-forming food, see pages 420–37). If you want to watch this destruction in operation, just juice up an apple and leave it to stand for a few minutes. The fresh, pale green very-good-for-you fluid will change extremely quickly into a brown, not-nice-to-look-at sludge.

# Versatile Vegetables

Vegetables and salads are probably the most versatile of food combining choices. One of the great plus points about food combining, apart from all the other plus points, is that it encourages us to eat more vegetables and salads. These **versatile** foods combine happily with either starches or proteins and make fabulously nourishing meals on their own. According to the feedback I've received from many, many food combiners over the years, even people who have hated their greens with a passion find themselves enjoying more fresh produce – and feeling better for it.

I've decided that, in most cases, enjoying vegetables is something that comes with maturity, and usually more quickly to women than to men or to children. I wonder if it is only as we age that we stop seeing vegetables and salads as some kind of poison. Perhaps if we were able to understand, early on, how deliciously nourishing these foods can be when they are imaginatively prepared and how we really can't live healthily long-term without them, we might see them in a different light.

Surveys show over and over again that people who eat plenty of fresh vegetables, salads (and fruit) every day have better general health profiles and, researchers are pretty sure, a significantly lower risk of cancer, heart disease and stroke than vegetable haters. But the very words 'five servings' can send a dyed-in-the-wool derider of anything grown in the ground scurrying for the nearest burger and bun.

A single serving sounds like heaps. But it really isn't that much. A tablespoon of peas, two or three small florets of broccoli or cauliflower, and a couple of small carrots is all that it takes to claim three daily portions. A side salad of a few lettuce leaves, a tomato, three slices of cucumber, a snip of cress and a bit of bell pepper is close to a whole day's intake. Add a glass of fresh fruit juice before breakfast and an apple or a banana mid-morning – and there you have it. Not bad for basics. If you manage to consume more than that, so much the better.

**! ESSENTIAL**

### Easy ways to up your intake of vegetables and salads:

▶ Make vegetables a main feature of a meal, not just a side item. Practise new ways of preparing, cooking and serving salads and vegetables to make them as tempting as possible.

▶ Not everyone enjoys crisp – al dente – vegetables. We've been told for years that overcooking depletes nutrients but nevertheless it's the case that 'softer' vegetables are sometimes more acceptable to the determined vegetable hater. And they're certainly better than no veg at all. In fact, new findings suggest that, because cooking helps to break down the vegetables into a more easily digestible form, more nutrients may be released for absorption.

▶ Stir chopped fried onion into green vegetables such as cabbage, kale or broccoli, before serving. It really lifts the flavour. All members of the onion family could be classed as superfoods. They are believed to be good for the heart and circulation, and for helping to keep colds at bay. And it's recently been suggested that onions may play an important role in keeping bones healthy and strong and preventing osteoporosis.

▶ Steam your Brussels sprouts, cabbage or broccoli and then put them through a food processor with a knob of butter and a little salt to make a palatable vegetable purée.

▶ Add extra flavour to cooked vegetables by chopping them and tossing them for a couple of minutes in a tablespoon of extra-virgin olive oil in a hot fry pan. Or try shaking a little dressing made with olive oil and balsamic vinegar over cooked vegetables just before serving – delicious!

▶ Make winter stews with less expensive cuts of meat or poultry and add parsnip, turnip, onion, carrot, baby tomatoes, bell peppers, broccoli and cauliflower stalks to the casserole dish. Or take the vegetarian option; leave out the meat or poultry altogether and add mixed pulses for a filling and nourishing meat-free casserole. The recipes in Part Three include some tasty vegetarian dishes for you to try.

▶ If you are serving fish, game, poultry or meat, why not skip the usual potato or rice and serve two or three vegetables instead? The meal will be just as filling, just as nutritious and may be better digested.

▶ If lunch is usually a sandwich, choose a variety of salad fillings – coleslaw, avocado, red cabbage, grated carrot, lettuce, skinned cucumber, tomato – instead of the usual cheese or ham. Or skip the bread and go for a really delicious tuna, prawn, chicken or bean salad. Remember that bread does seem to contribute not only to weight problems but also to that after-lunch energy slump. If you do eat bread, try to avoid sandwiches with protein fillings.

▶ Try to include at least one side salad and two servings of vegetables with your main meals each day. The list below and the recipes (pages 348–417) will give you plenty of good ideas. **The Quick Reference Chart** on pages 46–7 will show you which foods combine well and which ones are not so good.

▶ Always have a couple of different types of frozen vegetables stored in the freezer. Then, if you can't get to the shops, you won't miss out. While canned vegetables have significantly fewer nutrients than fresh equivalents (and often contain heavy doses of sugar and salt), frozen vegetables are a healthy option and are almost certainly more nourishing than wilted, allegedly fresh stuff that has been out of the ground and stored for a long time.

## Did You Know That?

▶ Dark green lettuce and dark green cabbage leaves can contain far more vitamins and minerals than most pale varieties.

▶ All vegetables contain valuable nourishment but the green, yellow and orange ones are tops for vitamins.

▶ Research shows that people who eat five or more servings of fresh fruit and vegetables every day have better health profiles than those who don't. Fruit and veg fans may also be reducing their risk of heart disease and cancer.

▶ Green leafy produce, such as cabbage, Brussels sprouts, broccoli and kale contains nutrients that, scientists believe, may have particularly special anti-cancer activity.

▶ Prepared salad foods can lose a whole day of shelf life for every half an hour that they are out of the cool cabinet or refrigerator. Save nutrients and improve shelf life by taking an insulated cold box or bag with you when you shop (in the winter as well as the summer) and pack it with all your chilled foods as you go through the checkout.

▶ Wash all fruit and vegetables really thoroughly to remove surface bacteria, moulds, soil, grit and grubs but don't leave foods soaking in water for long periods. Wash everything whether it's organic or not!

▶ Much of the dietary fibre in vegetables is to be found in the skin and stalks. Leaving the skins on seems to make sense. But the Catch 22 is that we then swallow increased quantities of pesticide residues. Many pesticides work systemically and any residues will probably affect more than just the outer surface. However, getting rid of the peel does cut down on the amount of chemicals ingested. There is no need to discard the peel on organically grown foods but do wash them well.

▶ Vegetables continue to breathe even after they've been harvested. They exhale carbon dioxide and another gas called ethylene which speed ripening and hasten deterioration. Asparagus, mushrooms and green leafy vegetables such as Brussels sprouts, broccoli and kale, age especially quickly. So store foods carefully. Vegetables are often better in a cool larder or shed than in the fridge. Keep bananas away from other produce. They give off a lot of ethylene which ripens everything else.

▸ If you live a long way from the shops or have problems getting fresh food every day, you can extend the life of vegetables and fruit by storing them in special stayfresh bags that slow down the natural ageing and ripening process. Available in the UK from Lakeland shops or by mail order (see page 440 for stockists).

▸ Soaking, chopping, slicing and boiling all cause vitamin loss. Maintain nourishment with the three Ms:

**1.** Maximum rinsing (no soaking)
**2.** Minimum cutting
**3.** Minimum cooking water – steaming is best.

# Pulses

Pulses (known in some countries as legumes) are the edible seeds from the *Leguminosae* family which includes lentils, beans and peas.

You might be forgiven for thinking that pulses simply don't fit with food combining because lentils, peas and beans contain a combination of protein and starch. Critics often use this as ammunition to shoot at food combining and suggest that the system has no merit. If nature produces foods that already have starches and proteins mixed together, they ask, then how can eating meat separately from potatoes make any difference to anything?

Sounds like fair comment until you examine the facts.

Beans are not, in fact, half starch and half protein.

More accurately, cooked soya beans are made up of around 14 per cent protein and 5 per cent starch. The protein portion is above my 10 per cent line (go back to page 19 if you missed this bit). This bias in protein's favour explains why soya usually appears on food combining's protein list. Most other pulses are the other way around – 6–8 per cent protein and anything between 15–25 per cent starch, which is why they are often found in the company of other starches.

## Dr Hay was Different – Again

On the matter of pulses, Dr Hay once again departed from the mainstream. He believed that the bean family were a troublesome lot. He reasoned that, because they were difficult for some people to digest and caused copious quantities of gas, they were best avoided. Some of the books that followed Dr Hay's ideas modified his original advice and suggested, probably sensibly, that pulses might produce less gas if they were eaten only with non-starchy vegetables and not with major proteins or starches. Others got around the question either by ignoring it or by simply repeating Dr Hay's advice to abstain.

A number of more recent writers have their underwear in a real old sheepshank over what to do. One reference I came across promised to explain everything the reader needed to know about the Hay diet and why it works. It then advised that all dried pulses could be combined as part of a protein meal but didn't explain why this was or why they had chosen this 'about turn'. Another recent publication tells us that lentils and chickpeas combine well with meat, poultry and fish but, on the very next page, 'lentils and beans' are no problem with rice! No wonder it's confusing.

I believe that Dr Shelton had it right by categorising soya beans as proteins and all other dried beans as starch. And that's how it is in *The Complete Book of Food Combining*.

---

### Don't give up on the bean

Beans, peas and lentils form part of the staple diet of many countries and cultures around the world and, of course, are an important source of non-animal protein for vegetarians and vegans. Because of their protein content, and the fact that they are used as a meat substitute, pulses are often listed on food combining charts as proteins. Soya beans are certainly rich enough in protein to warrant that category but, from a food combining perspective, other pulses are better classified on the starch and vegetable sides of the divide. See the chart on page 41. In other words, pulses are still an excellent protein source but careful combining can help to make them more digestible.

## Scientific Support for the Benefits of Beans

We now know a lot more about the nutritional status of beans than we did in the 1920s and 1930s. Research not available in Dr Hay's time shows us that beans, lentils and peas contain a particularly valuable type of soluble dietary fibre that helps to stabilise blood glucose; they are good for bowel and heart health and may even inhibit some types of cancer. All kinds of beans are delicious and nutritious if a little gassy for some of us. They are too good to avoid. Eat them and enjoy.

## Are Pulses Acid- or Alkaline-forming?

Now this is a tough one. Again, I can find no references that agree and, at the end of the day, I'm not sure it really matters. In my opinion, it really, honestly, isn't necessary to understand the chemistry of acid- and alkaline-forming foods to be able to food combine successfully. (For those of you, however, who are keen to understand the nitty gritty of food combining chemistry, see pages 420–37.)

There is a general consensus that soya beans are an acid-form-ing protein. But what about other pulses? Most often, they are listed as acid-forming. One book mentions 'beans' as alkaline-forming but doesn't say whether they are talking about green beans or pulses. Several others carefully avoid the question by making no reference. One tome promised it would provide 'a full explanation of the scientific evidence' then gave only a passing mention to acid/alkali balance and no guidance at all on pulses. Yet another suggested that butter beans and broad beans were acid-forming and everything else was alkaline-forming. In fact, young broad beans – such as those you might buy canned or frozen – have a similar starch/protein make-up to mangetout, and a slightly lower one than frozen peas! They are much lower in both starch and protein (only 5 per cent of each) than other pulses and, as such, can be treated as a non-starchy alkaline-forming vegetable.

You see how baffling this can be? To try to make sense of the muddle, I have taken what I hope is a simple, common sense view. We know that soya is a protein food and that other pulses are mostly starchy. Since most proteins and starches, generally, are acid-forming, I treat all pulses as acid forming too. So follow that lead. Again, you can find out more about the importance of acid/alkali balance on page 420.

## HERE'S A RECAP

▶ If you're into beans, use soya as a major protein and all other beans either with starches or with non-starchy vegetables and salads.

▶ And remember that non-starchy beans and peas (such as baby broad beans, French beans, green beans, runner beans, garden peas, mange-tout, sugar snaps, petit pois and beansprouts) are alkaline-forming, go-with-anything, non-starchy vegetables.

## But What About All That Gas?

There is no doubt that pulses can be difficult to digest and are infamous for their gas-producing properties! But that beans cause flatulence has nothing to do with food combining *per se*. Particular proteins and starches found in pulses don't get digested properly because we don't have the enzymes to deal with them. Some experts have suggested that, through evolution, we may have lost these enzymes – or it may be that we never had them in the first place.

Bacteria that live in the large intestine enjoy feeding off beans and, in doing so, help to break them down. This applies especially to two starchy molecules called raffinose and stachyose which can't be broken down in the usual part of the digestive system so have to wait until they get much further down the tube before those busy bacteria get to work on them. Unfortunately, in the process, they do produce rather a lot of gas! But, as I've explained above, because beans are good for us, it really is worth including in them in our diet.

**! ESSENTIAL**

## Four ways to improve digestibility:

**1.** If beans have caused you discomfort in the past, give them another go but, this time, try combining them only with salads or vegetables, rather than with other starches or proteins.

**2.** If you are using canned pulses, such as red kidney, black-eyed or flageolet beans, tip the contents of the can into a sieve, pour off the liquid from the can and rinse the beans really well with filtered water before using.

**3.** If you are cooking beans from raw, do ensure that they are cooked thoroughly. Undercooked beans can, at best, be uncomfortably indigestible and, at worst, could be poisonous. And did you know that the foamy residue that bubbles round the pan during cooking is what we affectionately call 'flatulence foam'? Scooping it off and discarding it, and changing the water several times during the long cooking process reduces the levels of those gassy starches, raffinose and stachyose. Adding pieces of fresh root ginger to the final cooking water may also help digestion.

**4.** It really does improve digestibility if pulses are chewed very thoroughly before swallowing. This helps to break down the starchy components and reduces some of the gas.

### Green Beans

Long green beans such as French or runner beans have a very low starch/protein content and can be treated as non-starchy vegetables.

### Pulses

Once pulses are sprouted (i.e. as mung bean sprouts or alfalfa) they are no longer starchy. They become alkaline-forming, non-starchy vegetables.

## Hummus

Hummus is made with chickpeas, a starchy pulse, so it does not combine well with protein foods. Use hummus with starchy foods such as jacket potatoes, as a spread on rice cakes, bread or savoury biscuits, on its own with salad, or in the hollow of half an avocado.

## Peas

Peas get starchier with age. Mangetout, sugar snaps, petit pois and fresh or frozen garden peas are classed as alkaline-forming, non-starchy vegetables – not pulses. They will combine comfortably with either proteins or starches and any other vegetables. Dried, processed, mushy and marrowfat peas are starchy and so are best eaten with other starches or vegetables.

## Soya Beans

Soya beans are acid-forming but once they are formed into beancurd, they are considered alkaline-forming.

## Peanuts

Peanuts are not nuts but belong to the pulse family. They are very rich in protein (25 per cent), so you'll find them listed with other proteins. They should also be considered acid-forming. Peanuts are a common cause of allergic reaction and, for some people, extremely difficult to digest. Nevertheless, they are a nourishing food, high in potassium, magnesium, vitamin E, vitamin B1, folic acid, biotin, and with worthwhile traces of zinc, selenium, iron and manganese. If you have no problem with peanuts, they make a nutrient-rich snack. Look upon salted peanuts as an occasional treat and go for unsalted whenever possible.

## Pulses and legumes to choose from:

| Acid-forming protein pulses | Alkaline-forming peas and beans | Acid-forming starchy pulses | |
|---|---|---|---|
| Peanuts | Beansprouts | Adzuki beans | Lupin beans |
| Peanut butter | Broad beans | Black kidney beans | Marrowfat peas |
| Soya beans | French beans | Black-eyed beans | Mushy peas |
| TVP (textured vegetable protein) | Garden peas | Blue peas | Mung beans |
| | Green beans | Borlotti beans | Pigeon peas |
| | Mangetout | Brown beans | Pinto beans |
| | Petit pois | Butter beans | Processed peas |
| | Runner beans | Cannellini beans | Red kidney beans |
| | Sugar snaps | Chickpeas | Split peas |
| | | Dal | |
| | | Ful medames | |
| | **Alkaline-forming pulses** | Haricot beans | |
| | Black bean sauce | Hummus | |
| | Salted black bean | Hyacinth beans | |
| | Tofu (beancurd) | Lentils | |
| | | Lima beans | |

For easy food combining, treat **SOYA** as a major protein food and **ALL OTHER PULSES** as starch. If you find them difficult to digest, combine them with vegetables or salads only

## You've got it!

# Nuts and Seeds

## Nuts

Even if you enjoy their taste, nuts are not always a popular food. Nuts in general – and peanuts and walnuts in particular – are a common source of allergic reaction, sometimes so serious it can be life-threatening. Nuts are also notoriously difficult to digest and so tend to be de-listed by anyone with digestive problems. In addition, many people are so concerned that nuts are rich in fat that they think they should avoid them because of concerns about gaining weight or about heart disease.

In fact, nuts are extremely nourishing, most having high levels of magnesium, potassium, folic acid and vitamin E. They are a good source of dietary fibre – and the natural polyunsaturated or mono-unsaturated oils they contain are protective. Research suggests that people who include nuts regularly in their diet have less incidence of heart disease.

If you like them – and are not allergic to them – but find they disagree with your digestion, an option is to try crushing or grinding them and chewing them *really well* before swallowing. This means that the stomach doesn't have to do so much work and the digestive juices can

---

**Coconut**

Coconut is so low in both starch and protein that it combines very well with most foods. Coconut milk is a nutritious substitute for cow's milk or soya milk where a non-protein liquid is needed. Concern has been expressed that coconut milk and cream are both high in saturated fat. However, there is no evidence that either contribute to heart or artery disease. Coconut fat differs from other saturated fats in that it is liquid at room temperature, not solid like other saturates. In the Far East, where coconut is widely used (for example in Thai cooking), it has attained an almost superfood status.

reach a greater surface area of the food, creating a far better chance of complete digestion.

Nuts are probably the most difficult food to put into food combining categories. Some types (almonds, Brazils), are rich in protein, one or two are quite starchy (chestnuts, tiger nuts) and several are comparatively low in both (macadamia, coconut, pine nuts, pecans, hazelnuts, pistachios, walnuts). So it can be difficult to know how best to combine them.

Experience shows that most nuts combine in small amounts with either proteins or starches but that they are digested most easily when mixed with only vegetables or salads. A large serving of nuts may cause indigestion, whereas a few may not. If you want to be more precise, keep almonds and Brazils on the protein side, chestnuts and tiger nuts for starchy meals, and treat the rest as **versatile**. Or do what I do and eat nuts in small amounts either on their own or with salads or dried fruit.

---

**Peanuts are pulses**

As I explained in the previous section, peanuts are not, in fact, nuts but pulses. They belong to the same family as peas, beans and lentils. Peanuts are very high in fat and contain around two-thirds protein to one-third starch. If used, they are best combined with vegetables or salads or eaten separately.

---

## Seeds

Most seeds have a similar nutritional make-up to nuts but, happily, seem much easier to digest than nuts. They are nutritious and the oils they contain are believed to be beneficial for heart health. Seeds are especially good sources of zinc, iron, magnesium, calcium and vitamin E. Although most seeds contain quite large amounts of starch and protein, they are usually only eaten in quite small quantities and do not appear to present any dilemma with regard to particular combinations. The food combining recommendations on seeds are that they are **versatile** and go with anything.

### Nut and seed oil products

Nut and seed oils, such as walnut, sunflower and sesame, are classed as fats and, as such, combine with starches or proteins. The same applies to tahini paste (made with sesame seeds) and pesto (made with pine nuts) which are just as **versatile** and combine with anything. If you are choosing ready-made pesto to use with starchy foods such as pasta, make sure it doesn't contain Parmesan – some brands do.

### Nuts and seeds to choose from:

| Nuts | | Seeds | |
|------|------|-------|------|
| Almonds | Macadamia | Caraway | Poppy |
| Brazils | Pecans | Celery | Pumpkin |
| Cashews | Pine nuts | Dill | Sesame |
| Chestnuts | Pistachios | Linseeds | Sunflower |
| Coconut | Walnuts | Melon | |
| Hazelnuts (filberts) | Water chestnuts | Mustard | |

## QUICK REFERENCE CHART

**Use this quick reference chart to check which foods combine with which.**

Combine any of the foods in Column B (the centre section) with either the left-hand column (Proteins) or the right-hand column (Starches). But don't mix the proteins in Column A directly with the starches in Column C.

| Column A | Column B | Column C |
|----------|----------|----------|
| **PROTEINS** | **VERSATILE FOODS** | **STARCHES** |
| Free-range poultry | Any non-starchy vegetables (so not canned corn or corn-on-the-cob, potatoes, sweet potatoes or yams) | Potatoes, yams, sweet potatoes and corn |

| Column A **PROTEINS** | Column B **VERSATILE FOODS** | Column C **STARCHES** |
|---|---|---|
| Fish and shellfish | | Oat porridge, Breakfast cereals, All grains (including barley, buckwheat, couscous, oats, quinoa, rice and rye) |
| Quorn and TVP | Any salad foods | |
| Soya milk | Herbs and spices | Bread |
| Tofu (beancurd) | | Buns |
| | Yoghurt | Soda bread |
| | | Pitta bread |
| | | Matzos |
| | | Crackers |
| Free-range eggs | Nuts and seeds | Pastry |
| | | Flour |
| | Salad dressings | Biscuits |
| | | Cakes |
| | Coconut milk | |
| | Coconut cream | |
| | Buttermilk | |
| | Cream | Maple syrup |
| | Butter | Molasses |
| | Vitaquell | Honey |
| | Spreading fats | (and anything sweet) |
| Cheese | Olive oil | |
| | | All pulses except soya |
| | | Hummus |

# CHAPTER 3

# Frequently Asked Questions about Food Combining

The questions in this chapter are ones that I've collected over the years from new and practised food combiners alike. I hope they will help clarify any issues you may have, too.

- ▶ I want to try food combining because I heard it was a great way to lose weight. Is that correct?

- ▶ So what's wrong with mixing proteins and starches at the same meal?

- ▶ How long should I leave between a protein meal and a starch meal?

- ▶ Where does sugar fit in to food combining?

- ▶ What about desserts?

- ▶ Does food combining allow alcohol?

- ▶ Where do fats fit in to food combining?

- ▶ Can you explain about milk and cream?

- ▶ I love porridge made with milk on a cold winter's morning, so I'm mixing protein and starch. Does that mean I have to give up my favourite breakfast?

- ▶ How do I get over the problem of putting milk on to breakfast cereal?

▶ Yoghurt is a protein food, isn't it?

▶ Pasta is shown as a starch but some types of pasta are made with egg. Doesn't that make it a food combining no-no?

▶ What about sauces and gravies?

▶ What do I do about salad dressings when I'm food combining?

▶ I read recently that marrow is a starchy vegetable. I'm confused. Don't I remember my home economics teacher saying that marrows were 95 per cent water?

▶ Why is it that corn-on-the-cob and corn from a can is starchy, but baby corns are not?

▶ Are peas listed with pulses (legumes) or with vegetables?

▶ What do I do about tomatoes?

▶ Are avocado pears listed as fruits or vegetables?

▶ Can you explain the term 'neutral'?

▶ I tried food combining once before but gave up because I wasn't sure how to plan my meals. Can you help?

▶ Several books on the Hay diet say that we should eat one protein, one starch and one alkaline-forming meal per day. What do you think about that?

▶ Sandwiches seem to be the biggest food combining nightmare. Have you any suggestions?

▶ How do I ensure that I eat enough vegetables and fruit?

▶ What about preserves?

▶ How do I food combine when I'm eating out?

▶ What about tea and coffee?

▶ Is food combining suitable for everyone?

**?** **I want to try food combining because I heard it was a great way to lose weight. Is that correct – and can you tell me how much weight I should expect to lose?**

Food combining has certainly proved itself to be a sensible and safe way to lose weight. One of the greatest plus points is that you don't need to count calories or weigh portions. If you food combine every day or if you follow the diet for five days each week and don't pig out at weekends, you should expect to lose weight at about 2 pounds (just under a kilo) every seven days. This may not seem very much compared to some diet programmes but, from experience, it seems to be a very effective method. Remember that weight lost slowly in this way tends to stay off. Weight lost quickly usually creeps back. Starting on page 112, you'll find a whole section of really useful information on the best way to balance your bodyweight.

**?** **So what's wrong with mixing proteins and starches at the same meal?**

To understand why combining proteins and starches may not be the healthiest option, it's important to know a little about how the digestive system works. I've explained this in the chapter entitled **Food Combining for Good Digestion** which begins on page 167.

**?** **How long should I leave between a protein meal and a starch meal?**

This is one of the most frequently asked food combining questions and causes unnecessary concern. In an ideal world, it is better to leave three or four hours between the two categories. If food is eaten at normal mealtimes, this gap is going to occur more or less automatically. Although food combining purists would not agree with me, I have found from my own experience that any gap is better than none. So if you find yourself eating protein only a couple of hours after starch – or the other way around – it is still going to be better than mixing them at the same sitting.

**? Where does sugar fit into food combining?**

Sugar is, in fact, a refined carbohydrate so should be treated as a starch. Keep sugar intake to an absolute minimum. See the **Swap Sheet** on pages 80–1 for sweet alternatives.

**? What about desserts?**

If sweet puddings (remember sugar is a carbohydrate) are eaten after a protein meal, they will interfere with stomach acid. All sweet foods are best kept to a minimum. Treat them as occasional treats and try to leave at least an hour between your main course and dessert.

**? Does food combining allow alcohol? If so, how is it combined?**

If you enjoy a glass of wine with a meal, don't worry about which foods you are eating at the time. Once again, I can hear the purists shaking their heads in disbelief and cautioning that wine, because it is made with grapes, shouldn't be taken at a starch meal. My attitude is a little different as I have not found that small quantities of alcohol disturb a food combined meal. At the end of a stressful day, a single unit of alcohol can be a real lift. And a little wine or beer added to a recipe gives flavour and interest. Research suggests that, in moderate amounts, alcohol may be a healthy addition to the diet. In excess, of course, it is a dangerous drug. Avoid cheap wines – they can upset the stomach. Keep fortified wines, beer, lager and spirits to a minimum, and avoid them altogether if you are trying to lose weight.

**? Where do fats fit in to food combining?**

Treat fats as versatile. They combine with proteins or starches. But use them wisely. Fats can be divided roughly into good and bad. *The Complete Book of Food Combining* includes only small quantities of butter, cream, crème fraîche, extra-virgin olive oil and other cold-pressed oils, and treats these as versatile. Lard, dripping, processed, margarine-type spreads and ordinary mass-produced cooking oils are not recommended. Follow the advice on pages 69–71 of the chapter **Eating for Better Health.**

**?** **Can you explain about milk and cream? Milk is supposed to be a first-class protein and yet you have it listed separately. And then you have cream as a versatile food. I thought they would both be under the protein section.**

The first thing to say is that, although we always think of milk as a protein, from a food combining perspective it has quite a low protein content (only about 3 per cent). It is, in fact, high in lactose (milk sugar), a carbohydrate which can be difficult to digest. Milk is also very mucus forming and, in some people, can aggravate sinus problems, catarrh, bowel discomfort and bloating. For this reason, I usually suggest that it is either avoided altogether or used in very small amounts, say in tea or coffee, but not added to other foods. On the subject of cream, some people find it easier to digest than milk possibly because we tend to use cream in much smaller quantities. The protein content is even lower (only between 1–2 per cent) but the fat content is high, so treat it as a fat and use it wisely. It combines with most protein or starch and makes a tasty extra added to porridge or soup.

**?** **I love porridge made with milk on a cold winter's morning, so I'm mixing protein and starch. Does that mean I have to give up my favourite breakfast?**

No, don't give it up. The answer to the previous question should answer part of your query. Make porridge more compatible and more digestible by preparing it with water instead of milk. Once it's cooked, serve with a drizzle of cold-pressed raw honey and chopped banana if you like it. For an occasional treat, add a teaspoonful of organic cream or crème fraîche. Delicious.

**?** **How do I get over the problem of putting milk on to breakfast cereal?**

If you eat breakfast cereal, adding ordinary cow's milk can make it very indigestible. I think this probably has more to do with the fact that milk is, for some sensitive stomachs, indigestible in the first place. Useful alternatives to cow's milk include rice milk, oat milk or almond milk (from health stores). Soya milk is very definitely a protein so doesn't mix well with starchy cereal. Yoghurt (especially sheep's yoghurt) and buttermilk are low in protein (see next question) and, for some people at least, seem to cause no problems when added to breakfast cereal. The answer is probably to experiment and see which alternative suits you best. Can I suggest that, if you find cereal difficult to digest, you avoid any that contain wheatflakes or wheatbran. See page 61 for more on wheat.

### ? Yoghurt is a protein food, isn't it? But I've also read that it contains starch.

Yoghurt has always been classed, officially and dietetically speaking, as a first-class or high-class protein. Until recently, I have always listed it as a protein. But, as a result of experience and experimentation over the years, I've found that it works well as a versatile food. This may be because most yoghurts contain only 5 or 6 grams of protein – well below that 10 per cent threshold. In addition, the actual process of making yoghurt renders it a much more easily digestible food than milk. So, although food combining books usually put yoghurt up there with the major proteins, consider it as a useful mix-with-anything food. The same rule applies to buttermilk.

### ? Pasta is shown as a starch but some types of pasta are made with egg. Doesn't that make it a food combining no-no?

The nutritional make-up of pasta is almost the same whether or not it has egg in its recipe. For the purposes of food combining, all plain pasta, whatever shape or colour, comes under the heading of starch. Herbs, spinach, tomatoes, garlic, vegetables or salads combine well with pasta. However, pasta with sauces or fillings made from meat or cheese are a mix of very concentrated starch plus protein and are therefore not compatible and best kept for non food combining days. See page 407 for ideas on pasta sauce.

### ? What about sauces and gravies?

Nearly all kinds of flour, such as wheat, potato, corn, chapatti, millet and rice flour, are a very concentrated form of starch. So, strictly speaking, any sauce that is made with flour (starch) and milk is an unacceptable combination. For the same reason, gravies and sauces that are thickened with flour are not ideal accompaniments for a protein meal. Pulped and puréed vegetables can make an interesting and nutritious alternative to gravy or sauce.

### ? What about salad dressings when I'm food combining?

Most dressings appear to combine well with protein meals. If a dressing contains lemon juice or vinegar, it is usually considered too acid for mixing with starch meals. Egg-based mayonnaise wouldn't be recommended with starch because of its protein content. However, (purists please put your hands over your ears) my experience has been that a drizzle (as long as it is a drizzle and not a huge dollop) of any kind of dressing is fine with proteins, starches, vegetables and salads. In other words, the quantities are usually too small to make any significant difference to the digestion of the main ingredients. Use your dressing and enjoy it.

### ? I read recently that marrow is a starchy vegetable. I'm confused. Don't I remember my home economics teacher saying that marrows were 95 per cent water?

You're quite right. I think you must have come across a book with a misprint. Marrows are mostly water and contain only a miniscule amount of starch, so low it's not even worth considering. Page 22 tells you which vegetables really are starchy.

### ? Why is it that corn-on-the-cob or corn from a can is starchy, but baby corns are not?

Corn becomes starchier as it ages. For example, baby corns are hardly starchy at all so you can combine them with starches or proteins. Once baby corns have grown large enough to be called cobs, or the kernels are removed from the cob and put into cans, their starch content has rocketed from 2 grams to around 20, so they need to be considered as a starchy vegetable.

### ? Are peas listed with pulses (legumes) or with vegetables?

Like corn, peas get starchier with age. Mangetout, sugar snaps, petit pois and fresh or frozen garden peas are classed as alkaline-forming, non-starchy vegetables – not pulses. They will combine comfortably with either proteins or starches and any other vegetables.

Dried, processed, mushy and marrowfat peas are starchy and are best served without proteins. Green beans, French beans and runner beans go in the non-starchy vegetable list.

### ? What do I do about tomatoes?

Strictly speaking, tomatoes are fruits not vegetables but they are so much part of our salad eating habits that, when it comes to food combining, we usually consider them as a salad item and say that they are versatile enough to go with anything. However, it is worth bearing a couple of things in mind. First of all, tomato juice can be very acidic and, as such, is best taken on its own and not with protein or starch. Second of all, tomatoes, once cooked, become extremely acidic and are not really suitable for mixing with starches. If you want to add tomatoes to pasta, the best way is to skin and pulp fresh ripe tomatoes into a sauce, heat the pulp very quickly and serve immediately, before it has a chance to acidify further.

### ? Are avocado pears listed as fruits or vegetables?

Like the tomato, avocado is really a fruit. However, because of its blandness and high levels of monounsaturated oils, it mixes comfortably and happily with absolutely anything. Avocado is an extremely nourishing food and also very easy for most people to digest.

### ? Can you explain the term 'neutral'? In some food combining books it seems to be used for two different things, one to refer to foods that are neither protein nor starch (such as vegetables) and also when talking about acid- and alkaline-forming food.

The word 'neutral' must cause a huge amount of confusion to anyone who has read more than one book on food combining. When I wrote my first food combining book, I was put under considerable editorial pressure to use the word 'neutral' when referring to anything that wasn't a protein or a starch in order to comply with an already published book on the Hay diet. I recognised quickly the error of my naivety and realised that I should not have allowed the mistake to be repeated. In subsequent books, I have interpreted the term, I hope, correctly. Neutral indicates anything with a pH of 7 – in other words, neither acid nor alkaline (see page 426). It is used as such in this book.

Water has a neutral pH. Unfortunately, the same word 'neutral' is still used by Hay followers to describe foods that are neither protein nor starch, in other words, vegetables and salads. This isn't really the correct use of the term but I presume it is chosen on the basis that, if a food is not a protein or a starch, then it must be somewhere in between. From a food combining point of view, vegetables and salads are not, in fact, 'neutral'. Once digested, they are, mostly, alkaline-forming. If you're confused, can I suggest that you forget about the word 'neutral'. You can follow the simple food combining system in *The Complete Book of Food Combining* very successfully without it. The best thing to do is to dismiss all the chemistry and just follow the charts on pages 46–7.

**?** **I tried food combining once before but gave up because I wasn't sure how to plan my meals. Can you help?**

Planning a food combined meal is not difficult. Simply imagine what you would have eaten before you chose to food combine and adapt it accordingly. And make sure you eat enough. Don't be afraid to increase portion sizes to compensate for the fact that you are no longer mixing proteins and starches on the same plate. Don't just skip the potatoes from a meal of, say, chicken, turkey or fish and leave it at that. Replace the spuds with extra vegetables or a generous side salad. If you're choosing a jacket potato as a main item, make sure it's bigger than usual. Top it with coleslaw, baked beans, hummus, grilled mush-rooms, or salad – or choose one of the alternative toppings on page 375. If you're used to eating your scrambled eggs (protein) on toast (starch), forget the toast and scramble an extra egg to make a bigger serving. Add a generous portion of sautéed mushrooms, or stir in some chopped smoked salmon, smoked haddock or grated cheese. If your chicken (protein) was going to be with rice (starch), prepare a slightly larger portion of chicken with at least three servings of vegetables. Plan to eat rice at another meal with beans and vegetables instead.

**?** **Several books on the Hay diet say that we should eat one protein, one starch and one alkaline-forming meal per day. What do you think about that?**

The idea behind this advice is to encourage a balanced intake of starch, protein, vegetables and fruit. It's a good way of ensuring a high intake of fresh produce and makes sure that we don't eat too much protein or too much starch. If we have, say, fruit for breakfast, that would be an alkaline-forming meal. A chicken salad would make a good protein lunch. A jacket potato with vegetables serves as an excellent starch-based supper. Alternatively, you could go for cereal and toast at breakfast (starch), a mixed salad at lunchtime (alkaline-forming) and a turkey stir-fry or fish dish in the evening (protein). These are good healthy guidelines, of course, but they don't always work in practice, especially if you are rushed off your feet and haven't had time to shop – or if you are eating out. Fortunately it can be just as healthy to have two protein meals and one starch meal per day – or two starch meals and one protein – as long as you include plenty of fresh vegetables, salad and fruit along the way. Don't forget that every time you add vegetables or salad to a protein or starch meal, you're adding alkalizing foods (for more information on acid- and alkali-forming foods, see pages 420–37). Do try to avoid having three starch meals or three protein meals a day and make sure that the starchy foods you choose are whole foods such as brown rice, pasta, whole oats and jacket potatoes. The recipe section, which begins on page 348, will guide you. So will the **Quick Reference Chart** on pages 46–7.

**?** **Sandwiches seem to be the biggest food combining nightmare. Have you any suggestions?**

It's easy to see that protein fillings such as ham, turkey, tuna, cheese and egg aren't going to combine with bread. Even some types of bread on their own can leave us feeling heavy and lethargic. If you're a sandwich fan, choose a close-textured soda bread, matzo cracker or rice cake and pile high with sliced avocado, tomato, red or yellow bell pepper and skinned cucumber. Potato salad, pasta salad or hummus (chickpea paste) make great toppings and fillings too.

**?** **How do I ensure that I eat enough vegetables and fruit?**

The simplest way is to count to five because you're aiming for five servings of fresh fruits and vegetables each day. Every glass of juice, piece of fresh fruit, side salad or heaped tablespoon of vegetables counts as one serving. So a banana, an apple, a tablespoon of peas, two or three good-sized florets of broccoli or cauliflower and a couple of small carrots is all that it takes to make up five daily servings. A slice of melon, a kiwi fruit, a vegetable stir-fry and a side salad of lettuce leaves, watercress, tomato and beetroot add up to another whole day's intake.

### ? What about preserves? Jam and marmalade are made from fruit so does that mean they don't combine with bread?

Acidic preserves do seem to cause indigestion in some people what-ever they are eaten with. Spreading them on to bread or crackers means you are mixing them with starch and this could be an indi-gestible combination for some people. However, I can only quote from experience which seems to suggest that jam and marmalade cause little or no difficulty if used on close-textured breads such as rye bread or soda bread. If you're crazy about preserves, enjoy them occasionally and don't worry about the combination. An even better alternative is to use cold-pressed raw honey instead.

### ? How do I food combine when I'm eating out?

Food combining in restaurants, at work, or at a dinner party in someone else's home isn't quite as simple as when you have direct control over your own menus. But if you can't food combine every single day of the week, don't be concerned. Eating out is, for some people, one of life's great pleasures. Don't spoil a special occasion by worrying about whether or not you are food combining. If you want to food combine away from base, here are a few ideas:

▶ Go for simple dishes, such as a fillet of fish with green vegetables or chicken breast with salad, so that you can see what's on the plate.

▶ Avoid foods that you can't directly identify, such as complicated dishes with a lot of ingredients hidden in a sauce.

▶ If you are ordering meat, poultry or fish, ask for an extra serving of vegetables or a side salad instead of potatoes or fries.

▶ Say no to the bread roll.

▶ Choose fresh fruit salad, melon or vegetable soup as an entrée instead of having fruit as a dessert.

▶ Allow time between courses.

▶ Avoid pizzas. They usually have protein toppings on starch bases.

▶ Avoid pasta with cheese or meat sauce or sprinkled Parmesan. Pasta with fresh vegetables, tomatoes or mushrooms, or tossed in olive oil and herbs would be fine.

▶ If someone offers you potatoes or rice with your protein, just say no thanks. If the plate arrives as a mixed meal, just enjoy it all and forget about food combining for this meal – or simply eat the protein and vegetables and leave the starchy foods to one side.

**? What about tea and coffee?**
Whether you choose to food combine or not, drinking too much coffee and tea can upset your absorption of some vitamins and minerals. There's no need to give up these beverages forever – there is some evidence that a cup or two each day can be uplifting and enjoyable – but it is best to drink them away from main meals.

**? Is food combining suitable for everyone?**
My experience is that food combining, if correctly followed, suits most people extremely well. None the less everyone has individual tastes and preferences and there is no diet in the world, however good, that will suit everybody. I usually suggest that newcomers to food combining try the system for one day a week or one meal a day to begin with, working up to five days (or, if you want to, seven days) a week. Write down any particular health problems before you begin and note improvements or changes as you progress. If it's working for you, you'll soon become aware of the benefits. If, after a month of regular food combining, you don't feel any benefit, then don't continue. If you are under the regular care of your doctor, dietitian or hospital specialist, are pregnant, or have any serious condition such as heart disease or diabetes, you should consult your medical adviser before commencing any new diet programme. If he or she hasn't heard of food combining, you may like to show them the sources of reference (pages 448–56) that relate to this book.

# CHAPTER 4

# Eating for Better Health

'It is not only the birds that have vanished. The wild flowers have gone from hillside pastures, while the heather and bilberry have been stripped from the upland plateaux. The diversity of life has been replaced with the gaudy bright green . . . of a snooker table baize.'

Graham Harvey, *The Killing of the Countryside*, 1997

Whether or not we choose to separate proteins from starches and go the food combining route, one of the most important aspects of any healthy eating programme should be to include a goodly proportion of unadulterated, fresh wholefoods. Unfortunately, many of the foods available to us are so heavily refined and denatured that most or all of the nutrients are lost during processing, in some cases requiring manufacturers to add back basic nutrients before they are allowed to sell the product. A great many items are also loaded, some might say over-loaded, with artificial additives, or sprayed liberally with pesticides. Although, individually, these chemicals may be classed as safe for human consumption, no one knows how trace amounts of lots of different ones might affect us in the long term.

One way to improve our nutrient intake and, at the same time, reduce the chemical overload that our bodies have to cope with every day, is to look a little more carefully at the food we eat and, whenever we can, choose chemical-free alternatives. In this chapter, I'll be looking at some of the problems associated with common foodstuffs and how we might overcome them. A useful way of keeping track of the changes you make is to tick them off as you go. Why not introduce one significant change each week?

## Bread

### Problem

**?** Bread is usually considered a dietary staple, an important source of B group vitamins and dietary fibre. Unfortunately the squashy, lightweight loaf that has become the standard bearer of British bread-making is not as nourishing as you might imagine. Fast-track bread production means that manufacturers need to add chemical improvers, emulsifiers and other additives to increase shelf life and replace the flavour lost through mass production. It also seems likely that increasing numbers of people are becoming sensitive to major ingredients such as wheat, gluten and yeast. A growing number of health practitioners now believe that the type of wheat used in commercial bread-making is not digested properly and, as a result, could actually be contributing to weight problems. I have seen many patients who found their digestive problems disappeared, their weight problems resolved and their energy levels soared when bread was reduced or removed entirely from their diet.

### Solution

Instead of regular sandwich bread, choose close-textured varieties such as soda bread or a wheaten loaf that is made using traditional methods. Or, if you are wheat-sensitive, avoid bread altogether and make rye bread, rye crackers, oat biscuits or rice cakes regulars on your shopping list.

All kinds of bread, biscuits and crackers are food combining starches.

# Breakfast Cereals

## Problem

? As with bread, sensitivity to the type of wheat found in breakfast cereals can be the sole cause of weight problems. Wheat is also rich in gluten, a gluey protein substance that, experts used to believe, only affected people with coeliac disease. Gluten can cause permanent injury to the intestinal wall and, recent figures suggest, may cause side effects in as many as four out of every ten people. In addition, many packaged cereals (even some that are marketed from a high-fibre or otherwise healthy standpoint) contain lots of 'hidden' sugar.

## Solution

Steer clear of those cereals that are obviously sugar-coated. Check the list of ingredients and avoid brands that have wheat and sugar (this could be sucrose, maltose, dextrose or glucose) near the top of the list. Unfortunately, this is an area that might require some dedicated sleuthing since the vast majority of supermarket cereals are wheat-based and sugar-rich. You could try oat-based cereals which contain much less gluten than wheat and do not appear to cause the digestive distress associated with wheat products. Or go for gluten-free muesli, or rice or millet cereals, usually available from health stores and becoming more widely available in supermarkets. If you suspect a gluten allergy or intolerance, simple blood tests should be available through your surgery or health centre.

All kinds of cereal are classed as food combining starches.

# Cheese

## Problem

? Cheese is generally high in fat and, as such, is often delisted from weight-loss diets as well as being a no-no for those with high cholesterol. In addition, cow's milk cheese is known to cause catarrh, skin eruptions, digestive discomfort and flatulence in some sensitive individuals. The cheese sandwich, a real heavy dude of a protein/starch mixture, can be a common cause of after-lunch lethargy and poor digestion. To cut down on chemicals, it's also worth steering clear of any cheese that is smoked, artificially coloured, processed or that contains artificial additives.

## Solution

Go for properly matured, unadulterated cheeses. Good-quality cheese is an important source of calcium. If you love this food but find that it doesn't agree with you in some way, then try goat's milk or sheep's milk cheeses (such as Feta, Roquefort, Peccorino or Halloumi) for a change. They are just as flavoursome and often easier to digest.

Cheese is a food combining protein.

# Chocolate

## Problem

For many of us, chocolate is an irresistible indulgence. What isn't so well known is that the commercial cocoa plantations that supply the raw material for chocolate-making are often sprayed with a particularly toxic cocktail of chemicals. Although this doesn't make chocolate an unsafe food, chocolate samples have been found to contain pesticide residues. In addition, environmental groups are concerned about the devastating effects of these sprays on the (predominantly female) plantation workers in developing countries who suffer severe health problems as a result of inhaling sprayed chemicals.

## Solution

Chocolate does not fit comfortably into food combining rules, so regard it as a treat and eat it separately from other foods. If you're a chocaholic, try to ease up but treat yourself to the occasional bar of organic chocolate which is grown without the use of pesticides. My favourite brand is Green & Black which comes in a variety of flavours. It's sold in nearly all supermarkets and health stores and tastes delicious! Green & Black also make an absolutely mouth-watering drinking chocolate powder which can be made into a hot chocolate treat using rice milk and, if desired, a little cold-pressed raw honey.

Chocolate doesn't fit well with food combining. Enjoy it as a treat but don't combine it with proteins or starches.

## Coffee

### Problem

**?** Caffeine is only one of several hundred chemicals in coffee and yet it's the one we seem to worry most about. A cup or two of coffee per day can be a useful 'pick-me-up'. However, too much can leave us feeling fidgety and unable to concentrate. Clinical observations suggest that coffee may also play havoc with female hormones, aggravating pre-menstrual problems, and menopausal symptoms such as hot flushes. A possible link has also been suggested between excessive caffeine intake and an increased risk of osteoporosis, infertility and cot death.

### Solution

For the first few weeks of your new food combining diet, try to avoid coffee altogether. Then, when you are feeling well and happy with your bodyweight, you can reintroduce it. But do enjoy coffee in moderation and use real ground coffee beans rather than instant powder or granules. Research suggests that coffee that is allowed to boil may increase the risk of furred arteries; so filtered coffee may be a better bet than percolated. Experiment with caffeine-free beverages such as herbal and fruit teas, savoury herbal drinks, dandelion coffee and grain-based coffee substitutes – all available from health stores.

Try not to take coffee or tea with a meal. These beverages may affect the absorption of some vitamins and minerals so they're best enjoyed away from mealtimes.

## Cow's Milk

### Problem

**?** Although seen as the ultimate calcium provider, milk is also a sensitive indicator of pollution levels. Dairy cattle pick up pesticide residues and other pollutants and pass them on via their milk. Even at levels deemed by the government to be 'safe', no one knows what – if any – long-term effects there might be. In addition, sensitivity to cow's milk appears to be on the increase, causing symptoms such as catarrh, sinus problems, irritable bowel, eczema, acne, digestive discomfort in adults and colic in babies. If you suffer from what one of my patients referred to as a 'gluey throat', feel mucousy or have difficulty swallowing, milk can sometimes be the cause.

Clinical observations also suggest that sensitivity to cow's milk can make it more difficult to lose weight. A magazine article I saw recently suggested that 'a glass of skimmed milk can curb the appetite and make a nutritious alternative to fizzy drinks'. Some may see it as better than soda pop, but others view skimmed milk as denatured, lifeless, boring and, like its semi-skimmed and full-fat relations, a troublesome allergen.

## Solution

Use small amounts in tea and coffee if you want to, but otherwise keep your intake to a minimum. For those who are not milk-sensitive, organic milk is an option that will reduce exposure to pesticides and hormones; it is available in all major supermarkets. Soya milk is not good in beverages as it can curdle. Although not compatible with starch from a food combining perspective, people with cow's milk allergy might use soya milk as an alternative on cereals. If you are concerned about genetically modified (GM) soya beans, ask your local store if they have organic non-GM soya milk. Almond milk – from health stores and some supermarkets – can be used for cold drinks and cooking, and can be added to coffee. Rice or oat milk are versatile alternatives that combine well with breakfast cereal. Surprisingly, yoghurt works well with cereal, too. This may be because yoghurt is already a very easily digestible food and has a protein level well below 10 per cent.

Cow's milk and soya milk are both classed as food combining proteins. Rice milk, oat milk, almond milk and yoghurt are **versatile** foods that go with anything.

# Crisps

### Problem

**?** Crisps (called chips in America, Australia and New Zealand) are a snack that most of us enjoy. They are classed as a starch but, because most tend to be high in fat and salt and are usually produced using hydrogenated vegetable oil (see **Margarine**, page 69), they are best kept to a minimum.

### Solution

A real treat but not very nutritious so only indulge occasionally. It could be worthwhile checking out your local health store for other healthier organic snack options. Organic crisps/chips are becoming more widely available.

Crisps/chips are definitely starchy.

# Eggs

### Problem

**?** Battery- or barn-raised eggs can contain artificial colourings (some colours are made from coal-tar dye) and residues from a number of different medicines, including antibiotics. As this book goes to press, there are moves afoot by a number of egg and poultry producers to stop using antibiotics as growth promoters. However, campaigners are still concerned about other aspects of feed quality, overcrowding and restricted movement, and of the stress and pain caused to a barn or battery bird during its short life. Standard free-range birds may have a less limited lifestyle, but could still be fed the same diet as a battery- or barn-raised hen. And remember that 'farm fresh' does not necessarily mean 'free-range'.

### Solution

Get the best eggs and poultry by choosing products that give you the maximum amount of information on welfare and feed content. Pack labels that don't tell you anything will almost certainly mean that the eggs they contain are battery or barn eggs. Some shops now stock organically fed, free-range eggs and poultry. Or you could buy from a local free-range farm that will let you see how the hens are kept. And by the way, contrary to common belief, there is no evidence that eggs raise cholesterol. There is no reason to avoid eggs unless you are vegan or unless eggs upset or disagree with you.

Where do eggs fit into food combining? Eggs (whites as well as yolks) are a food combining protein.

# Fish

### Problem

**?** Is fish polluted? For some time, experts have been advising us to eat fish, especially the oily kind (e.g. mackerel, sardines, herring, salmon) two or three times a week, mostly because they found that fish oil helped to reduce clogged arteries. Unfortunately, it has now been publicised that some fish is high in dioxins (page 251). As a result, the original recommendations have been changed to 'eat fish just once a week'. This is one of those Catch 22 situations where whatever we choose seems to be hazardous. There is little doubt that our food supply is increasingly contaminated in one form or another and, as a result, it's all too easy to become paranoid about everything we put in our mouths. Fish from the sea is very likely to be contaminated from polluted waters. Fish from farms may also be suffering from problems associated with toxicity or disease. Do we eat the food for its nourishment value or avoid it because of the chemicals it contains?

### Solution

The only real answer is to clean up the planet and reduce pollution levels but, in the meantime, it's worth sleuthing for good-quality fish. It's a quick-to-cook food that contains lots of valuable nourishment. My fishmonger tells me that fish from southern oceans (now also sold in many northern hemisphere supermarkets) and fish from good local fish farms may be the best options. Talk to your supermarket manager or local fishmonger, voice your concerns and get their advice.

Fish is a protein.

# Fresh Fruit and Vegetables

### Problem

 It is an unfortunate fact of modern intensive farming that the majority of crops are dusted with pesticides, herbicides and fungicides; some produce is doused many, many times during its growing cycle. Pesticide residues are a particular cause for concern. Staples, such as bread, milk and potatoes, have been shown to contain levels considered well above safety limits. In 1995, excesses of organophosphates were found in carrots; in 1998, levels of pesticides that exceeded safety limits were found in peaches and apples. And this doesn't mean that all other foods tested were pesticide-free, only that they were within the maximum limits allowed!

### Solution

Whenever possible, go for produce grown without chemical sprays. Organic potatoes, onions, mushrooms, lettuce, tomatoes, carrots and apples are widely available. Where organic alternatives are not around, don't give up on vegetables and fruit. Buy the best quality you can find and keep in mind that a slug, insect or blemish might indicate that a particular fruit or vegetable has been subjected to fewer chemicals than perfectly formed produce! Wash all produce thoroughly before use to remove dirt, bacteria, parasites and as much of the surface sprays as possible. Discard peel unless it's organic.

Non-starchy vegetables will combine successfully with either proteins or starches. Potatoes, sweet potatoes, yams and corn are starchy enough to be listed with other starch foods and so do not combine well with proteins. Fruit should be eaten separately from proteins and starches.

# Ice Cream

### Problem

 Avoid those brands that contain long lists of artificial additives and chemicals.

### Solution

Indulge as a treat but don't eat to excess. Choose quality brands with natural ingredients.

Not a good food combining item. Some ice creams contain dairy products (proteins) together with modified starches.

## Low-fat Foods

### Problem

**?** Low-fat cheese, low-fat ice cream, low-fat yoghurt, low-calorie mayonnaise and low-fat spread may sound better for us than the full-fat versions, but they can contain a whole stack of artificial additives; yet more chemicals to add to our toxic overload.

### Solution

Check labels and avoid those that contain obviously artificial additives. If the full-fat version is additive-free (they often are), then go for that but buy it in smaller quantities and eat less of it.

## Margarine and Butter

### Problem

**?** Low-fat spreads and margarines are promoted as healthier alternatives to butter because they are said to be 'rich in polyunsaturates', 'low in cholesterol', or have less saturated fat. All three attributes are supposed to be better for our heart and arteries. But I would advise caution. The majority of these fats are made from liquid vegetable oils that are heated under high pressure and mixed with hydrogen gas, chemical solvents, deodorisers and bleaching agents. This process, known as hydrogenation, alters the natural structure of the oil and changes some of the beneficial *cis* fatty acids into something called transfats. Some scientists have expressed concern that transfats may actually contribute to raised cholesterol or even heart disease. Hydrogenated vegetable fats turn up in a whole range of other foods too, including biscuits, cakes, crisps, doughnuts and oven chips.

Hydrogenation removes nutrients such as vitamin E, beta-carotene, lecithin and beneficial essential fatty acids. It's worth knowing that low-fat spreads go through a similar process but can also have emulsifiers, stabilisers, flavour enhancers, colours and plenty of water added to replace the fat.

And what about olive oil spreads? Well, although extra-virgin olive oil is believed to be very good for us, the olive oil used in spreads is still processed and, in any event, is unlikely to be the best quality oil. Extra-virgin olive oil is an excellent salad and sauté oil but, according to margarine manufacturers, its flavour is not suited to margarine-making.

### Solution

Why not go back to butter? Used in sensible quantities as part of a healthy balanced diet, there is no evidence that it causes heart disease. It's natural and, apart from a little salt in some brands, contains no additives. Or choose a spread made from unprocessed, non-hydrogenated oils – available from health stores and some supermarkets.

Good fats combine happily with protein or starch foods.

## Oils

### Problem

Nearly all the cooking oils that we see on the shelves are highly processed. The raw material (seeds, nuts, corn, etc) is treated in much the same way as it is for margarine-making. After being crushed or pressed, the extracted liquid is heated, bleached and deodorised using chemical solvents. Nutrients, including vitamin E and some essential fatty acids, are destroyed.

### Solution

A better-tasting alternative is to use extra-virgin olive oil. It costs more, but you'll use less. It's a good oil for stir-frying and for making dressings. And, even if it isn't good for manufacturing margarine, it's delicious spread on to or soaked into soda bread. Good olive oil thickens up if kept in the refrigerator. Go for bottles marked 'extra-virgin' or 'first pressing'. 'Pure' olive oil is cheaper but is often refined and not the best quality. The word 'pure' in this case usually indicates 'stripped' rather than its inferred definition of being something good. There are plenty of top-quality oils available in health stores and delicatessens, and some very good-quality 'own brand' labels available in most supermarkets.

Good fats and oils are compatible with proteins and starches.

## Red Meat

### Problem

**?** Putting moral issues aside, beef, pork and lamb are not always easy to digest and can take a longer time than most other foods to pass through the system. As a result, they can putrefy in the gut and give off toxins. If they are combined with starchy foods, digestion will be impaired even further. Concern has also been expressed that many sources of non-organic and intensively farmed meat (and poultry) contain antibiotic and hormone residues that pass into the food chain. A 1999 Food Commission report reminds us of some of the alarming ingredients that find their way into livestock feed. In the US, for example, animals have been fed cement dust, newspapers and cardboard. In the UK, an outbreak of botulism in cattle was traced to the use of chicken waste that included manure, feathers and decomposing carcasses being spread on to grazing land. And, as recently as June 1999, the Department of Agriculture in Dublin, Ireland, admitted that carcasses from abandoned and destroyed dogs were being processed into meat and bone-meal.

### Solution

If you enjoy your steak, chops or Sunday roast, check out a local supplier of organically reared meat. Instead of potatoes, which are of course, starchy, serve extra non-starchy vegetables. If you prefer to cut down on meat or avoid it altogether, replace some or all meat meals with other proteins such as fresh fish, organic free-range poultry and free-range eggs, non-GM soya, etc.

Red meat is a protein.

## Salt and Salty Snacks

### Problem

**?** Numerous research reports have confirmed that we should limit the amount of salt in our diets but this can be easier said than done. Sprinkling salt – and that added to vegetables during cooking – accounts for only around 10 per cent of our daily intake. A whopping 75 per cent comes from packaged foods such as biscuits, breakfast cereals, bread, bacon, stock cubes, soups, sausages and ready meals, and we don't always realise it's there. Just four slices of bread, two sausages and a couple of rashers of bacon would exceed the recommended maximum intake of 6 grams per day. Excess salt is associated with heart disease, strokes and a number of other serious disorders. Estimates suggest that 70,000 deaths per year in the UK – and much disability – could be prevented if less salt was added to processed food. In studies where salt has been reduced significantly in the diet, the number of strokes has declined by as much as 60 per cent.

### Solution

There are several ways to cut down on salt intake:

1. Keeping an eye on labels can make you more aware of what is in the food you are buying. The ingredients may not list the word 'salt' but might say sodium or sodium chloride, the chemical name for common salt. Avoid pre-packaged foods wherever possible and go for those that you know are low-sodium or sodium-free. Bread, breakfast cereals and biscuits are big danger zones.

2. Quit buying salty snacks. Look upon them as occasional treats instead. When you do indulge, make sure you drink extra quantities of water.

3. If you tend to use a lot of salt at the table, try to reduce it gradually over several weeks. It's worth knowing that if your system already has a high level of salt, you will be less able to detect a salty taste and be inclined to add still more to your food. The body does develop a kind of immunity to the flavour. Remember that it can take anything

from one to six months to adjust your palate away from salt. Once you've done it, you're likely to appreciate other, more subtle flavours.

**4.** Add new and interesting seasonings using fresh and dried herbs and spices such as ginger, curry, chilli, coriander, black pepper, parsley, mint and mustard. Include onions, shallots and chives, too – and garlic if you like it.

**5.** If you have seriously salty leanings, why not try shoyu or tamari – Japanese soy sauces – which can be less salty than regular dark Chinese soy. Or grey sea salt – said to be the best-quality sea salt – and more concentrated than regular salt so that you need to use less.

Be especially vigilant about your salt intake if you suffer from cardio-vascular problems, osteoporosis, asthma, or if there is a family history of heart disease or stroke. Unless you suffer from any of the above conditions, a little salt in the diet is unlikely to be harmful and can improve the flavour of some foods. Reducing salt during very hot weather can actually be dangerous to your health. The chapter on **Food Combining and Fluid Retention** (pages 156–66) has more information about salt.

As a condiment, salt can be used on proteins and starches.

---

**IMPORTANT NOTE**
Never give salty foods or add salt to a baby's or toddler's diet. At that age, their kidneys just can't cope with excess sodium.

---

## Soft Drinks

### Problem

**?** Those soft drinks that are sold as 'diet' or 'one cal' options usually have artificial sweeteners added to replace some or all of the sugar. It has also been suggested that some of the ingredients in canned drinks might be associated with hyperactivity or other behavioural difficulties in children. Fruit-flavour drinks contain only token quantities of fruit juice or, sometimes, none at all. Some 'energy drinks', juice drinks, soda pops, mixers and lemonades, may also include artificial flavours, sweeteners, sugars, colours and/or preservatives (see also page 76 on artificial sweeteners).

### Solution

In small amounts, canned and bottled fizz is unlikely to do us any harm, but they have little or nothing beneficial or nutritious going for them. They are best avoided by children who suffer with Attention Deficit Disorder (ADD) or who have problems with hyperactivity. Freshly squeezed juices, bottled organic juices topped up with carbonated water, and additive-free herbal drinks are delicious and a much healthier option. Several new brands incorporate natural sweetening in the form of real juice and plant extracts that are said to offer health benefits. Fresh lemonade and real ginger beer are also widely available.

Avoid drinks with additives – or keep them to a minimum. The high sugar content of many brands means that they are best taken on their own away from other foods.

## Sugar

### Problem

**?** Once referred to as 'pure, white and deadly', sugar really is a lifeless food. It contains no nourishment and, in fact, can actually rob the body of vitamins. Sugar stockpiles the calories and rots your teeth. It can also pickle your pancreas and upset the levels of glucose in your blood, increasing the risk of diabetes and cardiovascular disease.

Sucrose, maltose, dextrose and glucose are all forms of sugar produced by an industrial refining process that filters and boils the liquid extracted from sugar cane or beet into crystals using gases such as sulphur dioxide and carbon dioxide. Milk of lime together with charcoal – sometimes made from charred beef bones – have also been used in sugar production.

Sugar can provide instant energy but the effect is only short-lived. The absorption and metabolism of sugar puts enormous strain on the system, using up valuable reserves and overworking important organs such as the adrenal glands and the liver – and, of course, the aforementioned pancreas. Lots of refined sugar in your diet can cause the levels of natural glucose in the blood to fluctuate wildly, affecting the mechanisms that control hunger and increasing the risk of cravings, bingeing and putting on extra pounds. In fact, keeping blood glucose levels properly balanced is probably one of the most important factors in keeping your weight where you want it. And – sorry to have to tell you this – most ordinary brown sugar is merely white sugar plus colouring.

## Solution

Real brown sugar, which does contain trace amounts of a number of different vitamins and minerals, will tell you on the label if it is unrefined or 'raw'. Cold-pressed raw honey, available from health stores, is a healthier alternative to white sugar and can be used in beverages, and on yoghurt and cereals. New Zealand Manuka honey is especially flavourful and nutritious. Other useful sugar substitutes for occasional use are real maple syrup, barley malt, rice malt and blackstrap molasses – good because they tend to release their sugars more slowly into the system.

Keep sugar to a minimum and treat it – and other sweetenings – as starchy foods. They do not combine well with proteins.

# Sweeteners

### Problem

**?** Don't be tempted to use artificial sweeteners as a sugar substitute. Although sweeteners are essentially calorie-free and are to be found in an ever-increasing number of processed and packaged foods and drinks, medical experts can't agree whether these chemicals are a healthy alternative to sugar or a potential health risk. In fact, scientific and medical journals are peppered with less-than-encouraging reports about sweeteners. One study suggested that sweeteners can actually *increase* the appetite; and there are reports elsewhere of side-effects such as waterworks problems, headaches, visual disturbance, nervous-system disorders, nausea, bloating, and weight gain! Whatever the eventual outcome of the research, sugar substitutes are a relatively new introduction into the chemical cocktail of modern-day living.

### Solution

My advice would be: don't add them to your tea or coffee and avoid packaged foods that already contain sweeteners.

Sweeteners are calorie-free chemicals which are best avoided.

# Tea

### Problem

**?** Tea has less caffeine than coffee. However, too much tea can rob the body of iron. If you drink tea with – or immediately after – a meal, it may impair the absorption of iron. It's also worth knowing that overdoing the number of cuppas per day can aggravate constipation. However, in moderate amounts some research suggests tea may offer valuable health benefits.

### Solution

If you want to stick with your usual brew, try it weaker, with a slice of lemon instead of milk. People who give up milk in their tea often find that they then don't need the brew to be quite so strong. What about alternatives? According to research, green teas are believed to have potent health-giving properties and may also be of value to anyone trying to lose weight. Herbal tisanes are also healthier than caffeine-rich beverages. Peppermint and ginger teas can help to calm the digestion; camomile soothes anxiety and nervous tension and makes a good bedtime drink. Rosehip is gently detoxifying and helps to neu-tralise and remove waste products. Rooibos is a low-tannin substitute for ordinary tea. Jasmine tea is delicious with lemon. Fruit teas are refreshing, too. Most supermarkets now sell specialist teas as well as herbal variety packs that contain six or more different flavours in one box. Useful if you want to try before buying larger sizes. Health stores usually have a wide range of really interesting teas. See also page 440 in the **Resources** section.

Try not to drink tea or coffee with a meal as this could hinder absorption of some nutrients.

## Water

### Problem

**?** Water is even more essential to life than good food. Unfortu-nately, most of us don't drink enough of it. Even if we remember to drink it, we can be easily put off by the taste of tap water.

### Solution

I make no apologies for nagging on about water throughout this book. I would very strongly advise everyone to invest in a water filter. Sophis-ticated plumbed-in, under-sink units are the ideal option but not all of us can afford them. A good-quality jug or portable unit is a much cheaper alternative and can improve considerably the quality of drink-ing water. I've used a jug filter for many years and found it to be excellent. Fill your kettle from your filter jug and use freshly filtered water for cooking and drinking. In fact, every-thing except washing yourself, washing clothes and washing up! You'll find good-quality filter jugs in most supermarkets, hardware stores, kitchen shops, chemist shops and health stores.

One very important rule: Remember to change the filter cartridge frequently and wash the jug thoroughly between each change. Neglected jugs and old cartridges will breed bacteria very quickly and the cartridge may not be effective if it is allowed to dry out. During use, keep the jug topped up so that water is always available. If filtered water is not available, then choose non-carbonated bottled water. Unfiltered tap water is not recommended.

## A Note about Organic Foods

There is no doubt that organic meat and poultry tends to be more expensive than mass-produced 'equivalents' but, with a little planning, your food bills don't need to be higher. Because of the groundswell of public opinion in the UK and some European countries against genetically modified foods, supermarkets have responded with much larger stocks and wider ranges of organic produce, including such items as sauces, chutneys, juices, cereals, olive oil, baked beans, all kinds of pulses, milk, butter, eggs, soya milk and nuts – to name just a few. There are lots more organic vegetables around which, in many stores, cost only slightly more than commercial produce. Test this for yourself by checking the cost of, say, regular commercially grown carrots against that of organic carrots. If you do spend more on organics, balance your budget by replacing one or two meat, fish or poultry meals with less expensive options. Make good use of cheaper ingredients such as beans and rice, pasta and salad, and mixed vegetable dishes. In Part Three of this book – from page 348 – you'll find plenty of recipes for tasty budget meals.

## Be Well Informed

One of the best ways of improving the quality of the food available to us is to be as well informed as possible and, if you're not happy about something, to make a noise about it. Write to the head office of the supermarket you shop at most regularly and ask to see local managers. If you want fewer pesticides, no genetic modification, better food labelling and more organic produce, tell them. Write to MPs, MEPs,

Senators, Congressmen and tell them the same thing. Politicians and retailers do respond if they are put under enough pressure.

You can also learn more about food and keep up to date with the latest information if you:

1. Subscribe to *The Food Magazine*. This journal is published six times a year by the Food Commission (UK), an independent, non-profit-making organisation that campaigns for safer, healthier food. They receive no government subsidies and are not supported by advertising or by the food industry. Write to: The Publications Department, The Food Commission (UK) Ltd, 94 White Lion Street, London N1 9PF. Tel: 020 7837 2250; fax: 020 7837 1141; e-mail: foodcomm@compuserve.com and website: www.foodcomm.org.uk

2. Send an s.a.e. to The Soil Association, Bristol House, 40–56 Victoria Street, Bristol BS1 6BY. They can provide information about suppliers of organic meat and produce in your area including doorstep deliveries. Or visit their website at www.soilassociation.org

## ESSENTIAL READING

▶ Joanna Blythman's excellent book *The Food We Eat* (Michael Joseph). Very highly recommended.

▶ *Secret Ingredients – The essential guide to what's really in the products you buy*, by Peter Cox and Peggy Brusseau (Bantam Books).

▶ *Hard to Swallow – The truth about food additives* by Doris Sarjeant and Karen Evans (Alive Books).

▶ *Foods Matter at The Inside story*, a quarterly publication aimed primarily at people with food allergies and sensitivities but also an informative source of relevant health information and allergen-free recipes. For subscription details, send a large s.a.e. to Berrydales Publishers, Berrydale House, 5 Lawn Road, London NW3 2XS.

## SWAP SHEET

Whether you decide to food combine or not, you can improve the quality of your diet – and reduce the risk of food sensitivity – by taking a few tips from my specially devised Swap Sheet.

| SWAP THIS | FOR THIS |
|---|---|
| anything deep-fried | grilled, baked or casseroled |
| the chip pan | the wok |
| ordinary processed cooking oils | extra-virgin olive oil |
| ordinary salad oils | cold-pressed oils |
| hydrogenated and low-fat spreads | a little butter or Vitaquell |
| chips | scrubbed sliced spuds, sautéed in a pan or drizzled with olive oil and baked |
| instant mash | organic jacket potatoes |
| sweets and cakes | wholegrain cereal bars, dried figs, dried apricots, fresh fruit, natural liquorice, sesame halva |
| packaged orange juice | apple, cranberry or grape juice; better still, juice your own (see page 30) |
| chocolate | organic chocolate – truly delicious and chemical-free |
| coffee, strong tea and cola | weak tea, green tea, Bambu, savoury beverages, herbal teas, fruit teas, soup, fresh vegetable and fruit juice, lots of filtered water |
| red meat | fresh fish, especially salmon, sardines, mackerel, tuna and trout |

| SWAP THIS ➡ | FOR THIS |
|---|---|
| battery- or barn-raised eggs and poultry | organic, free-range eggs and poultry |
| cow's milk | organic soya milk, almond milk, rice milk or oat milk |
| cow's milk cheeses and yoghurt | those made from sheep's or goat's milk |
| wheat-based and sugar-heavy cereals | check pack labels for sugar and wheat; go for oat cereals, porridge and wheat-free muesli instead |
| mass-produced bread | yeast-free soda bread, pumpernickel, rye bread, rye crackers, oat biscuits, rice cakes, matzos, pitta bread |
| salt | fresh herbs, sun-dried tomatoes, garlic, ginger |
| vinegar | cider vinegar, balsamic vinegar, Molkosan |
| ordinary brown or white sugar | cold-pressed raw honey, real maple syrup, organic Demerara, blackstrap molasses, barley malt, rice malt |
| ready meals and takeaways | if possible, home-prepared meals from basic ingredients so you know what goes into your food |
| commercially grown fruit and veg | organic fruit and veg whenever you can |
| foods containing artificial additives | foods that don't |

# The Importance of Exercise

'Exercise in the open air is of the first importance to the human frame, yet how many are in the manner deprived of it by their own want of management of their time!'

Hints on active exercise, taken from *Enquire Within Upon Everything*, London, 1906

Everyone intends to do it, all the experts recommend we should do it, we all know it's good for us but we still make excuses for not doing it. I don't need to tell you that regular physical activity is great for boosting general health and well-being. So much so, say researchers, that it could help you to live longer. But only if you *don't* overdo it. Too much could be as bad as too little. And exercise doesn't need to be complicated, costly or time-consuming to be effective. Food combining is well known for its ability to help weight loss, but in order to lose weight and keep it off, you really need to exercise too.

Most people concentrate on the weight-loss aspects of exercise but regular activity has lots of other terrific health benefits. Apart from helping to tone muscle and speed up the metabolism, moderate aerobic exercise strengthens the heart and lungs, strengthens the bones, improves the circulation, helps to reduce cholesterol levels, and increases the production of chemicals that enhance our mood and our tolerance of stress. Exercise improves the way our bodies eliminate waste, and is especially good for the lymph system and for toning up a sluggish bowel. And, because it stimulates production of natural painkilling chemicals called endorphins, exercise can actually help to relieve pain. Moderate and sensible levels of exercise are great for the immune system, enhancing our resistance to infection.

## No Need to Overdo It

Too much exercise can have the opposite effect. So please take care. Over-exercising can put strain on all body systems, in particular the immune system.

Over-training can be a real risk for professional dancers, sports stars and athletes. While they have to be dedicated to rigorous schedules and strict diets if they are to succeed in their chosen field, there is a down-side. Excessive activity can lead to health problems such as lowered immunity, muscle fatigue, hormonal imbalances and, in some cases, weakening of the skeleton. The same dangers apply to anyone who works out to extremes.

## Easy Does It

The good news for exhausted executives, busy parents and couch potatoes everywhere is that exercise doesn't need to be an endurance test. The official recommendation is to do some form of aerobic exercise for 20 minutes a day or 40–45 minutes three times a week. But if you are really, seriously and honestly pushed for time, a minimum of just three 15-minute sessions each week is a good beginning. Quarter of an hour's brisk walk round the houses or across the park every other day is likely to be better for your bones than an every-now-and-then, all-day hike across the hills and just as good as a regular aerobics class.

## What's the Best Type of Exercise?

The best type of exercise is any regular, low-impact, weight-bearing activity. 'Weight-bearing' simply means that your skeleton is support-ing your bodyweight against the force of gravity, usually while you are moving the whole weight of your body from one side to the other. Such activities include keep-fit sessions, stepping, rebounding (mini-trampoline), brisk walking, badminton, tennis, squash and cycling.

## What can exercise do for you?

The following are just a few of the comments collected from people suffering a range of health problems who have taken up and now enjoy regular exercise:

'Exercise gives you more energy.'

'Exercise keeps my weight where it should be.'

'Exercise feels like it's made my heart and lungs stronger.'

'It just makes you feel better.'

'Exercise keeps me warm.'

'I've meant to do it for years. Now I wish I'd started earlier.'

'It's good for the bones. That's why I do it.'

'I couldn't walk, the pain was so bad. Now I walk every day.'

'It's the best stress-buster ever invented.'

'Exercise makes me sleep better.'

'Exercising is good for you.'

'It's licked my depression. I just don't get down any more.'

'Since I started walking I've learned so much more about wildlife and the countryside.'

'I loved it after I'd made the move.'

'Exercise helps you to enjoy life more.'

'I thought I'd hate exercise but I love it.'

'Exercise? What do you want me to say? It's just great.'

'Exercise is one of those wonderful things that, once you have put your proverbial toe in the water, you want to jump right in and do more.'

## Exercise and Detox

Exercise helps to detoxify the body and reduce acidity in the tissues. Some research suggests that the sweating associated with exercise may enhance the removal of carcinogenic chemicals from the body. Rebounding (exercising on a mini-trampoline) is an excellent way to encourage lymph drainage and so is an added bonus to detoxification. During any detox programme, it is wiser to take a little less exercise. Fresh air, sunlight, a short brisk walk every day (or gentle rebounding and simple stretching if the weather is inclement), together with plenty of slow, steady breathing, are all highly recommended. But don't jog for miles around the park or work out until you drop. It simply isn't necessary.

## Exercise and Weight Loss

Weight gain especially past the age of 30 can have a lot to do with lifestyle. We get to the point in our lives where leisure time is thin on the ground and workload increases. We're impossibly busy, we give everyone else priority, and have no space to look after ourselves. And yet, together with a healthy eating programme, regular exercise is a vital force for weight control. So it really is important to maintain the effort.

### Get yourself moving

If you've always thought that exercise was too difficult, sweaty and time-consuming, you might be surprised – and pleased – to discover that regular, sustained, low-impact activity such as brisk walking, rebounding, keep fit or cycling can be better for weight loss than strenuous aerobics or jogging.

When you sit still, you burn only between 75 and 100 calories an hour. Compare this to vigorous activity such as cycling or dancing which can use up anything from 250 to 500 calories in an hour. To get rid of fat, you need to push up your pulse rate and get a bit sweaty and a bit out of breath. The speed and intensity of the activity you choose will determine how much fat-busting you achieve. At first, your stamina may seem quite low. Endurance and staying power comes with practice and it can take time. So don't be disappointed or expect too much all at once. And don't try to 'go for the burn' (silly expression) or push yourself into strenuous work-outs that aren't suited to your level of fitness. Take it easy and you'll get there just the same.

## But you've tried it already?

It's a common cry from people trying to lose weight that exercise 'didn't work either'. That's usually because they start a programme, stick with it for a while, think it isn't working and so give it up. There are several reasons why this is set up to fail.

Exercise on its own, without the benefit of dietary improvement – may not be all that successful in the long-term weight-loss war. It's great for building and toning muscle. On the other hand, if you shun activity and try to lose weight just by dieting, you could lose muscle as well as fat. And less muscle means a slower metabolism. Exercise *plus a great diet* encourages muscle building – and muscle uses up more calories than fatty tissue.

In addition to the regular aerobic stuff, strength-training also builds muscle; new research suggests that it could play a useful role in speeding up the metabolism. But don't waste time checking yourself on the scales. When you exercise, muscles get toned as the flab decreases so weighing machines don't always register any immediate weight loss.

## Exercise and Mood

Exercise doesn't just make us physically fitter and healthier. It also increases the production of brain chemicals that make us calmer and happier. It lifts our self-esteem and adjusts our perspective so that we not only feel good about ourselves but also feel better about our surroundings. Exercise is good for the brain in other ways, too. With age and inactivity, brain cells die and the brain itself shrivels. Some experts have suggested that regular activity could help to reduce this cell degeneration by improving blood and oxygen flow.

## DON'T FORGET

Regular exercise should be as important to a healthy lifestyle as healthy eating. Think of them as two sides of the same coin. One side doesn't work too well without the other.

If you work out, or are involved in any other kind of vigorous exercise, running or sports on a regular basis, here's some important advice.

▶ Make sure that you're eating a varied diet that contains plenty of orange, yellow, purple, blue, red and green plant foods – a real 'rainbow' menu of fresh fruits and plenty of green and root vegetables, rich in antioxidant vitamins A, C and E. Heavy exercise can deplete the body of certain nutrients, leaving it more susceptible to opportunistic infections. The powerhouse of nutrients in fresh produce not only helps to boost the immune system, it is also needed for repairing sprains and strains, for healing cuts and grazes, and for protecting the skin against UV damage.

▶ Take a once-daily antioxidant multi-supplement to boost your dietary intake. Page 438 has information on the best brands to look out for.

▶ After training, our muscles need refuelling. Sports drinks are an ideal solution because they replace carbohydrates, water and electrolytes (mineral salts that are lost through profuse sweating), and supply readily usable energy. However, don't rely on them as a regular fluid when you are not exercising.

▶ On the days when you work out, aim to drink at least 2 (3½ pints) litres of water in addition to other fluids. On other days, 1–1½ litres (1¾–2½ pints) of water is about right. Failure to replace vital fluids can lead to cramps, fatigue and, especially in hot weather, heat stroke and heat exhaustion. Be aware that it's possible to get dehydrated without feeling thirsty so make sure you drink plenty in winter as well as in summer. Water is essential not only to prevent dehydration during hot weather; at any time of year, loss of fluid causes the blood to thicken and can increase the risk of a heart attack.

▶ Wear strong, supportive but supple and well-cushioned footwear.

▶ Women should wear a supportive and well-fitting (that doesn't mean tight) sports bra.

▶ Choose comfortable, roomy clothing, layered so that you can remove items as you begin to warm up.

▶ Always replace your track-suit top or jacket at the end of an exercise to help prevent chills and muscle spasms.

▶ Don't forget to stretch gently before and after exercise to maintain mobility and reduce the risk of injury.

## Exercise in Later Life

What about people who are older, less mobile, have sight problems or are simply not well enough to take their trainers round the block? Inactivity causes muscle loss and weakness, and slows up the circulation. Chair-based exercises, especially stretching and gentle arm and shoulder movements, and lifting small weights, can maintain muscle strength, keep the circulation going, help to keep joints flexible, and reduce the risk of cold, stiff limbs.

The pain and inflammation associated with arthritis is a very justifiable reason for moving around as little as possible. Movement causes discomfort, which can sometimes be extreme and almost unbearable. In rheumatoid arthritis, the breakdown of muscle tissue also hinders physical activity. But if moving worries you, not moving should worry you more.

It's true that, for many years, people with arthritis were told they shouldn't exercise because it might damage their joints. Now experts know the opposite is the case. What's really interesting is that, while overdoing it can cause even more discomfort, inactivity actually increases the likelihood of stiffness and immobility.

But how can you exercise when you're stiff and in pain? At the outset, exercise can seem a daunting prospect. But the benefits are so great that, believe me, the effort *really is worth it*. Yes, it can hurt to move but if you're consistent with your exercise programme, whether it's your twice weekly keep-fit class, a daily walk to the shops, simple stretching or dancing while you dust, the body's natural painkillers – known as endorphins – kick in and keep you going.

## Getting help to find out about exercise options

First of all, talk to your doctor, practice nurse or health visitor and find out about local exercise classes. If you can't drive and have no other transport, are there any local organisations or day-care services that could take you to a class? What about your local physiotherapy department? Your doctor should be able to refer you for assessment and help with a basic stretch and strengthen programme. If severe and chronic pain is preventing you from exercising, ask your doctor to refer you to the nearest pain clinic. Pain Management Programmes are run at a number of hospitals around the country. They provide an absolutely excellent service – including exercise, relaxation, occupational therapy assessment, advice on medication and plenty of other support for anyone who is immobilised by chronic pain. You'll meet other people with similar difficulties and share knowledge. For some people, it can be the beginning of a rewarding social life. You don't have to be wheel-chair-bound to qualify.

## Surf the net

If you're not up to surfing the waves, you could try surfing the net. The internet has a fabulous wealth of information on exercise for all age groups and abilities. One particularly helpful website is that of the American Arthritis Association which can be found at www.arthritis.org. In the UK, useful leaflets on exercise are available from The Arthritis and Rheumatism Council, 41 Eagle Street, London WC1R 4AR. Please send a large s.a.e. and two first-class stamps.

# On Your Marks, Get Set, Go

It's all too easy to make excuses for not exercising. Even the able-bodied among us – who really have no excuse – will turn up chestnuts such as 'I'm far too busy', 'I really don't have the time', 'I don't have the space', 'Exercise is boring', 'I don't need to exercise, I feel ok', 'I can't afford all that equipment', 'I don't have the right gear', 'There aren't any classes near me', 'It's dark', 'It's too cold', 'I'm too tired', or 'I'm too old for exercise'.

So you'll be pleased when I tell you that:

▶ A simple exercise programme really doesn't take up a lot of time.

▶ Or a lot of room.

▶ Exercise definitely isn't boring as long as you choose an activity you really enjoy.

▶ Everybody needs to do it however fit they think they are.

▶ You don't need any special equipment.

▶ Or special clothing.

▶ Classes can be helpful – and great fun – but aren't essential.

▶ You don't have to exercise outside if it's dark or the weather is bad.

▶ Exercise can give you a real energy boost even when you're feeling jaded.

▶ No one is ever too old to begin exercising.

## MY TIPS FOR GETTING STARTED

### Choose an activity that you really enjoy

What about cycling (moving or static), rowing, rebounding, walking the treadmill, walking the dog, swimming, skipping, stepping or aerobics? Lifting sensible weights or doing yoga are both great for strengthening muscles. Or how about Pilates, a programme of strengthening exercises, breathing, and posture techniques that incorporates elements of yoga, t'ai chi and the Alexander technique.

## Be creative

If the usually recommended types of exercise don't appeal, go for other options. What about ballroom dancing, line dancing or dancing around the house to your favourite music? Take a brisk walk down a country lane or go a few times round the block. Walk up and down stairs 25 times.

## Start slowly

Whatever you choose, start slowly and work up to a regular 20 minutes a day or 40–45 minutes three times a week. A five-minute stint is quite enough to begin with, if you're not used to exercise. Trying to do an hour's walk on your first day is almost bound to put you off going again because you'll feel sore the next morning.

## Always warm up first

Cold muscles are tense muscles and more prone to injury. Before you begin, reduce the risk of injury or pain by walking up and down on the spot, gently stretching the arms and legs.

## Make sure you're comfortable

You don't need special clothing but do wear comfortable clothes and sensible shoes, and make sure you aren't likely to get chilled.

## Pace yourself

Never exercise to the point of unbearable pain or discomfort. If, at any point, you are feeling uncomfortable, stop. And don't get to the point where you are so out of breath that you can't speak. It's fine to be puffed but you should be able to speak (or sing) while you are exercising.

## Think twice about jogging

Pounding the tarmac can cause more health problems than it solves. Unless you are really fit and have good impact-absorbing footwear, you are probably going to be jarring your spine. And if you are running near traffic, you will almost certainly be breathing in unacceptable levels of pollution. It seems to me that jogging is not the most enjoyable pastime. When I see runners huffing along the highway, I always wonder why so many of them look drained, exhausted, unwell and unhappy.

## Don't set unrealistic goals

If you tell yourself that you are going to exercise for 20 minutes and then you can't do more than 15, you give yourself the message that you failed. If you find it helps to set yourself a target, start with one minute, two minutes or five minutes and increase on that over a period of a few weeks.

## Be patient

If you've been overweight for years or have a lot of weight to lose, don't expect to shed it in just a week or two. Be patient. Remind yourself again that crash dieting hardly ever succeeds in the long term. Weight lost quickly nearly always creeps back. Weight lost slowly and naturally, stays lost.

## Plan your walks

If you decide on walking as part of your regular exercise routine, why not plan a new route each day and focus on a destination? It doesn't have to be miles away. It could be as far as the church door, the other side of the park, the trees by the lake, two tube stops or a few bus stops away, the war memorial at the other end of the village, the post office or the shops. If you really are under pressure at work and have to leave home early and get back late, could you go for a walk at lunchtime? Is there a park nearby? Or, if you use public transport, could you get off before your stop and walk the rest of the way?

## Make time

If time is at a premium, it can help to exercise in shorter bouts. For example, could you do ten minutes twice a day? Once you establish a routine, you'll probably find you want to make more time. What's important here isn't so much the amount of time you spend but the regular commitment.

## Ring the changes

You don't have to do the same type of exercise each day. Ring the changes. Anything that gets the heart rate up a bit and makes you puff will do.

## Exercise to music

For many people, music makes exercising easier. Choose something that has a good rhythm. Slow stuff won't encourage you to move and anything too fast could make you overdo things without realising it.

## Find a buddy

If you aren't motivated to exercise by yourself, find a companion. With a work-out partner, you'll be much more likely to motivate each other.

## Join a class

If you're better working in a group, make enquiries about local classes. They are usually very inexpensive and sometimes free. Ask at your local health centre, council offices or library. Or look in the local paper or community newsletter. Make your class into an enjoyable outing and get involved.

## Don't let age stop you

You're never too old to begin. One of the problems of ageing is that we swap muscle for fat. This is especially true if you haven't exercised regularly throughout life and have a sedentary job. It should encourage you to know that, the more regularly you exercise, the more flab you will whittle away, the more muscle you will build, and the stronger you will feel.

## Give yourself incentives

Tell yourself you can't read that book or article or watch television until you have done your daily exercise.

## Praise yourself

Congratulate yourself on your achievements, however small they may appear to be. Tell yourself out loud 'I did it' and then keep up the good work.

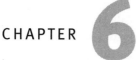

# Food Combining – Then as Now

'History does not repeat itself. Historians repeat each other.'

Arthur James Balfour, Scottish statesman and philosopher, 1848–1930

I've deliberately left the history of food combining until the end of Part One. I felt it was important for you to get to grips with the nitty gritty of how to food combine first. But let's step back for a moment and take a look at the history of food combining and how things have developed over the years. If you're familiar with food combining you'll probably have read a lot of conflicting information regarding its origins and who was responsible for what. This chapter will set the record straight.

## The History of Food Combining

The history of food combining is fascinating – and it's full of surprises. If you've already read any books or articles about it, you'll no doubt have discovered that its invention and subsequent success is usually attributed to an American doctor, William Howard Hay. Dr Hay's name is now forever associated with food combining. But that he invented it is a myth perpetuated by modern books and articles that keep the legend alive through repetition and hearsay. The truth has been exaggerated so much in the telling that nearly all UK publications on food combining credit Dr Hay with all kinds of discoveries that belong, indisputably, to others. In fact, the foundations of food combining were conceived many centuries before Dr Hay was even a twinkle in his father's eye.

Dr Hay was born in Hartstown, Pennsylvania, in 1866, and began his medical practice in 1891. By the time he reached his forties, his penchant for fine food had pushed his weight up to an uncomfortable 16 stone (224 lb or just over 100 kg), and, as a result, his health began to fail.

A vigorous exercise programme was initiated. The upside was that it greatly increased Dr Hay's endurance. But there was a downside. It did absolutely nothing to diminish his already admirable appetite. And the weight simply wouldn't shift. When he was diagnosed with high blood pressure, an enlarged heart and a serious kidney complaint, his medical colleagues were gloomy about his prospects.

In desperation, Dr Hay turned his attention to nutritional therapy and put himself on a diet, which he came to describe as 'eating fundamentally'. Over the ensuing months, he lost 3½ stone (49 lb/22 kg) and, to the amazement of his pessimistic peers, his symptoms gradually resolved.

Dr Hay's dietary changes were almost certainly inspired by a group of American nature-cure practitioners, in those days known as 'natural hygienists' who, during the nineteenth century, discovered that digestion and absorption could be seriously impaired if certain types of food were eaten together. The resulting toxicity caused by the inadequate elimination of wastes, they suggested, could lead to a lowering of vitality, loss of energy and an increased risk of disease.

The first really important research on the subject is attributed to Dr Isaac Jennings, a qualified medical man who, after becoming more and more disillusioned with the 'pills, plasters, powders and potions' of saddle-bag medicine, began – in 1822 – to recommend what were seen back then as radical dietary ideas. His success in healing the sick was remarkable and his fame extended far and wide. Ten years on, another advocate of natural dietary reform, Sylvester Graham, also set about overturning the long-held view that fruits and vegetables were dangerous foods and that meat and wine were the only means of escaping terrible diseases. In those days, most doctors believed that fresh produce was poisonous! Yes, really. A talented orator who was credited, rather grandly, with 'knowing more about the human body than any man who had ever lived', Graham gained a massive following, and 'Grahamism' became a byword for healthy living reform.

At around the same time, similar work was being undertaken by another 'trailblazer', Dr Russell Thacker Trall. After 12 years in regular practice, he became 'tired of writing prescriptions in Latin' and increasingly disenchanted with drug medicines – which he believed generally hindered rather than helped recovery. In the late 1840s, he decided to turn his back on orthodox methods and dedicate the rest of his life to researching and teaching the natural dietary principles that are the basis of today's food combining. In 1852, he founded the New York Hydropathic and Physiologist School, one of the first to admit both male and female students – a very daring thing for a medical school to do in those days.

As the nineteenth century progressed, other leading medical men – and women – including Drs Emmet Densmore, Felix L Oswald, Susanna Way and Mary Dodds, and Dr John H Tilden, all famous in their day, furthered the work of Jennings, Graham and Trall. It was the teachings and writings of these experts – and particularly the contribution made by Dr Tilden – that attracted the attention of Dr Hay.

As a result of Dr Hay's inquiries, and his own personal triumph in beating a thoroughly dismal prognosis, he began to look more closely at how the hygienists' radical ideas might be able to improve the health of others. He found that the vast majority of patients, many with supposedly incurable illnesses, 'recovered completely' when they followed certain guidelines.

The recommendations included eating food in its unadulterated form, increasing the intake of fresh fruits and vegetables, and not mixing proteins and starches at the same meal. And, in language rather quaint by today's standards, they also encouraged 'abstinence from all alcoholic and narcotic liquors and substances and observance of a correct general regime in regard to sleep, bathing, clothing, exercise and [I love this bit] the indulgence of natural passions and appetites'.

During the 1920s and 1930s, Dr Hay expounded what were very

much his own interpretations in a number of articles and books. *Health via Food* was published in February 1934 and was followed by *A New Health Era* which became a bestseller. The Hay diet was born.

Although Dr Hay was an American, his particular dietary philosophy eventually became better known on the European side of the Pond than on his home ground. At Ohm, in Germany, just after World War II, Drs Ludwig and Ilse Walb introduced the Hay diet as a standard treatment in their clinic. They observed some impressive improvements in conditions such as heart disease, arthritic and rheumatic disorders, digestive problems, asthma and kidney disease, and wrote a bestselling book based on their findings, *Die Haysche Trennkost (The Hay Food Separating Diet)*.

Whether or not Hay's diet would have stayed the course in UK without the intervention of his protégé, Doris Grant, is questionable. Like the Walbs, Grant's writings interpret Dr Hay's work very precisely whereas nearly all others, especially those published by American authors, follow a food combining system that, interestingly, hardly ever involves Dr Hay at all.

## A Wealth of Research

Arguably the most important researcher of modern food combining was another American doctor, Herbert Shelton. Although regarded by many practitioners as the ultimate guru of the art, he is hardly ever credited for the colossal contribution he made to its study. He was a prolific researcher and writer, publishing many articles and over 40 books on food combining, nutrition, natural hygiene and related subjects. The majority of these are still in print.

Herbert McGolphin Shelton was born in Wylie, Texas, on October 6 1895. He was two months premature, very frail and not expected to survive. 'I was born in a storm and for the most part I have lived in a storm all of my life,' he once said, hinting at the flak so often fired at his (then) controversial views. In fact, he lived a long, eventful life and died at his home at Alamo, Texas (also during a storm) on New Year's Day 1985, at the ripe old age of 90.

In 1920, at 35, Shelton received a doctorate in physiological therapeutics from the International College of Drugless Physicians in

Chicago. And, in 1924, he completed another doctorate at the American School of Chiropractic and a third at the American School of Naturopathy in New York City where he went on to teach courses in dietetics and naturopathic principles. From 1928 – until his death 57 years later – Dr Shelton headed three health schools based in San Antonio, Texas. He is said to have seen in the order of 30,000 patients and also found time to publish his own monthly health journal, as well as carrying out detailed research into the function of the digestive system and how different food combinations affected health and well-being. His work was continued there by another lifelong advocate of food combining and natural hygiene, Dr Virginia Vetrano, until her retirement in the early 1990s.

## A Medicine for the Future?

You may wonder why, if the recommendations of those early food combiners were so effective, their methods were not accepted into the mainstream medicine of the time and are not embraced wholeheart-edly by doctors today. Instead of receiving accolades from their fellow physicians for their amazing successes in treating resistant or challenging conditions, those pioneers and their unorthodox methods attracted much criticism. A quote from a food combining book published in 1934 gives us an inkling. 'Medical men in those days [referring to the mid-1800s] were no different in their intolerant attitude towards the ideas of others than they now are.' Whoops, how things haven't changed!

Like Dr Hay, much of Herbert Shelton's teaching was derided by the medical profession as quackery. His strong view that 'physicians were often blinded or brainwashed with an array of unfounded theories about sickness and disease' did not endear him to his peers. He acknowledged the need for skilled surgeons but believed that many physicians were preoccupied with too many 'wonder drugs' and 'revolutionary procedures', which inclined them towards *inter*-vention rather than *pre*-vention. He was convinced that, whilst a few types of drugs were of value, most were unnecessary. The public distrust of modern medicine and its practices was proof enough, he said, of something rotten much closer to home than the State of Denmark. As long as prescriptions were for medicines instead of natural healing, nourishing food, water, fresh air, exercise, sunshine, warmth, and mental, physical and psychological rest – lives would be shortened. He believed that 'physicians often bury their mistakes', a conviction supported by more recent statistics that show how significantly death rates drop when doctors go on strike! When this happened in Los Angeles in 1976, there were 18 per cent (that's almost one in five) fewer deaths while the doctors were out. Figures increased again to 'normal' when the strike was over. Comparable statistics, gathered by morticians, have been quoted during similar actions in Israel and Brazil. In one national study of more than 2,000 autopsy records (reported in the *Journal of the American Medical Association*, June 17, 1987), 34 per cent of patients were found to have been misdiagnosed before death, and, as a consequence, some may have also been prescribed the wrong medication. In another example, from the Boston University Medical Center, 36 per cent of patients were found to have 'iatrogenic' (doctor-induced) illness, although this figure included only medical, not surgical procedures.

Shelton never suggested that physicians have less compassion or integrity that the rest of humankind. Such an assumption would be unreasonable, unfair and inaccurate. But he was not the only one to be dismayed by a certain arrogance, endemic amongst some doctors, that they already know everything there is to know and that no one else could possibly be intelligent enough to have a valid opinion. He acknowledged that they do, of course, save many lives but he argued that they are at their best when challenged with emergency situations. They tackle the symptoms of chronic (long-term) illness 'like a captain lost at sea, groping in the dark without a compass'. Shelton's experience – and that of other doctors who had turned their attention to more natural methods – was that an improved diet and other lifestyle changes could knock spots off standard medical treatment, relieving symptoms and, in many cases, healing the condition completely, without any adverse side-effects.

## The medical lag factor

As many of us are only too well aware, the medical profession is supremely talented at dismissing, censuring or ignoring obviously beneficial treatments, for apparently no good reason, even if well-researched or tried and tested over many years. Known as the medical lag factor, there are endless examples of this throughout history.

▶ In 1747, Captain Surgeon James Lind carried out tests on 12 sailors and proved that lime juice prevented scurvy, at the time the major killer disease of seafarers. His findings were published in 1753. Fifteen years later, Captain Cook's ship, the Endeavour, became the first vessel to complete a scurvy-free voyage as a result of carrying citrus fruit in its rations. Medical experts and Admiralty officials were apathetic and clearly not impressed. As a result of their intransigence, thousands of sailors continued to die unnecessarily from the disease. Another 48 years were to pass before the authorities sanctioned limes aboard all Royal Navy vessels, and more than a century before the then Board of Trade agreed that merchant ships deserved equal dietary status.

▶ Nearly every woman knows, or should know, that the B vitamin, folic acid, prevents neural tube defects, such as spina bifida, in babies. The first study that turned up this truly important discovery was published in 1976. Another 16 years went by before the need for folic acid was taken seriously. A health education campaign commenced in 1992 but, a year later, researchers were expressing concern that only around two in every 100 women making their first antenatal visit were advised about the importance of folic acid. Most of the mums-to-be that were supplementing did so because they had read about the need for folic acid in a magazine or newspaper, not because they had heard about it from their doctor. The situation has improved, but only minimally. In 1999, the *British Medical Journal* reported that only 30 per cent of prospective mothers were taking this important vitamin.

▶ In the 1980s, Australian doctor (now Professor) Barry Marshall was subjected to a barrage of abuse and ridicule from highly qualified medical colleagues when he suggested that the majority of ulcers were caused by bacteria. Some doctors were so firmly wedded to the idea that ulcers could only be caused by stress – and, anyway, everyone knew that bacteria would be killed off by stomach acid, didn't they? – that the wrong medicines continued to be prescribed for several years after Professor Marshall's work had been proven and published. It is now completely accepted that the majority of ulcers can, in most cases, be eradicated by a short course of antibiotic therapy, and that a lifetime of antacid medication is unnecessary.

## Ancient Legacy

Those nineteenth century and early twentieth century researchers of natural diet therapy were not the first to spot the benefits of healthy eating practices. The first recorded information on what became the hygienist diet is said to come from a religious group called the Essenes who lived in Palestine at around the turn of the first millennium and who are believed to have written the Dead Sea Scrolls. The Essenes were an austere group who, it has been suggested, were not given to enjoying life. Their diet, it seems, was as rigid as most other aspects of their existence. It followed closely the teachings of Jesus, taken from the *Essene Gospel of Peace*, recommending that we should eat 'all foods prepared and ripened by our Earthly Mother,' in other words, vegetarian. These foods included 'all the grasses and grains of the fields, the fruit of trees, the honey of bees, and milk of beasts clean for drinking'. There was a great deal of raw food, extended periods of fasting, and little in the way of what we would call indulgence. Nevertheless, it was claimed to be extremely healthy; most Essenes lived to an average age of over 100. 'Rawfooding' principles are still embraced by today's Essene descendants.

## Raw Diets – Too Extreme?

Although I respect the views of those who believe that, to remain healthy, we should be eating a completely raw diet (they do, after all, have plenty of evidence that it works), my experience has been that a balanced intake of raw and cooked foods can be just as healthful.

Raw foods are often claimed to be superior to cooked foods in that they contain natural enzymes and vitamins that are lost when heated. Raw-food diets can be extremely valuable for cleansing and detoxifying. However, a completely cold, uncooked menu doesn't suit everyone nor is it compatible with every climate or every lifestyle. In the middle of winter, for example, most of us, especially in more temperate areas of the world, are much more likely to feel sustained by hot nourishing soups and stews than by chomping a raw carrot or a chilled salad.

## Absorption is the Key

Raw-food nutrients are only going to be of value to the body if the digestive system is able to latch on to the nutrients they contain. I can remember a college tutor telling me years ago that a grated carrot yields far more carotene than a chopped carrot. Some scientists also believe that a similar theory applies to cooked foods. Cooking softens the walls of plant cells, allowing the gut to absorb more vitamins, especially those all-important carotenoids that are being researched as a possible protection against cancer and heart disease. Even overcooked vegetables, it seems, may be better than no vegetables at all.

## Chinese Philosophy

The view of Traditional Chinese Medicine, a philosophy also many thousands of years old, is that an excess of low-calorie, raw vegetables or salad has no substance. The Chinese view the stomach as a kind of cooking pot which simmers food to digest it. Too much cold and raw food inhibits the 'simmering' and disturbs the digestive process, clogging the system with water and hindering weight loss. Lightly cooked food (e.g. the stir-fry) is considered a better option.

## Opposites Provide Balance

I believe we should be wary of any kind of dietary extreme. Like the shady side and the sunny side of the hill (the original definitions of the Chinese philosophy of yin and yang), there is equilibrium to be had by including both raw food and cooked food in our diet. Our bodies need other kinds of dietary balance, too: protein and starch, acid and alkaline, sweet and salt, bitter and bland. Such opposites are complementary and necessary to each other. It's not cooking *per se* that is bad for our health but meals that lack variety and balance, that consist of *too much* of anything; in most cases it's usually too much protein, fat, sugar or processed food.

Whilst hardly anyone eats enough fresh produce, and almost everyone knows that eating more fresh vegetables, salads and fruits is believed to reduce the risk of many of the serious diseases that plague Western civilisation, too much of it can create a sense of 'spaciness' and of not being quite grounded. To balance a high intake of fruits and vegetables, we might choose beans and grains – not usually included in a raw food diet – but valuably rich in B vitamins and vital both for keeping us calm and for giving us energy. Proteins such as cooked fish or eggs are warming, energising and another kind of balance for cooling alkaline-forming vegetables and salad.

Raw fooders base their philosophy on the fact that man has only relatively recently (probably by dropping his food into the fire by accident) taken to eating cooked food. They say our natural diet is raw and vegetarian. But needs and times change.

## Hunter-Gatherers

Our primeval ancestors were, initially, frugivorous – that is, fruit eating – although man is now considered to be naturally omnivorous (eating meat and vegetable foods). Today, fruit-only diets can be very valuable for helping to cleanse and detoxify the body and rest the digestion but would not fit, practically, into everyday lifestyle or our present nutritional needs. The ultimate hunter-gatherer diet, cited by many modern-day nutritionists as one of the best examples of an optimally healthy diet, was approximately one-quarter game and three-quarters vegetarian, in other words, predominantly lean protein and vegetables.

## Native Americans – Natural Food Combiners

Many tribes throughout history have been food combiners, often by default since they didn't consciously separate particular food groups.

Like all our hunter-gatherer ancestors, they were not given to eating several foods at one sitting as we do today. They would eat meat only when they had had a successful day's shooting or trapping and the rest of the time enjoyed gathered foods such as berries, roots, shoots, nuts, seeds and other vegetarian foodstuffs.

Native American tribes were, essentially, hunter-gatherers who were also involved in agriculture. Their lives were simple and largely spent in the open air. Health profiles were generally considered to be good. According to H B Cushman in an 1899 book entitled *History of the Choctaw, Chickasaw and Natchez Indians*, the author tells us that 'the Choctaws were erect, well-formed and vigorous mental and nervous diseases were unknown'.

The tribe ate well when food was plentiful and endured hunger when supplies were scarce. A white man who is said to have advised the practice of economy by saving superfluous food against the scarcity of winter, was asked by a tribesman 'Will I let my brother suffer when I have plenty?'.

Meals were uncomplicated and usually consisted of only one or two ingredients at a time. Food choices depended upon availability and climate, with fruits and vegetables predominating over meat. Hunting formed an important part of their way of life although deer, wild turkey and other game did not figure principally in the diet. Some meat was dried, but most was eaten at the time of the kill. Their diet contained such a wide variety of fruits, nuts, tubers and grains that, according to researchers it would have required 'an entire volume' to name them all. Prominent among these foods were artichokes, avocados, blackberries, blueberries, cabbage, cherries, eggplant (aubergines), grapes, pawpaw, peppers, pineapples, raspberries, melons, mulberries, sunflower seeds and sweet cassava. Most Indian tribes also had a vast knowledge of medicinal plants such as aconite, arnica, ipecacuanha, wintergreen, bonset (comfrey), ginseng, viburnum, tansy, yarrow and echinacea. They gathered wild fruits and nuts like acorns, pecans, walnuts and hickory nuts, and cultivated 'little fields' of beans, squash, pumpkin, chayote, sweet potato, beans and corn (maize). Maize was a staple because it was in plentiful supply.

It's interesting to note that the type of maize that is such a familiar part of our modern diet is, according to many practitioners and allergy specialists, a common cause of allergic reaction. One has to wonder if the problem of allergy, which was apparently unknown to hunter-gatherers, has anything to do with the fact that today's corn crops are so thoroughly hybridised, chemically sprayed and mass-produced.

## The Anglo-Saxon Diet

Consisting of proteins such as game, sheep's milk, goat's milk and curd cheeses, starches like rough bread, wild fruits, herbs and green leaves the Anglo-Saxon diet was another ancient diet where different foods tended to be consumed separately, in other words, as and when foods were available. Even at banquets, when there was a plentiful supply and greater variety, foods would be served separately and individually with considerable gaps between courses. It is only in the past few hundred years that the idea of serving several items on one plate has become commonplace. Even that favourite British protein/starch combination, fish and chips, has only been around for a little over a century. Fish used to be served with versatile vegetables, such as swede (rutabaga), not with starchy potato.

# Food Combining Brought Up to Date

Dr Shelton took a distinctly different approach to food combining than Dr Hay by following these early and unrefined dietary approaches far more closely. Dr Hay did it rather differently, although nothing that I can find in my extensive researches gives any clues as to why he decided to develop his own ideas in a potentially more complicated direction.

Because of fundamental differences between them, two basic 'varieties' of food combining have emerged into the new millennium; one based on the Shelton version, and another that remains devoted to Hay. This is not to say that one method is necessarily better than the other. However, my experience – and that of a number of other practitioners – has been that a simple approach can be just as valuable, perhaps more so, than a complicated one, and doesn't need to be bogged down by inflexible rules and regulations.

In recent years, many other experts and health writers have added their own ideas and experiences to the original naturopathic and hygienist philosophy, resulting in a miscellany of publications and, for better or for worse, a mishmash of maxims for the reader to unravel. Some use the words 'food combining' in their titles, some credit the whole thing to Dr Hay and some, although clearly based on Hay or on Shelton, don't mention either.

The fact that so many pretenders have jumped on to the food combining bandwagon could be taken as testimony to the success of the system and the need for more information, but the downside has been much confusion. Almost every author has a slightly different approach and there are wide-ranging views on where particular foods fit into the system. Some of the books are clearly well-researched and a few include a lot of scientific detail. But several books seem – to me at least – like slightly amended but otherwise parrots of previous work with little, if any, new material. Some information has been repeated, embellished and scrambled so often that it has, like Chinese whispers, become accepted, rather than actual, truth. A fair old smattering here and there is blatantly incorrect and described in such a way as to suggest not even the writer understands what they are writing about.

Because new discoveries are always being made and information changes all the time, no book is ever going to remain completely up-to-date for long. However, every author owes it to their readers to make sure, at the time of writing, that the material is as accurate as it can possibly be. Many of the flaws and fallacies that have grown up around food combining can be put down, simply, to shoddy research. I think that's a shame for the reader who, after all, deserves the very best quality and latest information.

## My Style of Food Combining

Not surprisingly, as a result of all this, food combining has attracted a reputation for being complicated and not compatible with a busy modern lifestyle. My own style of healthy eating advice has developed, over a number of years, along far simpler lines. I hope that, as a result of some extensive research and my experience in practice, I have given you one of the easiest, most enjoyable and most effective routes to follow.

# CHAPTER 7

# If You Do Nothing Else...

'We must learn to take responsibility for our own health.
Adopt a largely vegetarian diet of natural wholefood
products containing a preponderance of alkaline substances.'

Alfred Vogel, nutrition expert and pioneer in natural medicine, 1902–96

I hope I've convinced you that my style of food combining really is simple to put into action. If, however, you don't feel you can fully embrace it, for whatever reason, then do at least try to do the following. These suggestions alone could make a significant improvement to your general health.

▶ Promise yourself that you'll focus your diet on fresh and dried fruits, vegetables, salads, lean protein, yoghurt, beans, oats and brown rice.

▶ Plan to eat a piece of fresh fruit mid-morning and mid-afternoon instead of your usual coffee, tea and biscuits.

▶ Try to base at least three days' meals each week on the recipe ideas in Part Three.

▶ Drink plenty of water every day, preferably filtered.

▶ Make a real effort to bin the sweet and fatty foods.

▶ Become an avid label reader and avoid chemical additives (including artificial sweeteners and added salt and sugar) whenever possible.

▶ Go organic whenever you can.

▶ Give up margarine-type spreads and any foods that contain hydrogenated vegetable oils. Don't use commercially processed cooking oils. Instead, use extra-virgin olive oil for cooking and for salad dressings, and either small amounts of butter or a non-hydrogenated fat for spreading (check labels).

▶ Take a really good-quality, daily antioxidant multi-supplement with your breakfast or lunch, at least five days every week (page 257 has more information).

▶ Be sensible about alcohol.

▶ Make every effort to avoid wheat-based cereals, mass-produced breads, biscuits, pastry and cakes. I've found these foods to cause more digestive grief in patients than almost any other foodstuff. It can also make it much more difficult for some people to lose weight if their diets contain a lot of wheat products.

▶ Cut back on cow's milk. I don't recommend that anyone drink milk, apart from a small amount in beverages. I have seen this substance cause too much digestive distress in patients to favour it as a nutritious food for humans. It is, in fact, a common cause of intolerance and allergy, and a completely unnatural food for any creature but baby cows. However, if you enjoy milk by the glass and have no problem with it, follow the instincts of young mammals and take it on its own. For some reason, the dairy industry and the medical profession have persuaded us that we need cow's milk throughout our lives, making us the only species to drink the milk of another species and the only one to consume the stuff into adulthood. The inference has always been that it is the only worthwhile source of calcium. It isn't. Lots of other foods are calcium-rich. It has also been suggested that excessive consumption of dairy products might be linked to breast cancer. Milk is also recommended as a first-class protein but, in fact, contains only about 12½ per cent (one-eighth) of the protein of lean meat or poultry. The high proportion of lactose (milk sugar) means that there is actually more starch than protein in milk. Dr Shelton often wondered why we needed to remain 'unweaned sucklings all our lives'. I don't believe we do.

▶ Take regular exercise, even if it's only a brisk walk round the block every day.

▶ Smile more. I know this has nothing directly to do with diet or exercise but do please try it. Have you noticed how nearly all the people you see in the street, on the bus, in the shops or at work, go round with their mouths turned down at the corners. Smiling – at yourself, by yourself or with others – sends positive messages to your cells, enhancing your immunity and increasing your resistance to illness. And it still works, even when you don't feel like it, even when you smile at nothing. See how much better you feel inside yourself when you smile. Do it now. Do it more often.

▶ Read Chapter 4, **Eating for Better Health** (pages 60–81) and check out my **Swap Sheet** (pages 80–1). Both these sections should help you to improve the quality of your food choices and encourage you to eat more healthily in the long term.

# PART TWO

# Food Combining to Improve Your Health

Now that we've covered the basic principles of food combining, let's move on to see how it can help with some specific health issues, including weight loss, fluid retention, digestive problems, food allergies, eating disorders, low blood sugar, skin problems and stress-related illnesses. Of course, food combining is just one of the good practices which you can use to achieve better health, so you'll find plenty of other advice in the chapters that follow, too.

# CHAPTER 8

# Food Combining for Healthy Weight Loss

'Food combining makes so much more sense to me than dieting. I used to worry about everything I put into my mouth in case it made me fat. But with food combining, I don't starve and I don't overeat. I just get naturally full and then I stop eating. Food combining is liberating.'

26-year-old food combiner

Dieting isn't working.

You guessed already?

And most of the advice on how to lose weight isn't working either.

You knew that too.

If diets worked, we would surely all be svelte and healthy. Outsize clothing and diet foods would become obsolete.

Dieting can be successful for someone who has put on weight and has never dieted before. But if you have already dieted five, 50 or 500 times, it may no longer be the best approach.

Don't despair.

First of all, you're not alone, and second of all, help is at hand.

*The Complete Book of Food Combining* takes an entirely new approach and sets out to change your long-term eating habits for the better. It wouldn't be fair to call it a diet, not in the weight-loss sense of the word. Perhaps a more accurate term would be the one used by an American nurse I met at a lecture in Arizona who coined my kind of food combining 'a diet with attitude'. She had been using this simple formula for three months and had lost 21 pounds (9.5kg). 'This is great,' she told me, 'I'm on 7600 kilojoules (1900 calories) and I've gotten back to where I should be without really trying.'

**Food combining isn't a magic bullet but it does have a tremendously successful track record in helping people to achieve their target weight.**

Unlike low-calorie programmes that set you up to fail, *The Complete Book of Food Combining* sets you up to succeed by helping you to eat more healthily and to balance your weight in the long term.

'Balance' is a key word here. If followed according to the simplest of rules, food combining is about as close to a balanced diet as anybody could get. And it fits in with those all important official guidelines, too, on how much fibre, fat, fruit and vegetables we should be eating.

It is unfortunate that, as yet, funding has not been available to carry out a large controlled study of food combining. However, there are many individual examples reported by practitioners and patients, as well as a huge amount of positive feedback from people who have learned about food combining from books and articles. In addition, small trials have been carried out that show this system to be helpful not only as a weight-loss programme but also in relieving other health problems such as digestive discomfort, migraine, fluid retention, food allergies and hayfever.

## Why Diets Don't Work – In the Long Term

Obesity isn't a new thing, it's been a problem for centuries. Even Hippocrates, the acknowledged father of medicine, noticed that people who were heavier than average were more likely than their slimmer fellows to drop down dead without warning. Now, however, the situation has, officially, reached epidemic proportions. One in every five women and one in every six men in the UK are said to be clinically obese. A third of all women and half of all men are considered overweight. At any one time, around 20 per cent are trying to lose weight. Even worse, of those people that do achieve significant weight loss, 95 out of every 100 will put it all back on again. And yet we keep coming back for more. More dieting, more pain and, at the end of the next diet, lots more gain.

Being overweight or dieting to lose weight has become an all-consuming preoccupation for millions of people. And we're passing the obsession on to our children. Eating disorders and dieting dependence are now affecting youngsters at primary school. When mothers are always 'on a diet', it's not surprising that children hear the message.

## So What's Going Wrong?

Lots of things.

The biggest problem of all is that dieters have to cope with a colossal amount of misunderstanding, misinformation and misrepresentation that exists around dieting and bodyweight. Majoring in the deception is the notion that being overweight is linked, more or less exclusively, to eating too much and exercising too little. Sure, there are many situations where this rule applies. People turn to overeating for a whole variety of reasons. There's great comfort to be had from escaping into chocolate, cake or ice cream when life gets tough. For others, eating to excess may be a result of being simply unable to tune in to when their body is genuinely hungry or have had enough.

As a nutritionist and health writer, I've met hundreds of dieters. Many of them seem to have spent almost all of their adult lives to date trying to lose weight. Most said they were either on a diet, thinking about going on a diet, or had just finished a diet. Some had been on so many diets that they had given up trying. Others kept at it, even though they had lost count and knew they weren't going to get anywhere. And they usually don't.

## Deprivation Dieting

Anyone who has ever tried to lose weight will know only too well how difficult it can be to stick to a regime. Mealtimes are empty somehow. Not worth looking forward to any more. Many of the foods we love so much end up on the forbidden list. Instead – on the basis that it holds some health promise – we are persuaded to eat a range of plastic-tasting, low-fat, pseudo-food. The packaging plays on our emotions, exploiting the guilt trip, by telling us that it is better for our cholesterol levels, our heart or our hips. So we go for it, thinking we're doing the right thing. But some of the consequences of product loyalty can be disappointing. The flavour is no great shakes and we didn't lose any weight anyway. Low-calorie dieting that relies on manufactured and processed low-cal, low-fat products isn't just dull, it can be a complete waste of time.

Whichever way you look at it, dieting is a mug's game. It's so rarely successful that I'm surprised we have the courage and determination to keep on doing it.

Why do we?

Because we've been brainwashed into it. For years, the official rhetoric has been that weight increases when the number of calories consumed exceeds the amount of energy expended. *If you want to lose weight, you have to eat less; and once you've lost weight, you have to keep on eating less.*

## But Calories Aren't Always to Blame

I'm sure you have already decided this for yourself but, in case you don't already know, *calorie overload is not the only reason why weight can be so hard to ditch.* There are many other reasons that have nothing directly to do with food at all, and we'll be looking at these in some detail later on in this chapter.

### Overeat = overweight

Yes, it's absolutely true. Eating to excess without burning off the excess can lead to obesity – but to blame it all on the humble calorie is, in my view, far too simplistic. Metabolically, scientifically, physiologically and emotionally, the accusation is full of holes.

You and I have read many times that if you reduce your intake by 500 calories a day, you'll lose a pound a week. So far so good.

Presumably, after 14 weeks you'll have lost 14 pounds (6.3kg) and at the end of 28 weeks, you'll be 2 stone (28lb/12.5kg) lighter.

Wonderful.

Well, actually it's fantastic.

How long is this low-calorie intake supposed to go on? If you weigh 12 stone (168lb/76kg) at the start, you'll presumably disappear completely in just over three years' time.

Ok, that's facetious. When you've lost the excess weight, you're supposed to reach a natural normal weight and then stop.

But I have a point, don't I? They did say, 'once you've lost weight, you have to keep eating less'.

## All Right, Let's Look at this from Another Angle

You are eating a fairly average intake of 1800 calories a day. You're a tad too tubby around the middle so you decide to go on a diet. You cut your intake by the recommended 500 calories per day and you just about manage to cope on the 1300 that you're left with.

It's hard because you're always hungry.

You pull yourself together and muster every gram of willpower.

You tell yourself that you're not doing so badly.

Unfortunately, you soon find that you're tired.

All the time, in fact.

It's not surprising, if you think about it.

Not only have you cut your energy intake, you've cut your vitamins and minerals by around a third, too. Vitamins and minerals that you need to burn calories and keep your blood glucose balanced. See-sawing blood glucose levels are known to contribute to weight problems (see pages 300–28).

## Suppose You Have 28 pounds (12.5kg) to Lose

Well, don't even think about trying to get rid of it by cutting 500 calories a day. Twenty-eight weeks (half of a whole year!) on 1300 calories is simply not healthy.

Let's say that you follow this 500 calories-less-per-day idea and it works and, perhaps, after 9 or 10 months, you are down from 12 stone (168lb/76kg) to a deliciously trim 9 stone (126lb/57kg).

What now?

If you go back to your previous calorie loading of 1800, the whole situation goes into reverse, especially if you're not exercising and you haven't changed your eating habits. Chances are you'll put a pound a week back on. Which means that in another 42 weeks, you'll be back where you started.

## So Why Not Just Eat a Little Bit Less?

Here's an alternative. You've groaned your way to the end of your diet and reached your target.

Well done! That's quite an achievement.

Remember, only five people in every 100 actually manage this.

You're determined not to slip.

You promise yourself that you'll eat less and exercise more so that you maintain your 9 stone (126lb/57kg).

Great idea. It works well for some people.

But not for everyone.

If you're exercising more, the last thing you need to do is eat too little. Certainly not 1300 calories a day. You need those 1800 calories to maintain your energy and fitness level.

Perhaps you don't need to lose as much as 28 pounds (12.5kg) or even 42 pounds (18.75kg). Perhaps it's only 10 pounds (4.5kg) or 12 pounds (5.4kg)? Counting calories for a few months might just be enough to get you back to your normal weight.

But are you sure you're eating less? What about the official guff that so often reminds us that people who say they're eating less actually aren't?

We're all mistaken?

I don't think so.

You and I know different. We know, we *absolutely* know we are eating less but we still don't seem to be losing any weight.

As a practitioner, I've lost count of the number of people that I've seen who subsisted on a sparrow's diet and still couldn't shed that excess weight. And I'm not alone in this. I've talked with many practitioners who find the same scenario over and over again.

A good example is a letter I received while writing this chapter. A lady who had been diagnosed with a heart condition had been advised by her doctor to lose weight. She tried and failed. Several times. In desperation, she sent me a very detailed list of the food she had been eating for the past two months, asking if I thought she was doing anything wrong. Her calorie intake averaged only 1200 per day – and yet she hadn't lost a single ounce or gram in months. It was a good diet, low in fat and high in fruits and vegetables. But still it wasn't working. Her doctor, she told me, was convinced she was eating more than she said. The other symptoms she described indicated a possible thyroid problem so I suggested that she went back to her doctor and asked for further tests. A second letter arrived to tell me that the results showed she had an underactive thyroid. Bingo. It wasn't the calories at all.

## You Didn't Fail – The Diet Failed

If you've tried loads of times to slim down but not had much success, you may have wondered what went wrong. If you've lost weight but then put it all back on again, please don't imagine that you've failed.

You didn't.

*The diet failed you.*

So don't feel guilty.

Nearly all diets fail because they can't deliver what your body needs. They also change the way your body works. Research shows that dieting distorts natural weight regulation and upsets future eating patterns. Some researchers say that any disturbance to the metabolism quickly corrects itself but other experts believe that, when a diet finishes, *it can take a year or more for the metabolism to return to normal, even if that person doesn't diet again during that time.*

And there's more bad news.

During this period of readjustment, the weight lost is nearly always regained plus around *another ten per cent.*

Why does this happen?

The reason is that those ancestors of ours literally didn't know where their next meal was coming from. So their metabolism was pro-grammed to store extra calories to last them through times of famine. During the lean times, the body's calories-burning mechanism would slow right down to conserve fat stores.

Our lifestyles are totally different from theirs – and so is our diet. But evolution takes time to register the changes. When we modern-day humans cut our food intake significantly, the body still sees this as a threat of starvation and, to compensate, slows the metabolism so that we don't use up our reserves too quickly. You might be fortunate enough to lose half a stone (7lb/3kg) but when the diet is completed and calorie intake increases again, the metabolic rate is too idle to burn off the increase in food.

And the consequence is . . .?

## Weight gain!

---

**What is metabolism?**

Metabolism refers to all the chemical reactions that occur in all cells of the human body needed to support life; everything from the repair and renewal of tissue, the digestion of food and the production of hormones, to the excretion of wastes. All these reactions are fuelled by the energy that we convert from the food that we eat. The rate at which cells burn that energy is called the metabolic rate.

---

## Getting Back to Set Point

Over the next few weeks or months, *The Complete Book of Food Combining* aims to help you get back to your set point weight (SPW). This is the natural, normal weight that your body settles to when you are fit and well, eating healthily, and participating in regular physical activity.

If you've already tried dieting, ask yourself the following:

### Did your diet deliver?

To be successful, any healthy eating plan designed to bring about sensible weight loss needs to fit certain criteria. Ask yourself if the usual type of weight-loss programme you follow:

▶ Helps you to lose weight?

It might have done as long as you stayed the course.

But did it also:

▶ Satisfy your appetite?

▶ Guard against cravings?

▶ Ensure that you were properly nourished?

▶ Encourage you to eat more healthily in the long term?

and

▶ Help you to maintain good energy levels?

Are you sure that it was:

▶ Easy to follow?

▶ Enjoyable?

▶ Not stressful?

▶ Doing you no harm?

▶ Able to bring your body back into balance?

▶ Maintaining that weight loss?

Did it include recommendations on:

▶ Physical activity?

▶ Indulgences?

▶ Ways of coping with stress?

▶ Increasing the variety of foods in your diet?

**And most important of all:**

▶ Could you have followed it for life?

If the answer to any of the above, was 'no', then I encourage you to try the food combining route to weight loss.

## Willpower and Weight Loss

The paradox in all this is that *most diets do work*. If you can cope with the hunger pangs and the cravings, you can lose weight. Unfortunately, apart from your own willpower, there is little else in the way of support.

No after-sales service, you might say!

My ideas on food combining are there to support and encourage you while you're working towards permanently balanced weight and better health. What *The Complete Book of Food Combining* doesn't do is count calories, kilojoules or fat grams. What it does do is re-educate your eating habits in the long term, encouraging you to eat a more varied, nutritious diet. Meals are satisfying and snacks are allowed if you feel you need them. There are lots of treats and definitely no deprivation; indulgences are positively encouraged! And you don't need to food combine seven days a week, either. Follow the recommendations that begin on page 139.

## Before You Begin, Ask Yourself if You Honestly Need to Lose Weight

I know that your answer is almost certainly going to be a resounding 'yes' but please think about it for a moment. There's a good reason for my bringing this up. Although it can be difficult to accept, it's possible that you aren't actually overweight at all. Please don't dismiss the idea out of hand. Consider this:

Small increases in weight over the years are quite normal and can actually be a healthy sign.

We often expect to be the same weight at 50 as we were at 20. But this may not be as natural as we like to think. Putting on extra weight in our middle years has the naturally added benefit of making our bones work harder against gravity, helping to maintain bone density, and is Mother Nature's way of giving us some protection. If you are approaching or going through the menopause and have gained a bit here and there, then you might be comforted to know that small increases in body fat in your age group can actually be good for you. For example, a woman who accumulates a bit of extra padding during her forties and fifties can be better protected against one of the most serious conditions associated with the menopausal years, osteoporosis (brittle bone disease). That's because when the ovaries stop making the hormone oestrogen, small amounts are produced from the body's fat stores, especially abdominal fat.

The likelihood of brittle bone disease increases dramatically as we get older. It affects *one in every three women over 60 and half of those over 70*. If you are only 10 pounds (4.5kg) or less above what you considered to be your ideal weight, it could be healthier and more sensible to go up one size in clothes than strive to shed what Nature needs you to keep.

## How do You Know What Your True Weight is Supposed to be?

Height/weight charts – and other methods of calculating what your bodyweight is *supposed to be* – aren't always reliable and can mislead you into thinking you're overweight when you are not. There are so many of them, and most of them seem to disagree. In addition, they take no account of individuality, expecting everyone of the same height to be the same weight. And yet, as we can all testify, people of the same height can have totally different body shapes while those of similar body shape may be different in height. These kinds of charts are a guide, nothing more.

**TECHNICAL STUFF**

## So how do you calculate your ideal weight?

(Skip to page 125 if you don't need to know this.)

One of the most usual ways is to use a height-to-weight ratio called the body mass index or BMI. I haven't found this a very reliable system because it doesn't allow for differences in bone or muscle size or for fat distribution. For example, a sedentary office worker and a marathon runner might have the same BMI rating because the marathon runner's muscle weighs heavier than the office worker's fat. Or a thinner person with heavier bones might show the same BMI as a fatter person with small bones.

Like the height/weight charts, BMI can only ever be a guide. The results may be calculated from stones but aren't carved in stones. You don't have to live by them.

If you want to work out your own BMI, take your weight in kilograms and divide it by your height in metres squared (i.e. metres x metres). Here's an example.

Say you weigh 13 stone. Turn this to pounds by multiplying by 14. Then multiply those pounds by 0.45 to turn them into kilograms:

13 x 14 = 182lb
182 x 0.45 = 81.9kg

Next, work out your height in metres.

If, like me, you went to school in feet and inches, work out the metres by multiplying your height in inches by 0.0254.

Thus, someone of 5ft 10in is 70in tall.
70 x 0.0254 = 1.78m

Now you have your height and weight in metric measurements. If you're already familiar with metric measures, then start your calculations here.

Multiply your height by itself:
i.e. 1.78 x 1.78 = 3.168m$^2$

Then all you need to do is to calculate your weight by your height squared:

Your weight (81.9kg) divided by your height squared (3.168m$^2$) = your BMI (25.85)

If your BMI works out at between 20 and 25, that's considered normal. Between 25 and 30 means overweight, 30 to 40 is obese, and above 40 is seriously obese. So, 25.85 indicates that you are only slightly overweight. Let's look at another example:

Someone who is 10 stone 4lb (144lb) and 5ft 5in (65in) tall has a body mass index of 23.82.

1. Change pounds to kilograms:           144lb x 0.45 = 64.8kg
2. Change inches to metres:               65in x 0.0254 = 1.65m
3. Square the metres:                     1.65 x 1.65 = 2.72m$^2$
4. Divide the kilograms by the metres squared:   64.8 ÷ 2.72 = 23.82

This weight is within the normal range.

What's interesting here is that I've met many people of this approximate height and weight who have been convinced they are overweight.

## Check it another way

This was a method given to me by one of my college tutors. Again, it's a guide.

Take your height in inches and divide it by 66. Multiply the answer by itself and then by 100. Then add your age to the final figure. Thus:

65 ÷ 66 = 0.985
0.985 x 0.985 = 0.970
0.970 x 100 = 97
97 + your age = the pounds you should weigh
So 97 + 45 years = 142lb
142lb = 10 stone 2lb or 63.9kg

This result is very close to the BMI calculation above.

## Lose Weight, Gain a Healthy Shape

There are lots of incentives to get yourself healthily into shape. One of them has to do with living longer. Crash dieting isn't going to get you there. Extreme eating habits – whether that means eating to excess or not eating enough – can lead to serious health problems with the strong possibility of, at best, upsetting your long-term health or, at worst, shortening your life.

The key to predicting future health could have more to do with where the fat accumulates in the body than how much there is in quantity. The risk of serious disease (diabetes, heart problems and some cancers) may turn out to be less in women and men who are pear-shaped (bigger hips, bigger bottoms) than in those who are apple-shaped (more belly or upper body fat).

Once deposited, fat doesn't just sit there. It's picked up by the blood and circulated around the body, increasing the risk of fatty arteries and cardiovascular disease. Some fat, depending on its location, can also affect hormone production and may be a factor in some hormonally related cancers. It has been suggested that women with more upper body fat have a 70–100 per cent greater risk of breast cancer than the traditional pear-shaped women who accumulate fat on their lower bodies. It may be that apple shapes have lower levels of particular substances that bind to the female hormone, oestrogen, and prevent it from flowing freely in vulnerable tissues such as the breast and the lining of the uterus.

### Apple or pear?

Most people know if they are an apple or a pear. If you are unsure, however, do a little simple arithmetic.

1. Take your waist measurement (at belly-button level) and your hip measurement at the widest point.

2. Divide the waist figure by the hip measurement. For example, if your waist is 28 inches (71cm) and your hips are 40 inches (102cm), then your waist/hip ratio is 0.70.

   If you measure 30 inches (76cm) round the waist and 38 inches (96cm) round the hips, your ratio is 0.79.

Experts say that anything higher than 0.75 is an apple.

But they also say 'don't panic'. You can't alter your basic frame shape but you can go for a weight-loss programme that helps you to lose upper body fat and, as a result, improve your waist/hip ratio. Research results suggest that an overweight woman losing 10 pounds (4.5kg) or more could reduce her risk of breast cancer by as much as 45 per cent.

## Remember – Weight Problems can be Linked to a Whole Host of Factors

It's comforting to know that weight problems can be linked to many other things than just calories. Let's look at some of the other reasons why weight can be so stubborn to shift, and what to do about them.

▶ Blood sugar imbalances

▶ Fluid retention

▶ Food allergies, intolerances and sensitivities

▶ Frequent dieting

▶ Individual biochemistry, physiology and metabolism

▶ Genetic make-up and family history

▶ Fat distribution

▶ Thyroid problems

▶ Adrenal exhaustion

▶ Lack of exercise

▶ Low intake of vitamins and minerals

▶ Low self-esteem or emotional distress

▶ Overgrowth of yeast (candidiasis)

▶ Poor digestion

▶ If you haven't been well

▶ Poor general health

▶ Constipation

▶ Toxicity and poor elimination

## Blood sugar imbalances

Persistently low or wildly fluctuating blood sugar levels are one of the major reasons why people don't stick with low-calorie diets. Low blood sugar is a natural mechanism that tells your body you need to eat. But sometimes, the balancing apparatus gets screwed up, pulling you into a spiral of cravings and binge eating. Getting your blood sugar back on an even keel is a major step forward in long-term weight control. Turn to pages 300–28 for more information on how to balance blood sugar and beat cravings.

## Fluid retention

Sometimes we can feel podgier or more bloated than at other times, even though we know we haven't been overeating. We might find that clothes we can get into one day, suddenly don't seem to fit the next day. If your weight fluctuates by more than 4 pounds (2kg) between break-fasttime and bedtime, it could be fluid, not fat, that is responsible. If you're feeling swollen and uncomfortable, then the stuff on pages 156–66 could be useful.

## Food allergies, intolerances and sensitivities

If your efforts to lose weight have never been successful, even though you've exercised regularly *and* been careful about your food choices, it's possible that you could be allergic or sensitive to certain foods.

Some experts believe that certain common food allergens might be responsible for disturbing the way food is digested. Others say that they could cause an increase in appetite or slow up the metabolism, making it more difficult for our bodies to burn fat. Isolating and elim-inating problem foods – such as wheat-based or corn-based breakfast cereals, bread, cow's milk, cow's milk cheese, certain additives, gluten and yeast – may hold the key to successful weight loss for some people. One of the many things that is different about my own simple style of food combining is that it avoids the most common allergens. Pages 202–18 have more details on how food allergies can affect weight and general health.

## Frequent dieting

How fat we are, and how much fatter we become, can be closely connected to how often we diet. The more we diet, the easier it is to gain weight and the harder it is to lose weight. That's because the body burns less calories after each diet so when we finish a diet and return to our previous eating habits, we accumulate more fat. So then we go on another diet – and another – and so on.

But to stick resolutely to a reduced-calorie regime takes willpower. Stacks of it. Attempts to lose weight by reducing meal sizes are rarely successful because people need to be very disciplined and committed to ignoring increased feelings of hunger. And it rarely works anyway. For example, it's known that people who eat a light, low-calorie breakfast often compensate by eating more at lunchtime. Research also shows that many overweight people skip breakfast and lunch, only to pile on the calories at the end of the day.

Persistent on-off dieting is shown to increase the likelihood of a number of health problems, including hormonal imbalances, recurring infections and eating disorders. There are better and healthier ways of achieving your goal. The key to sustained weight loss is to change your eating habits. Success will come not from worrying constantly about calories or quantity, but by staying active and making sure that your food intake is varied, nutritious, as natural as possible and *digested properly*.

## Individual biochemistry, physiology and metabolism

Everybody looks different. That's how we recognise our friends, work colleagues and members of our family. They have distinct physical characteristics that make them individual, and known to us. Hair colour, eye colour, shape of nose, long face, round face, voice, length of neck, inside-leg measurement, shoe size, body shape and manner-isms, etc. Nobody looks, sounds or behaves exactly the same way as someone else. Even identical twins have different natures. We all have varying tastes in food, drink, music, art, the colours we like, the car we drive, the television or radio programmes we prefer and the newspa-pers or magazines we read. Our constitutions are all individual too. So are our personalities. We accept all this as completely normal. Not very likely then, is it, that our internal body chemistry, physiology and metabolism could be the same as everyone else's? All our internal organs have individual characteristics. No two digestive systems are exactly the same. And we all have different nutritional needs. Which is one reason why the diet that worked for your sister, your mother or your best friend might not work for you.

And yet we spend so much time striving to be slimmer, to alter our body shape, to be someone we are not. It's never going to work. It's important to make the effort to lead a healthy lifestyle but not to try to change yourself. Accept your own genetic make-up. Being so individ-ual is what makes you special.

## Genetic make-up and family history

If there is a history of obesity in a family, it can sometimes make it more likely that the next generation will be prone to weight problems. Hor-mones and other natural substances that are produced within the body as signals that it's time to stop eating may work more efficiently in some people than in others. It also seems likely that the type of fat cells that make up body fat (see **Fat distribution** below) could play a part in determining how successful we are at losing weight. This doesn't mean that there is no point in trying to lose weight. Nourishing your genes with the right kind of food really can make a difference to your own long-term health and well-being. Food combining will show you how.

## Fat distribution

One of the most fashionable excuses for remaining overweight used to be 'I don't have any brown fat' or 'I have too much white fat'. The ratio of brown fat to white fat (the 'white' is actually a rather nasty yellow colour) could, say scientists, explain why some people stay slim from the cradle to the grave and others spend their lives battling with bulges.

As a general rule, white fat is deposited nearer to the surface in places like the thighs, buttocks, hips and – guess where? – the abdomen. Brown fat tends to be tucked further into the body, as well as in the neck and the back. The brown fat differs from the white stuff in that brown fat cells hold a larger number of special energy production units within cells called mitochondria. These little 'power plants' or 'power houses' burn a great deal of energy. Inside each mitochondrion, complex processes extract energy from the nutrients absorbed from our food; energy which is then used for all the body's activities.

Brown fat is able to convert calories to heat by a process called chemical thermogenesis. The degree of thermogenesis (heat production) is, in fact, almost directly proportional to the amount of brown fat within the body. Because of its heat-making abilities, brown fat is warmer whilst white fat is cooler. White fat has less energy producing properties and so isn't able to produce much heat. Ever noticed how flabby bits are usually cold to the touch? That's probably going to be white fat.

People who stay slim all their lives appear to have more heat-producing brown fat cells – and so are able to burn energy more efficiently than those who gain weight easily. The brown to white fat ratio could also explain why weight increases with age (as we grow older, white cells take over and brown cells decline), and, perhaps, why young children don't appear to feel the cold (they have more brown fat cells than adults).

The distribution of brown and white fat cells is genetic, in other words, determined by our DNA. However, when we lose weight, especially if we try to do it too quickly, we get rid of a lot of both kinds of fat and a bit of muscle. When we regain weight, the unwanted extras come back as *more fat*. It's likely, although not yet proven, that the fat we regain may be white, rather than brown, and harder to get rid of than the fat we lost first time around.

## Thyroid problems

An under-active thyroid gland (known medically as hypothyroidism or myxoedema) is one that is not producing enough of the hormones thyroxine and tri-iodothyronine. Almost everyone knows that if someone has an under-active thyroid gland, they are likely to have weight problems. This gland, situated at the base of your neck, along with two other glands in the brain, called the hypothalamus and the pituitary, plays a key role in controlling your metabolism.

When the thyroid hormone (thyroxine) is in short supply, the metabolic rate nearly always decreases and bodyweight almost always increases. When no hormone at all is produced, metabolic rate can fall by as much as half the normal rate. Thyroid hormone is involved directly or indirectly in almost all aspects of carbohydrate and fat metabolism so if there isn't enough of it, the breakdown of fats and starches will be affected.

The chemical thermogenesis we talked about just now is, to some extent, affected by the output of the hormone thyroxine from the thyroid gland. When the thyroid is functioning properly, the body is usually warm – or at least is able to cope with changes in temperature fairly quickly without causing you any discomfort. When the thyroid is under-active, one of the major symptoms may be cold hands, cold feet and possibly even cold flabby bits.

---

### Symptoms of an under-active thyroid gland

Apart from weight gain, some of the many other signs of low thyroid function can include constipation, depression, dry skin, hair loss, headaches, infertility, lethargy, loss of sex drive, elevated cholesterol, high blood pressure, muscle tension, sensitivity to cold, and reduced immunity to infections.

---

An over-active thyroid (called hyperthyroidism or thyrotoxicosis) indicates an over-production of thyroxine or tri-iodothyronine. Greatly increased thyroid hormone production almost always decreases bodyweight by increasing the metabolic rate to anything from 60–100 per cent above normal.

---

**Symptoms of an over-active thyroid gland**

These include weight loss or inability to gain weight despite a normal diet, breathlessness, constant tiredness, difficulty sleeping, digestive disturbance, diarrhoea, muscle weakness, muscle tremors, palpitations, sweating, and scanty or absent periods.

---

No single cause has yet been found for thyroid malfunction. However, there are many contributing factors. Family history may play a part. Yo-yo dieting, extreme diets, smoking, certain medications, poor digestion, poor absorption of nutrients and low intake of certain vitamins and minerals, have all been linked to thyroid breakdown. Emotional reactions such as excessive anxiety, prolonged negative stress, unexpressed anger, frustration and feeling trapped by too many obligations, may also affect the output of thyroid hormones. The pituitary gland, situated in the brain, is responsible for producing thyroid stimulating hormone (TSH), the hormone messenger that stimulates production of thyroxine from the thyroid gland itself. If the pituitary is malfunctioning, the thyroid won't work properly.

If you have any kind of weight problem that has not responded to other forms of treatment, do please visit your doctor. He or she may suggest taking a blood sample for analysis, which should show the level of thyroxine circulating in the blood. Unfortunately, borderline thyroid problems are not always picked up by standard tests. If the results are inconclusive, it can be worthwhile asking for thyroid stimulating hormone (TSH) to be measured as well. If the result is still indecisive, you might discuss something called a basal temperature test (or BTT), devised by an American doctor, Broda Barnes. Basal simply means the base temperature measured when the body is resting.

All doctors in the US know about this test because it is listed in the US medics' bible, *The Physician's Desk Reference*, but not all doctors in the UK will be aware of its existence. It's a simple procedure that can be carried out at home. BTT results are calculated on the basis that body temperature in those with an under-active thyroid is, persistently, slightly lower than average and that an over-active thyroid results in increased body temperature. If you suffer with any of the symptoms I've listed above, and suspect you have an under-active thyroid, you could try this test for yourself. If the results appear to confirm your findings, then do go back to your doctor and discuss them.

## ! TECHNICAL STUFF

### How to Take the Basal Temperature Test

Basal temperature is taken once each day. Some practitioners suggest it is done for only three days but others recommend seven or ten consecutive days because this provides a better average. So let's do it for seven days.

Men should note their temperature first thing in the morning on any seven consecutive mornings. Women who are post-menopausal or not menstruating for any reason, should also take their temperature first thing in the morning for seven consecutive mornings. Otherwise, wait for your period and do the test from the morning of the second day of menstruation for the next seven days.

Have the thermometer on a bedside chair or table so that you don't have to get out of bed in the morning to go searching for it. On waking, lie still. Don't sit up or drink anything or go to the bathroom. With the display reading at zero, or the mercury well below 35°C (96°F), put your thermometer snugly under your armpit either for ten minutes (regular thermometer) or until it bleeps (electronic thermometer). Note down the reading each morning. After day seven, add the readings together and divide them by seven.

Normal basal body temperature is usually considered to be between 36.4°C–36.7°C or 97.6°F–98.2°F. So if you measured, let's say, 36.2 on day one, 36.0 on day two, 36.2 on day three, 36.3 on day four, 36.0 on day five, 36.1 on day six and 36.1 on day seven, you'd add them all together, divide the total by seven and the average will be 36.1, which indicates a low thyroid function. If you measured 36.3, 36.2, 36.3, 36.4, 36.4, 36.6 and 36.6, the average is 36.4, which is normal. Don't forget these are only examples.

Taking basal temperatures can be a useful guide but this is not a conclusive test. However, if your results suggest that your thyroid might be malfunctioning, I would urge you to talk again with your doctor and ask for further investigations to be carried out.

## Adrenal exhaustion

If your adrenal glands are overworked or under-functioning, for example as a result of stress, it may have an affect on your body's ability to burn calories. Most people don't realise that stress and weight gain can be so closely connected. Some of us eat far more when we are under stress – and usually not such healthy foods. Dealing with existing stress and helping your body to cope with future stress can ease the path to balanced weight.

It's also interesting to know that thermogenesis (see page 130) is also affected by two adrenal hormones called epinephrene (say e-pie-na-freen) and norepinephrene (they used to be called adrenalin and noradrenalin). Anxiety, panic and excessive negative stress states can cause an over-production of adrenal hormones and a decrease in the secretion of thyroid stimulating hormone, affecting metabolic rate and possibly leading to weight gain.

## Lack of exercise

There are no two ways about it. Inactivity can definitely contribute to obesity. Mostly thanks to technology and all those time-saving devices we have at our disposal, physical exertion is no longer a daily occurrence in most people's lives. In this era of washing machines, computers and motor cars, we're just not as active as we used to be. One statistic tells us that the average Brit spends 27 hours a week watching television, but it could be worse than that. They didn't ask me – and I know I only spend around two to three hours a week in front of the box, so somebody out there could be getting my viewing share on top of their 27-hour average. To get the body moving, exercise has to be introduced as a kind of discipline, something we have to find time for or force ourselves to do. Unfortunately, most of us don't. Perhaps now is the time to make that resolution. Exercise isn't boring – or time-consuming. It's terrific. Doing it can change your life. It might even *save* your life! Pages 82–94 have more information. *Please* read them.

## Low intake of vitamins and minerals

I have seen a number of patients who had been trying to lose weight for years but only succeeded when they improved their nutritional status; that is, increased their intake of vitamins and minerals. This doesn't mean popping hundreds of pills. But it can help enormously, in addition to improving the quality of your diet, to take a really good one-daily multivitamin/mineral or broad-range antioxidant complex with breakfast or lunch.

When your diet is short on vitamins and minerals, or if your body isn't absorbing them, your ability to burn fat is diminished, making it more difficult to lose weight. As I explained earlier, dieting itself can make matters worse because, as you cut calories, you also cut nutrients too, the very ones you need to burn off energy and keep your body fit and healthy. In particular, the B complex is vital for the breakdown of carbohydrates, iodine is needed for the healthy function of the thyroid gland, and chromium is absolutely essential for insulin production and balanced blood glucose.

## Low self-esteem or emotional distress

Most of the time, most of us aren't satisfied with ourselves. We complain that our feet are too large or too small, that we have a short waist, flat chest or big boobs. We're not tall enough or blonde enough or tanned enough or, the biggest complaint of all, not thin enough. Person A may think Person B has the most beautiful skin. Person B won't appreciate her lovely skin, but she'll wish she had Person A's lovely eyes. But you can bet that someone lucky enough to be born with a fabulous face will be unhappy about their hips or their fingernails. Tall people complain that extra height can be such a nuisance. Clothes are so hard to find. But be born beautifully petite, and we want to be taller. Overall, we don't like ourselves much. Yet most of us have so much to be thankful for. All we should desire is that we maintain our health and well-being. Never forget about the man who complained about having no shoes until he met a man with no feet.

But, sometimes, seeing someone else in a worse state than ourselves *doesn't* make us feel grateful or relieved or more pleased about the way we have turned out. No matter how talented, artistic, good-looking, good-natured or hard-working we really are, we may have lost much of our confidence and sense of self-worth. School can knock it out of us. Other children aren't always the kindest of people. Teachers can sometimes be brutal to our emotions without realising the lifelong damage they are inflicting. Bullying can leave us feeling small and alone. If we are struggling with excess weight, being branded 'fat' is a terrible insult. If we're underweight, names like 'skinny', 'beanpole' or 'lamppost' can be just as hurtful.

Families can destroy someone's confidence, especially if whatever you do never seems to be good enough. Harassment at work – innuendo, gossip, whispering, bitchiness and bullying – can leave someone feeling isolated and afraid. Teasing is only usually fun for those doing it, not those receiving it. If things aren't going well at any time in your life – as a young child, a teenager or an adult – and you hear the message often enough that you are useless, ugly or fat, you end up believing it.

Constant sniping plays havoc with your emotions, making it more likely that you turn to food for comfort. Anything that shocks the system, physically or emotionally, or causes us grief, can trigger a bout of bingeing. Once your self-esteem has taken a downturn, it can be difficult to convince yourself that you're worth bothering with. But you are worth it. Everyone is. You're no less special than anyone else. Why bother to take pride in your appearance? Because it matters to you. The time to make the effort is now. I did. You can, too. Be positive, not negative. Do it for me.

## Overgrowth of yeast

I have talked to many practitioners who are convinced that obesity can be aggravated by a condition known as candidiasis, caused by the yeast fungus *Candida albicans*. Candida is a natural inhabitant of everyone's digestive system and is kept in check by friendly intestinal flora. But, in some people, it can 'overgrow' and damage the lining of the gut, giving off toxins and increasing the risk of food sensitivities.

Antibiotics, high-sugar diets, excess alcohol, the contraceptive pill, hormone replacement therapy, an under-active thyroid, low immunity, poor liver function, unrelenting stress and poor-quality diet are some of the most likely causes or triggers. Candida can affect anyone, whatever their weight, but is also a common problem for dieters. The condition has so many different symptoms that accurate diagnosis is best left to a qualified practitioner. For more information, see pages 214–16.

## Poor digestion

The idea that some weight problems could be linked to poor digestion is not usually embraced by mainstream medicine. However, my experience suggests that this is a much ignored area that deserves more attention. Although there is very little research into the relationship between digestion and obesity, improving digestion does appear to have helped some people overcome their weight problems. Pages 167–201 have more information.

## If you haven't been well

If your health is under par, your body's instinct is to put the brakes on your metabolism and hold on to stored nourishment if there is any risk that food might be in short supply. This also applies if you are recovering from an accident or operation or are in pain. Although, in modern times, there is nearly always someone around to keep an eye on us and feed us if we are unwell, this very clever survival mechanism would have been vital to our nomadic ancestors when they were ill or injured and unable to gather food.

Of course, situations do arise when we go without sustenance for long periods of time because we are not well enough to eat. In such cases, the lack of food can cause us to lose large amounts of weight. When we begin to feel better and return to normal eating habits, it's quite likely that our metabolic rate will have slowed right down and we could find that we then gain weight that is increasingly difficult to lose.

Conversely, certain types of illness can cause us to lose large amounts of weight, and when we recover, we can sometimes find that lost weight is *very hard* to regain. As one senior registrar (intern) explained to me, 'The body won't be interested in accumulating extra padding until all the healing up is completed. Sometimes that can take months, or even a year or two.'

## Poor general health

Our state of health could determine how successful we are in beating the bulge. I have found, consistently, with my own patients, that weight loss only usually occurs when their general health improves. It seems as if the body has an innate intelligence that says 'I can't get around to sorting out my weight until I'm fit enough to cope'. You should not attempt any kind of weight-loss diet if you are unwell or are suffering from any medically diagnosed condition, unless you are being super-vised by a qualified practitioner.

## Constipation

Constipation can be yet another handicap to successful weight loss. A compacted, silted bowel leads to toxicity which, in turn, makes it more difficult for the body to maintain a balanced weight. When faeces sit for too long in the colon, water and toxins are re-absorbed through capillaries into the liver. Wastes dry out through lack of fluid and are more difficult to pass. The liver, which has probably already dealt with these same toxins and passed them to the colon for excretion, has to deal with them again. In addition to a whole variety of problems, such as stale breath, flatulence, lethargy, skin problems and headaches, major side-effects of an inactive colon are bloating and fluid retention. Pages 191–201 have tips on improving digestion and regularity.

## Toxicity and poor elimination

The suggestion that toxins and waste products might be responsible for weight problems has often caused heated debate among health experts. Some view the very idea as tosh while others believe that detoxification helps speed up the metabolism by cleansing the liver and improving absorption of vitamins and minerals. This idea is not a new one. The possibility that the body's ability to burn calories could be affected by 'internal pollution' was first suggested by doctors at the turn of the twentieth century. Remember food combining pioneer, Dr John Tilden (see page 97)? He published his findings on toxicity back in 1926.

When the systems responsible for collecting and processing wastes get overworked, or if the body is undernourished, debris isn't excreted and gets clogged up in the system. When toxins aren't released from the body, they accumulate. Guess where they take up residence? You got it. In your fat cells. Detoxification really does seem to be a good way to kick-start weight loss. Regular cleansing sessions can also help to lift lethargy and improve energy levels. *The Complete Book of Food Combining* has a whole section on detoxification starting on page 219.

# Do You Still Think You Need to Lose Weight?

If you've thought about everything in this chapter, have ruled out any medical problems, and are sure that you would benefit from shedding a bit of weight, there are healthier and safer ways of doing so than resorting to deprivation dieting.

## MY HOT HINTS FOR HEALTHY WEIGHT LOSS

### Always eat breakfast

Going from your previous evening's meal through to lunchtime or your next evening meal is simply not a healthy thing to do. Apart from playing havoc with your metabolic rate, running on empty seriously upsets your blood glucose levels and your nutritional status.

Pages 350–4 have plenty of sustaining breakfasts for you to choose from. If the thought of food is anathema first thing in the morning, eat some fresh fruit and then follow up an hour or so later with a generous-sized tub of plain yoghurt.

## Start the day with fresh fruit

How about half a fresh grapefruit? It has good soluble fibre, lots of vitamin C and can help to lower cholesterol levels. On colder mornings, drizzle the grapefruit with cold-pressed raw honey and pop it under the grill for a couple of minutes.

## Eat more fresh fruit

But don't eat it after main meals. If you haven't already heard about this, pages 23–33 have more info.

## Don't miss meals

Missing meals may seem like a useful calorie-saving exercise but if you go all day without food, your body thinks it's being starved and decides to store fat rather than burn calories. In addition, because lack of food has such a devastating effect on blood sugar balance, the body's emergency survival mechanism kicks in and could encourage you to eat more at the next meal.

## Eat more slowly

Chewing everything really thoroughly helps to prevent overeating and gives you a sensation of fullness before you get to that awful stage of having eaten too much. As food enters the stomach, a hormone known as cholecystokinin (CCK) is released into the blood from the lining of the duodenum (the upper part of the small intestine). Its primary purpose is to make the gallbladder contract and stimulate fat- and protein-digesting enzymes from the pancreas. CCK also sends messages to the brain to let it know that you are filling up and soon won't be able to eat any more. It acts rather like the mercury in a thermometer, except that it reacts to food levels rather than to temperature. When your stomach is empty, CCK stays low but, after a few minutes, levels rise, telling your appetite centre that you won't be able to manage that piece of cheesecake or helping of chocolate mousse. Because CCK isn't triggered immediately, it helps if you can slow down your eating pattern by chewing thoroughly and pausing between mouthfuls and courses.

## Include plenty of fibrous foods in your diet

Dietary fibre slows the rate of absorption of carbohydrates from the digestive system, helping to prevent fluctuations in blood glucose levels and reducing the risk of cravings and junk-food snacking. But be sure to choose the right type of fibre. Too much of the wrong kind could cause deficiencies of some nutrients. This is because insoluble fibre binds to certain minerals – in particular, calcium, magnesium, iron and zinc – and prevents them from being absorbed. Better types of fibre may come from vegetables, fresh and dried fruits, pulses, seeds, nuts, oats and brown rice than from wheat bran. Wheat-bran fibre can also contribute to weight problems because of its allergenic nature. If you don't know what's in your cereal, check the pack label.

## Try a new meal format

▶ Until you are back to a weight you are happy with, try this daily format. Eat a really good, sustaining breakfast (toast and coffee is not enough to keep you going through the morning), a substantial protein-based lunch with extra salad or vegetables, and a lighter starch-based meal in the evening. Proteins sustain the appetite and help to support blood glucose throughout the morning and afternoon, while starches are soothing at the end of the day, and could help you to sleep better.

▶ Go for fish or chicken with salad or vegetables at lunchtime. Overcome that 11.00 a.m. and 4.00 p.m. slump in energy by tucking into fresh fruit. Make supper a light one. A meal of complex carbohydrate, such as rice or pasta, with green vegetables or green salad in the evening is calming and unwinding and should be well digested before your head hits the pillow.

▶ Start a main meal with soup, fresh fruit or a green salad. Adding a starter to your meal may sound contrary in a world where so many health experts are telling us to eat less – but a healthy, light-weight entrée, such as a fresh fruit salad, green salad, vegetable consommé or soup, means you'll eat a smaller main course and probably forego the dessert.

▶ Balance a cooked meal with a raw side salad. I know I keep on about salad but there is a good reason. Not only does it add points to your daily vitamin and mineral score, but fresh salad provides dietary fibre and slows down the rate of absorption – so you feel fuller for longer.

## Try Quorn

Swap a red-meat meal for this myco-protein meat substitute. It's much more filling than meat or poultry, has plenty of B vitamins and is low in fat. I use it in stir-fries and curries, and it makes a great 'cottage pie' with a lightly buttered mashed swede (rutabaga) and turnip topping.

## Eat baked beans

Go for regular-style, organic if possible and not low-cal. Baked beans are very sustaining and good for keeping blood glucose balanced. Try them on wholegrain toast, over a jacket spud – or tip a small can of them into a bean stew. Canned beans can be quite high in sugar but the soluble fibre in the beans slows down sugar absorption.

## Avoid regular sandwich bread

Go for pumpernickel (black rye), brown rye, sourdough, yeast-free soda bread, rye crackers, rice cakes or oat biscuits as alternatives.

## Avoid these foods

Whilst you're trying to lose weight, don't eat or drink the following:

▶ Port, sherry, beer, lager and spirits

▶ Peanuts and salty snacks

▶ Artificial additives

▶ Flavour enhancers such as monosodium glutamate (MSG) or foods containing chemical sweeteners that can make you want to eat more

▶ Cow's milk, except a small amount in a cup of tea or coffee

▶ Cow's milk cheese

▶ Bread, except those recommended

▶ Deep-fried foods

▶ High-fat foods

## Reduce sugar and sugary foods

Not only does sugar use up large amounts of nutrients during its absorption, it also overworks the pancreas and can lead to insulin sensitivity (see page 308 for more information on this) and blood glucose imbalance. High-sugar diets have also been implicated in heart disease.

Although it can be difficult to say no to sugar, the effort should pay off. Don't be too hard on yourself. Begin by giving up sugar in tea and coffee. Instead, use dark, cold-pressed raw honey, available from health stores. Honey is high in fructose (fruit sugar) which doesn't call up the large amounts of insulin needed to process other types of sugar such as sucrose or glucose.

## Avoid artificial sweeteners

There is some evidence that chemical sweeteners may actually stimulate the appetite and encourage you to eat more. In addition, it has been suggested that sweeteners could add to the toxic load in the liver, making it more difficult to lose weight. If you are faced with a product that offers original or low-cal alternatives, either avoid it altogether or go for the original one in small amounts only, even if it contains sugar. It's a better option, in my view, than downing a cocktail of chemical sweeteners.

## Dump the chocolate

We all know it can make us feel good to eat chocolate – the natural chemicals it contains provide a similar buzz to being in love or taking drugs – but the effect is short-lived. The backwash brings guilt, remorse, unwanted weight and, for some people, skin problems and headaches. If you are desperate to indulge, do it and enjoy it but ration your intake and save some for another day. Eat a few chocolates or squares, not the whole box or bar. Forget the guilt. It isn't worth it. And choose organic chocolate. It is chemical-free and delicious. In the UK, my favourite brand is Green & Black, available in health stores and most supermarkets.

If hot chocolate is your thing, go for the organic Green & Black chocolate powder, now available in most supermarkets. Hot chocolate is not something I would recommend in large amounts to anyone trying to lose weight. However, it is much lower in caffeine than coffee and the organic brands are, of course, free of unnecessary pesticide residues and other chemicals.

---

### Essential fatty acids (EFAs)

EFAs (sometimes referred to as Omega 3 and Omega 6 fatty acids) are special nutrients needed for a whole variety of different body processes. They cannot be manufactured by the body and have to be provided via the diet. EFAs are vital for the production of biologically active messengers known as prostaglandins. EFAs form part of every cell structure and are essential for the regulation of the heart and circulation and to help maintain a healthy nervous system and strong immunity.

---

## Cut back on fat

But don't cut it out altogether. Although there is plenty of evidence that low-fat and fat-free diets encourage dramatic weight loss, eating too little fat can create other health problems too. The quality of fat is also important. Change the type of fat you use. Cook with extra-virgin olive oil, and use either a little butter or a non-hydrogenated spread (from health stores). Get plenty of those very important *essential fatty acids* by including foods such as pumpkin seeds, sunflower seeds, walnuts, almonds, pistachios and cold-pressed oils in your diet. From a food combining perspective, fats, oils, seeds and nuts can be considered as **versatile**, go-with-anything foods. Pages 69–71 has more information on how to balance fat intake.

## Beware of additives

Foods labelled low-fat may be high in artificial additives. There is a school of thought that suggests chemical additives might contribute to weight problems by congesting the liver and other tissues and hampering detoxification. Many so-called 'diet' foods are heavily laced with additives. Avoid them if you can. If this means choosing a full-fat, additive-free version of, say, cheese or yoghurt, then go for that but eat less of it.

## If you are eating out, go light

Avoid rich sauces, cheese toppings and desserts. Ask for steamed and non-fried vegetable dishes, fish and chicken. And say no to the bread roll.

## Don't overeat

▶ Don't destroy the quality of a nutritious meal by eating too much of it.

▶ If you are presented with a large portion, don't be afraid to say it's too much or to leave food on the plate.

▶ If you're inclined to overeat, why not try this idea: instead of a starter and a main course, or a main course and a dessert, go for two starters or order half-portions.

## Before you shop

▶ Eat. Shop after meals, not when you are hungry.

▶ Make a list and stick to it. That way, you are less likely to buy items you don't need.

## Before you eat

If you're tempted to eat outside normal mealtimes, ask yourself if you are really, honestly hungry. It is easy to reach for food through habit or boredom. Drinking a glass of water can help reduce hunger pangs.

## Eat sitting down

Sit at a breakfast bar or at the dining table. Do the thing properly. Set a place with a plate and eating utensils. Take your time over the meal and enjoy what you eat. Or take yourself outside to a seat in the garden or the park. Standing up to eat or eating while you are moving not only puts a huge strain on your digestion, it is also likely to be far less nourishing. Snacks grabbed quickly on the move are more likely to be of the junk-food variety rather than the kind of food your body really deserves!

## Sort out your stressors

Finding out what worries you or makes you anxious can be a real step forward in the fight against cravings. Under stressful conditions, it seems that people with weight problems eat far more than those who are a normal weight. Pages 329–47 have lots of tips on how to soothe away stress.

## Beat boredom

Tackle the tasks you don't enjoy all that much earlier in the day. Completing the potentially boring jobs in the morning means that you can look forward to things you do enjoy doing. This may sound simplistic but it really does seem to help. If you are stuck in a rut and think that your whole day is boring, or you are having to do a job you really hate and can't avoid, do whatever you can to improve your immediate environment. For example, you could:

▶ Play some favourite music.

▶ Open the windows.

▶ Place houseplants around your working area.

▶ Do the task outside. I know someone who always sits in her backyard to clean the brass and someone else who sets up her ironing board on the tiny patio outside her kitchen. If the weather is reasonable, I'll sit outside under a lean-to to tackle boring paperwork.

▶ Use daylight bulbs instead of ordinary bulbs or fluorescent tubes.

▶ Change your colour scheme. If you are easily depressed, don't wear blue or paint your walls blue. It could just make you even more blue. And don't use or wear anything that is red or orange – these two colours are known to stimulate the appetite! Instead, choose green, cream, pale peach, pale apricot, pale yellow, turquoise, lavender, purple or pink (please never all in black, except for parties).

## Change tack

If you are doing something that allows your mind to wander to thoughts of food, do something else until the moment passes. Cravings are not permanent; they do go away. Try the following:

▶ Move around

▶ Stretch

▶ Breathe deeply

▶ Get some fresh air

▶ Have a drink of water

▶ Empty your bladder

▶ Wash your hands and face

▶ Rub the backs of your ankles and soles of your feet

▶ Massage your ear lobes

▶ Change your shoes

▶ Comb your hair

▶ Freshen your make-up

▶ Go for a walk

## Go pamper yourself

Invest in regular sessions of reflexology or aromatherapy massage. Your local health centre should have details of your nearest therapist. If funds are tight, treat yourself to a luxurious bath (see below) and pamper your skin with a good-quality, body lotion or massage oil (made from natural ingredients) from the chemist, health store or The Body Shop. A bottle usually lasts for months. Why not get a partner, spouse, sister or girlfriend to give you a back and leg massage – and then do the same for them.

Buy (or borrow from the library) a self-help book on reflexology and teach yourself how to do a basic treatment. I especially like *The Family Guide to Reflexology* by Ann Gillanders (Gaia), a colourful book which has some excellent drawings to guide you and plenty of really sensible information about how to use reflexology to treat common ailments and help relieve stress or *Vertical Reflexology* by Lynne Booth (Piatkus).

## Take a deep, relaxing bath

Add two or three drops of beneficial essential oils and prepare to wallow.

▶ Lavender, chamomile, nutmeg and frankincense are soothing and relaxing.

▶ Grapefuit and geranium are good if you're depressed.

▶ Try sandalwood and orange if you're feeling dejected or despondent.

▶ Choose jasmine and neroli if your confidence needs a boost.

▶ Cypress oil can help if your willpower is weak.

▶ Go for juniper, orange and mandarin if your self-esteem could do with a lift.

## Stay mentally and physically active

▶ Take up a new hobby.

▶ Help out at your local charity shop.

▶ Join a local walking club.

▶ Or a local fitness club.

▶ Read – anything that you find absorbing as long as it's new to you. *Time, The Spectator, National Geographic, Hello!, Computer-Active,* a good novel, the latest bestseller, any kind of reading material that really grabs your attention. Listen to plays or books on tape. Anything from Jane Austen to Rosamunde Pilcher. My favourite escapes are such delights as Bill Bryson, Maureen Lipman, Peter Ustinov or Oliver Pritchett. They all make me smile and think.

▶ Learn a language. There are plenty of packages available that you can connect to a home computer or tapes that you can listen to on a walkman or in the car.

## Don't watch stressful television programmes

Avoid programmes that stress you unnecessarily, such as horror and action movies. Make a rule that you don't eat while you watch TV – under any circumstances. Don't have the TV on just for the sake of it. Boredom encourages impulse eating. Up comes the commercial break and it's loaded with ads for food and drink. No wonder you head for the refrigerator.

## Avoid temptation

If you find watching TV inclines you to nibble absent-mindedly, make sure that you keep only healthy snacks in the cupboard or fridge. If you don't buy crisps, biscuits, cakes or chocolate, you won't be tempted. If you're really suffering, snack on some fresh fruit or raw carrot or celery sticks.

## Instead of television

Do ten minutes of stretches and dancing to your favourite upbeat music. If family or flatmates are around and you don't want to be seen, escape to your room.

## Keep your hands busy

▶ For some people, hobbies such as knitting, sewing or embroidery help to reduce the risk of snacking while viewing TV.

▶ One of my former patients tells me that she has banished her cravings for snacks by altering her beauty routine. Instead of waiting until bedtime when she's too tired to be bothered, she takes her skincare routine to the television. One evening, she'll do her nails. The next, she'll massage her feet and legs. Or neck and arms. Or scalp. 'All I need is a small tray for bottles, jars and cotton wool, and a towel to protect clothing or furniture. The only rule I make is "no red varnish" in case of spills.' It's impossible to eat when you're covered in cuticle remover, or hand lotion, she tells me. 'The other benefit is that it's improved how I feel about myself. I never bothered before, never had time to look after me. Now I'm looking good.'

## Drink a glass of water

Sometimes, you can feel hungry when, in fact, you are thirsty. Drink a large glass of filtered or mineral water and wait ten minutes. Your hunger pangs may subside. If a mealtime is approaching and you're desperate, a glass of water can stop you nibbling.

## Don't store food where you can see it

For example, in glass-fronted cupboards, and don't store things in clear containers or polybags.

## Top up your vitamin intake

Take a top-quality, broad-range multivitamin/mineral or antioxidant supplement with your breakfast or lunch. Vitamins are vital in the weight-loss war. A whole range of nutrients are needed to convert food into energy. Unfortunately, cutting calories by, say 50 per cent, means that we will have cut our vitamins and minerals by a similar amount. Years of dieting can take its toll on our reserves and leave us with borderline deficiencies. Add to that the likelihood of poor digestion and absorption, and it could be that you haven't absorbed nutrients properly for years.

From now on, make a good-quality supplement part of your diet. There's no need to take it every day. Just five days a week will do. Choose a multi one-a-day that includes all the B complex vitamins and the minerals magnesium, manganese, zinc, selenium and, especially important, 50mcg–200mcg of chromium. All these nutrients are needed to convert foodstuffs into energy. A number of studies have shown chromium to be at lower than normal levels in vast numbers of the population.

## Give your digestion a boost

Follow a course of digestive enzymes for four months. You'll need 180 capsules (usually sold as a two-month supply). Take one with every meal for the first month (90) and one just with the evening meal for the next three months (another 90). Poor digestion is a common reason for weight problems. Short-term treatment with enzymes not only improves absorption but could also give stubborn weight a kick.

## Be careful about caffeine

Ease up on caffeine-loaded beverages such as coffee, tea and cola. They can give you a valuable emergency 'lift' but they're not a great way to sustain energy long term.

## Keep your fluid intake high

Drink plenty of filtered water, diluted fresh fruit juice and green teas such as jasmine. Herb teas are fine but don't overdo them. They are naturally diuretic – good for your kidneys and liver – but, if taken in excess, could cause you to lose some nutrients. Instead of ordinary tea every time, why not try green tea? Much favoured in China and Japan, green tea is believed to have a beneficial effect on fat and sugar metabolism, and its powerful antioxidant action may help to protect liver cells from damage.

## Eat as naturally as possible

Whenever you can, choose unadulterated, chemical-free, organic ingredients. Each time you go to put something in your basket or trolley, ask yourself if this is the freshest, least-processed option available. Ready-prepared packets may seem like a time-saving short cut but can also add up to more expense and less nourishment. And there's no way of really knowing what has been done to the food before you buy it.

## Aim for as varied a diet as you can

We all tend to rely on a relatively limited menu, often high in common allergens such as cow's milk, wheat, sugar and artificial additives. But a restricted or unadventurous diet means curbing our number of nutrients. Limiting our intake of vitamins, minerals, amino acids and essential fatty acids disturbs the production of enzymes, hormones and other natural chemicals needed to maintain good health and keep our bodies balanced. Instead of sticking with the same old meals, year in, year out, try to broaden your shopping horizons. Every week, promise yourself that you'll add extra variety and nourishment by introducing a new recipe, a new food, a different vegetable or a fresh fruit that you haven't tried before.

## Be wary of magic bullets and empty promises

There are many products on the market that suggest almost instant weight loss with little or no effort. None may be directly harmful but it is important to keep in mind that a single nutritional supplement or 'special' diet food is not going to be a long-term solution to weight problems in the absence of healthy food and a sensible exercise programme.

## Take regular exercise

I've heard all the excuses and sympathise, but exercise isn't boring and it isn't time-consuming either. Once you get started, you're bound to get the bug and want to keep at it. It gives you a real buzz and, apart from anything else, it's fun. Remember that 95 per cent of failed dieters we were talking about earlier? Well, studies show they're the ones who don't exercise. The 5 per cent who succeed in maintaining normal weight, stay active. Regular exercise needs to be done in conjunction with a healthy eating programme, though. If you exercise but stay with those old eating habits, weight is harder to lose. See pages 90–4 for some new ideas.

## Be patient and lose weight slowly

Don't try to lose a whole load of weight all at once. *The Complete Book of Food Combining* encourages slow and steady weight loss of 2lb (around 1kg) a week. It doesn't sound much but it's an effective way to reach your target weight. Everyone knows that weight lost quickly nearly always creeps back. By using my simple food combining system, your blood sugar, your appestat (your appetite control mechanism), and your metabolism stay balanced, so that weight lost stays lost.

## Forget about weighing yourself

Scales are notoriously inaccurate and are really not that helpful. Check your progress using clothes that don't fit you at the moment. Try them on again every few weeks, not every other day. It's important to understand that it can take around six weeks for real weight loss (as opposed to fluid loss) to register.

## Be committed

Introduce as many of the tips in this chapter as will fit comfortably into your lifestyle. Change your eating habits gradually over a period of several weeks. Promise yourself you'll make the effort (that's why you are reading this book) but don't try to do too much at once. This isn't a competition. Even the smallest step forward is an achievement, and brings you a little closer to your goal.

## Above all, enjoy

▶ Enjoy what you eat. Don't allow any kind of diet to take you over. Weight loss or not, if your eating habits have reached the stage where they are ruling your life, they are no longer any good for you.

▶ Enjoy your indulgences. There is good evidence that denying yourself a favourite food treat when you're already down in the dumps can lower your spirits even further. Remember the words of the French historian Voltaire (1694–1778) who said that 'pleasure is the object, the duty and the goal of all rational creatures'. According to Traditional Chinese Medicine, anything really enjoyable that gives you a psychological and emotional boost is considered vital nourishment for the *shen* or spirit, even if it is perhaps not all that nutritionally sound. On the other hand, ploughing through something you absolutely loathe just because you've heard it's healthy can have a detrimental effect on *shen*. Unless the particular food in question is causing full-blown allergy or intolerance, an occasional indulgence can be positively beneficial!

▶ Enjoy what you do. Count your blessings and see the positive side of every day. Boredom, depression and stress are the prime enemies of successful weight control. Pages 329–47 have more info on how to manage stress effectively.

## If, whatever you try, your weight problem is still not responding

▶ See your doctor and ask for a health check that includes thyroid function.

▶ See a qualified nutritional therapist who can carry out investigations for candidiasis. And get yourself allergy tested. Sensitivity to certain foods can increase the risk of blood sugar problems, fluid retention and weight gain. Pages 202–18 have more on how my particular kind of food combining can help relieve allergies.

CHAPTER **9**

# Food Combining and Fluid Retention

Remember in the previous chapter my mentioning that weight gain was not always the result of too many calories? For an estimated one in three people, those extra inches are due not to fat but to excess water; in some cases, as much as 7 pounds (just over 3kg). And the problem appears to be more common in women than in men. Unfairly, the female body actually has a slightly lower water content than the male because women have a higher percentage of fat-storing tissues that contain less water.

## What is Fluid Retention?

When the body accumulates water that it can't unload, we develop a condition called oedema, the medical term for fluid retention. This can vary from the uncomfortable and inconvenient to the serious and life-threatening, depending on the cause. Some, including kidney disease, heart disease, diabetes and liver failure, can obviously be very serious indeed. Not so complicated, but none the less troublesome, may be fluid retention caused by hormonal imbalances, constipation, toxicity, high salt intake, too much sugar, excessive stress, deficiencies of certain nutrients – especially magnesium and potassium – or food sensitivities.

The most visible symptoms of fluid retention are swollen ankles, puffy fingers, breast swelling and distended abdomen, all very familiar to many women around period time. This is because female hormones are closely associated with the balancing of body fluids. In particular, oestrogen increases the production of another hormone called aldosterone which enhances salt and water retention.

When blood vessels can't clear unwanted fluid, the blood stagnates, pushing water into the tissues, causing puffiness and bloating. The situation is made worse when arteries and veins become less elastic with age, allowing fluid to build up in the legs.

---

**Did you know?**

Localised oedema is the swelling that occurs following injury, such as a sprained ankle, a cut or insect bite. When part of the body is injured in any way, blood vessels and capillaries are damaged and become more permeable to water. This type of inflammation is the body's normal response to trauma, helping fluid to carry special cells to the injured site, which then gobble up bacteria and unwanted foreign material.

Oedema is also associated with more serious infections such as peritonitis (affecting the lining of the abdomen) or pleurisy (where fluid collects in the membrane between the chest cavity and the lungs).

---

## Diuretics

Diuretic drugs – commonly referred to as 'water tablets' – are often prescribed to treat the condition. 'Diuretic' simply means any substance – medicine or food – that increases the output of urine. Sometimes the level of fluid may not be serious enough to warrant the use of drugs or, alternatively, the side-effects may not be acceptable.

> **IMPORTANT NOTE**
> Diuretic drugs cause the body to lose potassium and magnesium. Medical checks usually take potassium into account but magnesium is often missed. Anyone taking diuretic medicines long-term should ensure that their doctor or specialist carries out regular tests for both these minerals so that deficiencies can be corrected. Don't be afraid to ask. Many doctors seem unaware that magnesium loss occurs and so fail to check for this important mineral.

# What Can You Do About Fluid Retention?

What you eat can have a major impact on how your body deals with water. Changing to a food combining diet, making sure that all the elimination processes are working efficiently and, where applicable, using herbal and nutritional supplements, can bring welcome relief.

Some foods are naturally diuretic, encouraging water loss; others may cause us to hold on to water. How well we digest can also determine how well our metabolism deals with fluid – which could be one of the reasons why food combining has shown itself to be so helpful for relieving mild to moderate fluid retention.

## MY TOP TIPS FOR FIGHTING FLUID RETENTION

### Food combine

I can't give you any scientific reason why food combining appears to help reduce the symptoms of fluid retention for some people. I have seen a great many patients with oedema and a considerable number have reported significant improvements in symptoms after a few months' food combining. Perhaps it's simply food combining's apparent ability to improve digestion and absorption so that minerals and fluids are better balanced. I should like to see more research carried out on this.

## Eat less salt

Excess salt means that the body will hold on to water. It's been esti-mated that if someone accumulates as little as four ounces (100g) of salt in the body, they will need to carry an additional three gallons (13 litres) of water. This means extra bodyweight close to 24 pounds (approximately 11kg).

We simply don't need sodium in the large quantities that most of us consume daily. It isn't so much the salt added to vegetables during cooking or a sensible sprinkling at the table that pushes up the sodium in our systems to dangerous levels. It's the almost unbeliev-able 75 per cent hidden in packaged and convenience foods that is said to cause the most problems. It's been suggested that tens of thousands of deaths and disabilities could be prevented if less salt was added to processed food. And it's everywhere, in sweet as well as savoury items – but it's also well concealed. Read the labels on breakfast cereals, gravy granules, stock cubes, biscuits, ketchup, pasties, pies, ready meals, salty snacks, canned and packet soups, burgers, bacon or sausages; the word 'sodium' is almost bound to be there. It is also high in smoked fish, any foods canned in brine, boiled ham, tinned meats and cheese. One of the largest single sources of hidden sodium is bread, which we don't usually think about (because bread is normally promoted as a healthy food) but it should concern us because we eat so much of it.

Sodium occurs naturally in fresh fish, raw meat, root vegetables, milk, cream, yoghurt, oatmeal and dried fruit. As a general rule, foods of fish or animal origin are usually higher in sodium than fruits, vegetables, juices and grains. But the amounts that nature puts into food are there for good reason, because we need them. The extras that manufacturers put into processed foods are there to titi-late our taste buds and make us buy more of this product.

I appreciate that cutting back on added or hidden salt isn't always easy. You'll go a very long way towards a safer intake if you do nothing else but abstain from those packaged and processed foods listed earlier. As an extra precaution, try introducing other flavour-ings such as herbs, Japanese soy, spices, olive oil and balsamic dressings, and seaweeds instead of salt. They can help to re-educate your taste buds away from salty foods. As well as being a great way to reduce salt intake, herbs and spices are also good for increasing magnesium and potassium.

!  **TECHNICAL STUFF**

### Working out sodium levels in foods

It's easy to confuse sodium with sodium chloride, the chemical name for common salt. If you're interested in sums, the amount of sodium in sodium chloride is around 40 per cent. For example, there are 2.5 grams (2500mg) of sodium in the recommended daily maximum of 6 grams of salt; a pack label that indicates 0.5 grams of sodium per serving would make up one-fifth of your daily intake. Put another way, the percentage of sodium (this is the part we need to consider when it comes to conditions such as hyper-tension) in common salt or sodium chloride is just over 40 per cent. So, if a label tells you the total sodium in grams per serving, you can calculate the salt content by multiplying the sodium (chemical symbol Na) by 2.4.

Here are a few examples. One serving of poppadums (2.85g Na 3 2.4) exceeds the limit at 6.8 grams of salt. A teaspoon of soy sauce (1.5g Na 3 2.4) weighs in at 3.6 grams of salt. Two sausages (1.4g Na 3 2.4) add up to 3.4 grams salt. Most bread contains between 0.5g sodium (1.2g salt) and 0.75g (1.8g salt) per 100g serving or 4 slices. The chances are therefore highly likely that if bread or other foods with a similarly high sodium content form a significant part of your diet, you'll be exceeding the recommended intake.

So, why has salt become such a problem? In the days of our hunter-gatherer ancestors, diets were naturally low in sodium (no packaged foods or salt on the table) and high in potassium (plenty of berries, roots, shoots and other vegetable matter). Because of this very natural state of affairs, the body was programmed to retain sodium and excrete potassium. But, as a result of dramatic changes in modern dietary habits, we now consume large amounts of salt-laden foods and much less in the way of fruits and vegetables. Unfortu-nately, evolution hasn't yet got around to mentioning this to our bodies so they still excrete potassium and hold on to sodium.

Find out the best ways to cut back on salt intake by turning to pages 72–3 in the chapter Eating for Better Health.

## Drink more water

This can sound a strange bit of advice when water is what we want to get rid of. But drinking more helps to dilute sodium salt in the system. How much water we take in is controlled, primarily, by our thirst mechanism. How we much we lose will depend upon other factors such as weather, body temperature, how much exercise we take, how much we sweat and how many times a day we empty our bladders. That lost fluid needs to be replaced.

Toddlers and young children respond to thirst naturally but soon get out of the habit. As adults, we don't always think to drink water, especially if our thirst control centre is not functioning as it should. Like most things, it tends to get sluggish and lazy with age. Cola, soda, squash, alcohol, coffee and tea don't hydrate the body as efficiently as unadulterated water. If the system becomes dehydrated, the body produces hormones that encourage it to hold on to water. It's a natural safety mechanism, which, unfortunately, can also increase the 'waterlogging' associated with fluid retention. Get into the healthy habit of increasing your water intake now. There is more information on water on page 77.

## Did you know?

In a newborn baby, three-quarters of its bodyweight will be water. In an adult, this averages at between 50–60 per cent, decreasing as we age. That's one of the reasons why things begin to sag, and our skin becomes drier and less supple. About half of our water stores are to be found inside the cells, and the other half in the bloodstream and cushioning the tissue spaces outside the cells.

## Careful on the caffeine

When it comes to working out whether you're having enough to drink, it's worth remembering that anything containing caffeine has a diuretic effect on the body. This means that, in larger amounts, it is potentially dehydrating rather than hydrating. There's no need to give up your favourite bevvie but, if you have a fluid-retention problem and are drinking more than three cups or glasses of coffee, tea, cola or hot chocolate per day, you could benefit from cutting back a little on the caffeine and upping your water intake.

And it's worth remembering that your body needs even more fluid than normal during times of infection, such as colds, flu and sore throats. It's easy to become dehydrated, even if you don't feel thirsty. So, if a bug gets you, drink lots of water, herbal and fruit teas, green tea, soups, and freshly squeezed lemon juice with honey in hot water.

### Skip the sugar

A diet high in sugary foods can cause an over-production of the hormone insulin which, in turn, can increase the body's tendency to store water and fat.

### Check for food intolerance

Some common foods can cause a condition known as allergic oedema. No one really knows yet why this happens but it may be the result of the body trying to dilute the tissues with extra water in an effort to dilute the irritation cause by the allergen. Yeast, wheat cereals, bread, cow's milk, cow's milk cheese, orange juice, sugar, artificial sweeteners and colours are all worth avoiding. It's been widely suggested that foods that aren't digested properly could cause irritation to the intestinal lining, allowing undigested residues to pass into the bloodstream. The body tries to wash out these residues by flooding the tissues with fluid. If the person continues to eat the offending food, the tissues stay flooded, adding fluid retention to the existing weight problem. More information on food sensitivity can be found on pages 205–10.

### Don't diet

I know it's difficult to resist the temptation. Apart from the discomfort caused by clothes and shoes feeling too tight, one of the greatest anxieties created by fluid retention is weight gain. Frustrating though it is, conventional dieting does not normally get rid of water weight. In any event, going on and off diets – and especially cutting calories before a period – can be seriously counter-productive. Firstly, eating less may appear to help you to lose weight but will also mean taking in less of the very nutrients you need to help keep your body fluids in balance! Secondly, missing meals or not eating enough can lead to a sudden drop in your levels of blood glucose (hypoglycaemia) which, itself, can increase the risk of cravings for sugary and salty foods so that you can, very easily, end up back where you started! If you need to get to grips with a weight problem, try food combining first.

## Increase your intake of alkaline-forming foods

Some experts believe that an over-acid system can lead to waterlogging. A diet that concentrates on cereals, sandwiches, meat, poultry, sugar, and foods high in fat is likely to cause the blood and lymph to be excessively acid, especially if intake of vegetables and fruits is low. Smoking, drinking and stress are also acid-forming. Food Combining Chemistry (pages 420–37) has more information on how to increase your intake of those beneficial alkalising foods.

## Up your magnesium intake

Ensure that your diet includes plenty of foods rich in magnesium – that means any kind of fresh or dried fruit, brown rice, fresh and canned fish, fresh root ginger, garlic, green vegetables, lettuce, potatoes, pasta and pulses. Magnesium helps to balance salt and water levels in the body.

When magnesium isn't supplied in sufficient quantities, the production of a particular hormone called aldosterone increases and, as it does so, it depletes even more magnesium. Aldosterone's job is to make sure that you hang on to some salt because your body can't function without a certain amount of it. However, if there is too much aldosterone, there will be an automatic increase in the amount of salt and, as a consequence, more fluid will be retained.

## Eat plenty of foods rich in potassium

This mineral sits on the opposite end of the see-saw to sodium salt. Whereas sodium makes us retain water, potassium makes sure we don't hang on to too much. We get potassium from all fresh and dried fruits, fresh vegetables and salad foods. Especially good sources include apples, apricots, artichokes (Jerusalem and globe), bananas, bamboo shoots, carrots, celeriac, celery, chard, courgettes (zucchini), cucumber, grapefruit, shiitake mushrooms, potato, sweet potato, watercress and all kinds of green vegetables. Notice that quite a few of these foods are also rich in magnesium too. Nearly all herbs and spices, such as fennel, garlic, parsley, sage and horseradish contain valuable amounts of potassium and magnesium.

## Choose naturally diuretic foods

Foods such as parsley, apples, asparagus, watermelon, cucumber and celery have gentle diuretic properties that don't disturb the natural mineral balance of the body. So, too, do many plant medicines, including dandelion, burdock, nettle, milk thistle, juniper berries, kava kava, liquorice, sarsaparilla and uva-ursi. They have the added benefit of being generally free of unpleasant side-effects.

▶ One of the most nutritious herbs with natural diuretic properties is **stinging nettle** (*Urtica dioica*), well known and much respected for its ability to cause that familiar red itchy rash. Nettle rash (or urticaria) is caused when an irritant is injected into the skin through the fine barbs on its hairy leaves. But nettle is also a therapeutic herb with many useful properties and doesn't, of course, cause any stinging sensation when it is taken in capsule form.

Traditionally a tonic used during convalescence, this nourishing plant is rich in vitamin C, B group vitamins, and a host of minerals including iron, magnesium, silica and zinc. Nettle has a stimulating action on the kidneys, helping to relieve fluid retention, ease bladder and vaginal infections, and cleanse the body of wastes and toxins. And it can have a beneficial action on the body's hormonal system, too. It is used as a pick-me-up during the menopause and may assist thyroid function and blood glucose balance.

> **Before taking herbal diuretics**
>
> If you have already been diagnosed with oedema, and are taking diuretic medication, you should talk to your doctor and ask to see a qualified medical herbalist before using herbal diuretics.

Fresh nettle leaves can be added to soups and stews and used as a vegetable in much the same way as we use spinach. Harvest with care, though, and don't pick them from the roadside or anywhere that might have been contaminated with exhaust fumes or chemicals. Never use uncooked plants. Apart from the obvious risk of severe irritation, they can cause kidney damage in their raw state. There is no sting, however, once the leaves are cooked.

Nettle tea and herbal supplements containing nettle are available from most health stores and some chemists.

▶ **Dandelion** (*Taraxacum officinale*) is a well-known garden weed with long and difficult-to-pull roots. One of the best liver tonics, a digestive stimulant and natural diuretic, it is often prescribed by herbalists to stimulate digestive juices, increase bile flow and help balance body fluids. Stashed full of vitamins and minerals, young dandelion leaves are particularly rich in potassium and, weight for weight, are richer in beta-carotene than carrots!

Freshly picked, well-washed, young leaves make a nutritious addition to salads. But, as with nettles, don't collect them from roadsides or anywhere else where they might have picked up pollution or weed-killer. Most people are able to recognise dandelion leaves without any problem, but if you're not sure, don't use them.

▶ **Milk thistle** (*Silybum marianum*) is known, primarily, as a liver cleansing herb, which is believed to protect and regenerate liver cells and help remove toxins. But it could be beneficial in the treatment of water retention too.

Among many other tasks, the liver is responsible for breaking down 'used' hormones. If the liver is overworked, this recycling and elimination process may be impaired, increasing the likelihood of hormonally related fluid retention. A course of milk-thistle capsules may help to ease symptoms, especially those associated with pre-menstrual weight gain.

## Increase your vitamin B6 intake

Vitamin B6 is often recommended to relieve the fluid retention associated with pre-menstrual tension (PMS). Some of the best food sources of vitamin B6 include bananas, lentils and beans, brown rice, dried fruits, green and root vegetables, free-range eggs, lamb's liver, nuts, oats, oily fish, potatoes and turkey.

If you choose to try B6 in supplement form, it's worth knowing that it usually works best if taken as part of a B complex or multivitamin, not on its own. Any nutrients that are taken in isolation, rather than together with other vitamins and minerals, could cause deficiencies or increase the need for other nutrients.

## Take more exercise

Regular exercise is known to improve lymph drainage and circulation, and enhance removal of wastes, including trapped fluid.

# Food Combining for Good Digestion

'If [understanding] the physiology of digestion can lead us to eating practices that ensure better digestion and better nutrition only the foolish will disregard its immense value to us, both in health and disease.'

Dr Herbert M Shelton *Food Combining Made Easy*, 1979

One of the major plus points for food combining is the way that it seems able to improve digestion. Digestion sounds a really boring subject – but when you realise how important it is to good health it begins to get really interesting. Understanding a little about how the digestion works allows us to see why it may not be in everyone's interest to eat concentrated proteins and starches at the same meal – especially if our digestive system is already grumbling, rumbling and complaining.

Many people have turned to food combining as a last resort when they hear how it has helped others to ease symptoms such as heartburn, bloating, flatulence and irritable bowel. But improving our digestion doesn't only make us *f-e-e-l* more comfortable, it's also vital for our long-term health and well-being. The information in this chapter has been accumulated not only from my extensive research into food combining but also from my years as a practitioner, specialising in the treatment of digestive disorders. I hope you find it useful, too.

If we don't digest and absorb vitamins, minerals and other nutrients from our food, every single bodily function can be disturbed. We don't sleep well, we're more prone to the effects of stress and we have less resistance to infection. Damaged or worn-out cells in the body can't be replaced, organs begin to degenerate and poisons and wastes won't be eliminated properly.

I have found the very simple system of food combining described in *The Complete Book of Food Combining* to be of benefit for a whole range of digestive malfunctions. It speeds up digestion time, relieves constipation, eradicates indigestion, reduces bloating, and helps ease the symptoms of more complicated gut disorders such as hiatus hernia, diverticulitis and irritable bowel syndrome. I have also recommended food combining to several patients diagnosed with ulcerative colitis and Crohn's disease who have reported significant improvements.

## Is Your Digestive System Struggling?

Look at the questions below and tick those to which your answer is 'yes'. All these things can contribute to poor digestion and absorption of nourishment, especially if they are a regular part of your weekly routine:

### QUESTIONNAIRE

▶ Do you miss breakfast more than twice a week? ☐

▶ Do you eat your mid-morning snack or lunch standing up? ☐

▶ Are you often too busy to eat lunch? ☐

▶ Does your work prevent you from taking proper meal breaks? ☐

▶ Do you often have to eat your evening meal after 8.00 pm? ☐

- ▶ Do you always finish your meal before everyone else? ☐

- ▶ Are your mealtimes regularly interrupted? ☐

- ▶ Do you get up from the table in the middle of your meal to attend to someone else's needs? ☐

- ▶ Do you get up to clear the table as soon as you have finished eating? ☐

- ▶ Do you eat one course immediately after another? ☐

- ▶ Do you suffer from ongoing daily stress? ☐

- ▶ Are you usually rushed and hurried? ☐

- ▶ Do you drink tea or coffee with meals or straight after meals? ☐

- ▶ Do you eat fruit as a dessert? ☐

- ▶ Do you eat fruit (say, an apple) after a lunchtime sandwich? ☐

- ▶ Do you drink fruit juice with meals? ☐

- ▶ Do you drink more than just a small glass of water or wine with a meal? ☐

- ▶ Do you like very hot spicy foods? ☐

- ▶ Do you eat spicy foods more than once a month? ☐

- ▶ Do you enjoy cold foods such as ice cream or chilled drinks? ☐

- ▶ Do you have to rely on ready meals or takeaways more than once a week? ☐

- ▶ Do you eat out in restaurants or cafés more than once a week? ☐

- ▶ Is eating out an inevitable part of your job? ☐

- ▶ Do you have to rely on motorway service areas or roadside cafés for your meals? ☐

▶ Are you more than a stone (14lb/6kg) overweight? ☐

▶ Do you suffer regularly with heartburn, bloating or flatulence? ☐

▶ Do you take indigestion remedies more than three or four times a year? ☐

I'm not going to ask you to score this questionnaire. You'll know, just by reading it through, if your digestive system is under strain. Even if you have no particularly troublesome symptoms but have ticked more than a couple of questions, it's likely that your digestion could do with a bit of nurturing.

## Eating Proteins and Starches Together Can Seriously Disturb Digestive Capability

As a rule, most of us sit down to mixed meals that consist of some kind of protein such as meat or fish, accompanied by a starchy food such as potato or rice, with, perhaps, a vegetable, and then, maybe, some fruit or a sweet pudding. We put it in our mouths, swallow it and then expect the stomach and intestines to take what it needs and discard the waste. Or we might choose a hamburger and bun. We don't eat the meat first and then the bread. We bite into both, chew up the mouthful and swallow. The stomach has no mechanism for separating these thoroughly mixed foods and partitioning them off into separate compartments. So it does what it can and leaves the rest undigested.

The only time we give thought to our stomach or intestines is when they cause us discomfort. Food combining takes the strain off an overworked digestion by separating the concentrated proteins from the concentrated starches and helping foods to be more thoroughly digested.

## Conflicting Views

This is usually the point at which food combiners, and the practitioners who recommend it, part company with those who believe the system has no value.

The critics do, however, make a number of credible points:

**1.** The body is designed to accept mixed meals – in other words, it is quite capable of digesting starches and proteins at the same time.

**2.** People have been eating the two together for a very long time and don't appear to have come to any harm as a result.

**3.** If proteins and starches together are such a bad thing, why isn't everyone falling ill?

**4.** Almost every food contains some protein and some starch so separating them simply isn't possible.

No disagreements there then!

Or are there?

Food combining experts have an equally plausible point of view.

### Our ancestors were natural food combiners

Anthropological and archaeological studies suggest that the human digestive system has not changed much in the past (at least) 10,000 years. It still works very much as it did in the days of our hunter-gatherer ancestors. Foods were usually eaten separately: meat (game) when the hunt was successful; wild fruits and vegetable matter within hours or just a few days after gathering. Our ancestors had no facility to store food for long periods as we do. There was no canning, preserving, freezing or refrigeration. It is only in the past few hundred years, due to the more plentiful supply of food and the way that we shop, that we have acquired the habit of serving more than one food at a time on one plate.

### We're not designed to mix protein and starch

It is a commonly held belief that we can take whatever foods we choose into our bodies, in any haphazard combination, and in any quantity, and expect them to be efficiently digested. Herbert Shelton was adamant that 'this is not good chemistry – and even worse physiology'. Indeed, he continued, 'Any professional who makes such a pronouncement should not pose as an authority in the field of human nutrition and presume to advise millions about proper eating.'

Shelton's conviction that the digestive system is not actually designed to eat protein and starch combinations at every meal seems to be backed up by the very science that conventional doctors and nutritionists learn during their training. Pick up almost any medical physiology textbook (the kind a student of medicine would use) and it will tell you that 'the activity of salivary amylase is blocked by the acid of the stomach secretions . . . for it is essentially non-active as an enzyme in an acid environment.' Or, put another way, the starch-digesting enzymes in saliva stop working once they hit stomach acid.

Essentially, then, if you eat chicken with rice, the breakdown of the rice (the starch) will stop as acid levels rise in response to the chicken (the protein). Similarly, if you eat fish with chips, neither one nor the other will be properly digested, and if you eat pasta with cheese sauce, the stomach acids will put paid to pasta digestion.

It's possible that we may have built up a tolerance to incompatible mixtures of proteins and starches but, if the medical textbooks are correct, it seems very likely that mixed proteins and starches are not dealt with as efficiently as proteins and starches that are eaten separately from each other.

## And as for symptoms?

Given the vast numbers of people who suffer constipation, flatulence, repeating, bloating, heartburn, halitosis and foul-smelling stools, it seems rather strange to infer that the body digests everything without a whimper. To quote Dr Herbert Shelton again: 'Less of a whimper, more of a loud national groan.'

One of the reasons that doctors don't always get to hear about minor symptoms of digestive discomfort is that we tend not to tell them. Most of us put up with lesser symptoms, sometimes for years, and only complain when they become incapacitating or intrusive. It is generally accepted that by the time serious problems manifest themselves, many diseases are well advanced.

'That digestion is not very efficient,' says Dr Shelton, 'is shown by [the amount of] gas, discomfort and foul stools [containing] large quantities of undigested food.' In his own studies, he found that most people digest only about half their food, passing the other half as undigested waste. In other words, it's not just what we eat that matters, but what happens to it after it has been swallowed.

Foods that linger in the system for too long encourage fermentation, a build-up of gas and production of toxins. Not to put too fine a point on it, when foods hang around for too long, *they rot!* Hence the pong! Some digestion will take place but it will always be incomplete.

## It's mixing concentrated proteins and starches that causes problems

Let's pick up on the critics' gripe that most foods contain starch and protein together so it's impossible to separate them. It's true as it stands but it's a pretty unqualified statement. For example, asparagus, alfalfa, cauliflower, celery, spinach, spring onions (scallions) – nearly all vegetables, in fact – contain a few grams of protein and a few of starch but it's only a small percentage of every 100 grams of each vegetable. These amounts are not sufficient to trigger large amounts of stomach acid or to interfere with the digestion of starches. Digestive difficulties arise only when we begin to mix concentrated starches, like bread or rice, with concentrated proteins, such as poultry, fish or meat.

Once the starch or protein content goes above 10 grams for every 100 grams weight of food, then it is getting to the point where it needs to be combined more carefully. Or put another way, the higher the percentage of protein or starch there is in a particular food, the more likely it is that each will be better digested if eaten separately.

Let's repeat the example that I used earlier on. Brown rice, which is classed as a starchy food by food combiners and orthodox dietitians alike, has around 30 grams of starch for every 100 grams of rice.

But it also contains protein, carp the critics.

Absolutely right, but only around three per cent; not nearly enough to upset digestion significantly.

But hang on . . .

Starch digestion will pick up again once the stomach contents have passed through to the next section of the digestive system, the small intestine, so why worry if it doesn't get sorted in the stomach?

The small intestine?

That 20 foot or so of coiled tubing at the bottom end of the stomach, where almost all the nutrients from your food are taken up by the body?

Ah yes, you're absolutely correct.

Starches are processed here.

This is because the acidic semi-liquid that has just travelled from the stomach triggers a whole load of natural bicarbonates which neutralise the acids and allow more starch-digesting enzymes (similar to those in the saliva) to go back to work on the starches.

But it's no good saying that the small intestine will carry out any work that the stomach doesn't do. If the small intestine could carry out the digestive process all by itself from start to finish, why bother having a stomach at all?

In fact, the digestive enzymes secreted into the small intestine are not designed to break up complex starches or complex proteins. It is the stomach, a primary holding and sorting tank, that is supposed to deal with the preparatory breakdown of proteins and starches ready for more detailed processing in the small intestine.

So there are the pros and the cons in little more than a nutshell. I have made every effort here to give you both sides of the bivouac and leave you to make up your own mind.

Whoever in the end turns out to be right about the science, I think it is important to bear in mind that digestive function is incredibly complex; so complicated, in fact, that the more honest and accessible of today's health experts are prepared to admit that they are still learning how it works. The highly respected author of probably the best physiology text in the world today, Arthur C Guyton, had an open mind on this. In his preface to the eighth edition of his massive *Textbook on Medical Physiology* he tells us, 'Each time I revise this [book], I think that someday physiology will become a completely mature subject without change from year to year. However, this always proves to be far from the truth. Physiology is a vast discipline, and only now are we beginning to make inroads into many of its fundamental secrets.'

Not surprisingly, I support the pro-food combining camp because I have witnessed, at first hand, its therapeutic benefits more times than I can count. In addition, having studied the anatomy, physiology and chemistry of the digestive system, I find it hard to believe that mixed meals can ever be digested well enough for anyone to absorb optimum nourishment from them. Reading the following section on how the digestive system works will give you a clearer insight into why mixing proteins and starches may not be suitable for everyone. I hope you'll find the details helpful but if you want to skip them, go on to page 166.

## Understanding Basic Digestion

Digestion takes place in three main areas of the body: the mouth, the stomach, and the small intestine. Along the way, a variety of different juices are produced.

The process begins when we put food into our mouths.

We chew. Well, we're supposed to chew.

Unfortunately, many of us gulp – and far too quickly.

It's easy to forget that 'well chewed means half digested'.

The idea is that our teeth smash the food into smaller particles so that digestive juices and enzymes can get to a larger surface area of the food and begin to break it down.

### Mouth juices are alkaline

Saliva, which helps to lubricate food as we chew it and makes it easier to swallow, contains an enzyme known as amylase which splits complex carbohydrates such as bread, pasta and rice (also known as starches) into simpler components ready for more complete digestion further down the tubes. Chemically, saliva is what is known as alkaline – the opposite of acid. The membranes of our mouth and tongue are not designed to withstand strong acids. If our mouth juices were acid instead of alkaline, our teeth would crumble and fall out.

## Stomach juices are acid

The majority of stomach or gastric juices are completely different from saliva; they range all the way from nearly neutral (neither alkali nor acid) to strongly acid, depending upon the food that is being eaten. The stomach lining is tough and is coated with a protective mucus membrane so that acids attacking the food can't digest the stomach itself.

## Starch likes saliva, doesn't like acid

For starch digestion to continue in the stomach, food needs to remain in a relatively neutral environment for anything up to an hour after being swallowed, so that the amylase (the enzyme produced in the saliva) can continue to work and give the starch a real head start. Only after this should the acidity of the stomach begin to rise and the salivary amylase stop working. Nevertheless, on average, as much as 30–40 per cent of complex starches will have been broken down before the food becomes mixed with gastric acid.

## Proteins aren't digested in the mouth

Starchy foods begin their digestion in the mouth but proteins are treated quite differently. Proteins, such as meat, cheese and fish, are broken up into smaller bits and pieces by the teeth and are moistened by saliva to make swallowing easier, but nothing else happens to them until they reach that pouchy bag at the bottom of the gullet, the stomach. So, although proteins are broken down in a mechanical way, no actual protein digestion takes place in the mouth at all.

## Protein triggers stomach acid

Almost as soon as protein is swallowed, cells in the stomach wall begin to produce gastric acids which trigger an important enzyme called pepsin. Pepsin grabs hold of complex proteins such as cheese, fish, meat, soya or eggs, and divides them into simpler structures ready for more complete digestion later on.

These components are a bit like Lego™. With Lego, you could build a castle, then dismantle it and use the same materials to make a truck or a spaceship. In the same way, the building blocks that the body gets from protein foods are dismantled and rebuilt into other protein structures such as hormones and enzymes.

When it comes to the value of food combining in helping the digestion, here is the really significant point: once the stomach has become acidic enough to break down those protein-building blocks, **starch digestion stops**.

It is an absolutely unavoidable fact that the digestion of starches comes to an almost complete halt if there is protein in the stomach. That's because the stomach juices needed for protein digestion are so acidic that they inactivate the starch-digesting enzymes that began work on the food when it was in the mouth.

## Acids and alkalis cancel each other out

In the same way that stomach acids can put a stop to starch digestion by stamping out the alkalis, early food combining experiments have shown that starches can also curb protein digestion by cancelling out some of the acids. Pepsin, the protein-splitting enzyme, will work only in a strongly acid stomach and is completely inactive in an alkaline or neutral environment – so it won't do anything for starches and it won't even work on proteins if there isn't enough acid around. This means that, when we eat proteins and starches together, the passage of food from the stomach slows right down.

In addition, when proteins are only partially digested, the peptides and amino acids are not broken down properly either. This can, in turn, affect the body's ability to produce hormones, enzymes, and the new cells that are needed to make blood and to repair worn-out or damaged tissues. One essential amino acid, lysine (called 'essential' because it has to be provided by the diet and can't be made within the body), may be destroyed when proteins and starches are either cooked together or eaten together. A deficiency can lead to chronic tiredness, poor concentration and dizziness. Lysine is needed by the immune system to build antibodies. It is also used to ease the symptoms of the herpes virus and may have a role to play in the transport to the cells of nutrients known as essential fatty acids.

---

### Interesting experiments

Studies have been carried out to investigate the level of acidity in the stomach after protein meals, after starch meals, and after meals consisting of starch and protein together. When we eat complex proteins and complex starches at the same time, neither is properly digested. Results showed that there was enough acid to destroy the starch-digesting enzymes but not enough to allow the pepsin enzyme to properly break down the protein. In addition, digestion was much slower. However, when starches and proteins were eaten separately, digestion was speedier and more efficient.

---

## Transit time

The length of time that it takes to digest any particular food will vary from person to person, depending upon a number of factors including the general health of their digestive system and on how foods are combined. However, it is possible to make certain generalisations.

Most animal-based proteins can take up to eight hours to be broken down.

But, where digestive capability is poor, some experts suggest 72 hours may be required for some foods, such as pork and beef products, to pass from one end to the other! If you think this sounds healthy, consider this. Take a pork chop and an apple. Leave them both on a table in a warm room for 72 hours. When you return to them in three days' time, would you choose to eat the pork chop or the apple? A similar process takes place inside our warm bodies. Foods that hang around in there for too long get very nasty indeed; they go off, produce gases and toxins and become extremely smelly!

Starchy foods pass more speedily through the system than most proteins, requiring three to four hours. Fruit is fastest, making the trip through the stomach in about half an hour.

---

**HERE'S A RECAP**

**Time taken for digestion**

▶ Meat, poultry, cheese, fish, eggs:  4–8+ hours

▶ Potato, bread, rice, pasta:      3–4 hours

▶ Fruit:                20–40 minutes

---

When foods that need different transit times and different conditions are chewed up together, it is easy to see how the digestive process not only slows right down but also becomes inefficient.

---

**Pudding alert**

An added problem is that humans have acquired an unnatural desire for eating something sweet after a main meal. Unfortunately, sugary and refined foods interfere with stomach acid and increase the risk of fermentation. If you can't live without pudding, then it can help to leave a gap of an hour or more between main course and dessert.

---

# Digestive Problems that Respond Well to Food Combining

The best way to prove the matter one way or the other is to give food combining a chance, especially if you are plagued with any kind of digestive malfunction, such as simple heartburn or more complicated constipation, irritable bowel, diverticular disease or haemorrhoids.

I am quietly confident that the many people who suffer from acid indigestion following, say, a meal of steak and chips, would not experience the same discomfort after a food combined meal. Think how nice it would be to throw that antacid medicine away for good.

## Bowel Complaints

One of the most beneficial aspects of food combining is its ability to improve bowel function. I've had some of the most positive feedback from people suffering a whole range of small and large bowel problems including diverticular disease, constipation, anxiety-related diarrhoea, Crohn's disease, ulcerative colitis and anal fissures. No more abdominal gripe, no bloating, and going to the toilet more easily and more regularly are the major improvements often mentioned by patients. Two conditions that appear to respond particularly well to the introduction of food combining are irritable bowel syndrome (IBS) and piles (haemorrhoids).

## IBS

Until relatively recently, irritable bowel syndrome was believed by many medical experts to be a psychosomatic disorder. Stories of patients being referred for psychiatric assessment or counselling were not uncommon. However, IBS is now recognised as, essentially, a physical problem with some very real symptoms which, not surprisingly, can also cause depression and emotional turmoil.

IBS can, quite literally, get on your nerves. If your diet is lacking the nutrients needed to feed the nervous system, or if you suffer from any kind of nerve damage or nervous disorder, the nerves that control bowel function can send the wrong messages to the bowel, causing it to empty more frequently or suddenly.

Where constipation is a dominant symptom, psychologists say that sufferers may be reluctant to share their feelings. If diarrhoea is a persistent problem, this could indicate a subconscious or unexplained fear. Being 'put down' or feeling trapped or dominated in a relationship and unable to express anger or 'let go' are some of the emotions that have been linked to bowel disorders.

Where nervous stress or upset causes a rush for the loo, the condition may be diagnosed as performance-anxiety diarrhoea or PAD. Relaxing therapies such as t'ai chi, meditation, yoga, aromatherapy and simple deep-breathing exercises can provide valuable support.

IBS symptoms can be persistent or intermittent, and can include:

▶ Abdominal gripe

▶ Alternating constipation/diarrhoea

▶ Anal itching or soreness

▶ Bloated abdomen

▶ Constipation

▶ Depression

▶ Diarrhoea

▶ Hyperventilation

▶ Jaw clenching

▶ Lower back pain

▶ Mucousy stools

▶ Muscle spasm

▶ Rectal bleeding

▶ Rectal pain (called proctalgia fugax)

▶ Stress

▶ Teeth grinding (bruxism)

▶ Tiredness

▶ Urgency to visit bathroom

▶ Weight fluctuation

▶ Worry and anxiety

**Other names for IBS**
Colicky bowel
Colitis
Mucous colitis
Nervous bowel
Non-inflammatory
bowel disease
Spastic colon

No one knows what causes IBS, but possible triggers include:

- An overgrowth of the yeast, *Candida albicans*

- Food sensitivity, particularly to milk sugar (lactose), milk protein, gluten, wheat or yeasty foods

- Hormonal disturbance – IBS can flare up pre-menstrually

- Inadequate diet

- Intestinal parasites such as threadworm and Giardia

- Low levels of hydrochloric acid

- Nervous-system damage

- Nutrient deficiency

- Poor digestion

- Relationship conflicts

- Side-effects of some types of medication

- Stress

- Work pressure

## Treating IBS

Peppermint tablets are often prescribed for IBS because of their ability to help relax muscle spasm in the intestines. Also used are anti-cholinergic drugs that control gut contractions. Laxatives may be suggested where chronic constipation is the dominant symptom. Drugs to suppress diarrhoea can be a useful emergency measure if you have to travel or are in a situation where toilet facilities are not readily available. However, none of these medicines are recommended in the long term.

I have treated a great many IBS patients who have benefited from the use of diet therapy and natural remedies. The information in this chapter has helped many people to ease their symptoms.

## Check for food sensitivity

Sensitivity to certain foods can be associated with irritable bowel syndrome. Find out if this applies to you by keeping a food diary. Write down all the food and drink that you consume for, say, two weeks, and note alongside when IBS symptoms are most troublesome. Be aware that it may not be the most recent meal that causes problems. In addition, a particular food could trigger an attack when you are stressed or unwell but not at other times. Common culprits are cow's milk, cow's milk cheese, bread, wheat cereals, sugar and yeast, but other foods might also be indicated.

## Don't restrict your diet

Don't be tempted to remove more than one or two food groups from your diet at any one time. Severe restriction can lead to nutrient deficiency. The best plan is to avoid the suspect food for, say, four or five days to see if your symptoms disappear. If not, reinstate it in your diet and go on to the next suspect, giving up a food only if you are sure it's an IBS trigger. Sometimes, it's possible to reduce or relieve symptoms by simply eating less of a suspect food. In other words, where three slices of bread might cause an attack, one may not. A drop of milk in tea or coffee may be fine, but a glass of milk could cause pain, bloating or diarrhoea. And, unfair as it may seem, it could be a favourite food that causes most sensitivity.

## Eat the right kind of fibre

IBS sufferers are often advised to eat more fibre. Wheat bran doesn't work for everyone and, if your gut is very sensitive, it may actually make symptoms worse. The more gentle types of fibre, such as linseeds, psyllium husks, porridge oats and brown rice can be very effective at relieving diarrhoea and constipation.

## Keep fluid intake high but watch out for tea and coffee

They can be fine in small amounts, but excesses can aggravate both constipation and diarrhoea and upset the digestion if taken at mealtimes. Try to replace one or two cups with herbal and fruit teas, diluted fruit juices and, most important of all, water. Remember that fresh fruits, vegetables, salads, home-made vegetable soups and broths will add to your daily fluid quota.

### Try massage

Before going to sleep at night, massage the whole area of your abdomen with a little extra-virgin olive oil. Work from right to left and back again, using firm, circular pressure. Done regularly, this helps to release trapped gas and relieve muscle spasm (see page 182 for further instructions).

### Keep warm

Being tense with cold can increase the likelihood of muscle spasm. Standing or sitting in one place for several hours at a time can make you feel chilly. Take a brisk walk every day. If you can't leave your desk or work station, improve your circulation by swinging your legs and arms or walking up and down on the spot for a few minutes every hour.

### Check your posture

How are you standing and sitting? Check your posture and breathe more deeply. Standing or sitting in a cramped or slouched position can increase tension.

### Try natural remedies

▶ Bach flower remedies, from health stores and some pharmacies, can ease the emotional aspects of IBS. Try: **aspen**, for fears of unknown origin; **crab apple**, if you feel despondent, mentally or physically unclean or ashamed of your appearance; **mimulus**, for fear of known things, i.e. illness, people, darkness; and **scleranthus**, if you suffer from mood swings or extremes of emotion.

▶ If depression or stress are major symptoms, there are a number of remedies that can help. The herb **St John's wort** (*Hypericum perforatum*), sometimes referred to as 'Nature's Prozac', can improve mood and ease anxiety.

▶ If pressure at work or at home is causing undue stress, **evening primrose oil** taken together with **B vitamins** could be worthwhile.

I would suggest a three-month course of evening primrose oil and a good-quality, one-daily multivitamin/mineral supplement that contains all the B vitamins, plus the minerals calcium, magnesium, selenium, manganese and chromium.

▶ **Passiflora, valerian** and **kava kava** are three herbs that help to ease stress and encourage sound sleep. **Californian poppy** may also be helpful.

▶ If you are stressed or anxious during the day, add the herb **kava kava** to your daily supplement programme.

The chapter on **Stress** (pages 329–47) has lots more information on how to improve mood and coping skills.

---

**IMPORTANT NOTE**

If nothing works, talk to your doctor about tests to eliminate other possibilities. There are several conditions, including fibromyalgia syndrome, candidiasis and common intestinal parasites such as Giardia and threadworm, which can produce symptoms similar to those of irritable bowel syndrome. Bowel polyps, stalk-like growths that can become malignant and should always be investigated, give off a chemical that mimics IBS symptoms.

---

# Haemorrhoids

Haemorrhoids (or piles) are swollen blood vessels, similar in structure to varicose veins, which develop in and around the anal canal (back passage).The condition causes unnecessary but understandable embarrassment, is rarely discussed, and often looked upon by non-sufferers as a joke.

In fact, piles are incredibly common and can affect any age group. I have been unable to obtain figures for the UK but, in the US, it's estimated that around half the population of adults and children may be affected. Definitely not funny!

A pile, although desperately painful, is treatable so don't be nervous about asking for help. As one hospital consultant told me, doctors see patients' backsides every day. It's part of their job. A doctor I spoke to recently emphasised very clearly the importance of overcoming the embarrassment of discussing bowel disorders. 'It could save someone's life,' he said.

Our reluctance to discuss sensitive issues, such as piles, constipation or IBS, with a doctor means that a potentially serious bowel problem could become life-threatening before the doctor has a chance to check it out.

Internal haemorrhoids involve veins near the upper end of the anal canal. External haemorrhoids appear at the lower end, around the anus, just under the skin. The word haemorrhoid comes from the Greek *haimorrhoia* and means 'flow of blood'. Symptoms include bleeding, itching, pain and a feeling of incomplete evacuation when emptying the bowels. A pile is more likely to rupture and bleed when irritated or pressured.

## Treating haemorrhoids

If you are troubled by piles, see your doctor or ask your pharmacist for advice. There are several medicines, usually in the form of creams or suppositories, available both on prescription and over the chemist counter, that can ease the pain, inflammation and irritation caused by piles.

Where haemorrhoids have become entrenched and medication just doesn't help, surgery – although it sounds drastic – can be very successful. Known as a haemorrhoidectomy, a ligature or tight string is used to tie around the base of the pile which controls bleeding and cuts the pile off.

---

**IMPORTANT NOTE**

If you are suffering persistent indigestion, are severely constipated, or you notice either red or dark blood or dark stools when you go to the lavatory, visit your doctor at once for a consultation and check-up.

---

Prevention is always better than cure, so try out the following.

### Don't strain
The condition can be caused or aggravated by straining or trying to force bowel emptying and is very often – although not always – accompanied by constipation. Regular and easy bowel movements should reduce the risk of both problems.

### Answer the call of nature when it happens
Don't put it off, otherwise your bowel will go back to sleep. Holding on when you need to go is likely to aggravate the condition. Be prepared to sit, relaxed – and wait. Breathing deeply and slowly and massaging your abdomen, waist and lower back (just massage the bits you can reach) helps to relax the intestines. Lifting the arms above the head might also help trigger the bowel into action. However, if nothing happens within 10–15 minutes, give up and wait for the next call.

### Eat more fibre
Increasing your intake of dietary fibre from sources such as fresh fruits (apples and bananas are especially good), fresh vegetables, jacket potatoes, peas and beans, brown rice, oats, pumpkin seeds, linseeds and cereals, is an important first step. Help the fibre to work well by making sure your diet also includes plenty of fluid, especially water, herbal and fruit teas, home-made broths and soups. Fruit juices made from dark-coloured berries, such as cranberries, cherries, grapes, blackberries, bilberries and blueberries, not only add healthily to your daily fluid intake but also increase your levels of important nutrients, known as proanthocyanadins, that help to strengthen and tone the walls of your veins. If you are taking on board the right amount of fibre and fluid, you should experience two formed but strain-free bowel movements per day.

### Deal with stress and anxiety
Piles appear to be more common in people who worry or are under a lot of work or domestic pressure. On the psychological, symbolic and emotional side, there is the old folk-wisdom that connects mud, dirt or

excreta with money ('Where there's muck there's brass'). Some countries associate being hit by bird droppings as being a sign of good luck. Not letting go of waste suggests a reluctance to let go of material things: 'holding on' to unexpressed feelings; or an inability to 'open up' to new ideas or new thinking, Louise Hay, in her famous book, *You Can Heal Your Life* (Eden Grove), says that dealing with problems such as feeling angry, burdened or trapped are important factors in the treatment of piles.

### Taking warm baths

A daily soak in a warm bath, especially if taken just before bed, can encourage relaxation and relieve itching. Add three drops each of essential oil of lavender and juniper and wallow for ten minutes. Don't use soap, bubble baths, shampoo or anything else that might irritate the skin. Dry the skin gently but thoroughly and apply a witch hazel or horse chestnut cream to the affected area.

### Try visualisation

Some patients have found visualisation or imagery helpful. A basic exercise involves closing your eyes, breathing in and out slowly and deeply, and imagining that your piles are shrivelling up and disappearing. Then picture the walls of your anus being smooth, pink and healthy. Repeat the visualisation for at least two minutes twice a day.

### Use Bach flower remedies

Try these for four to six weeks; they can be just as helpful for haemorrhoids as for IBS. Add six drops of crab apple and six drops of rock water tincture to a glass of filtered or bottled (non-fizzy) water and sip at it throughout the day. **Crab apple** is the cleansing remedy. **Rock water** suits a taut, tightened-up person who has a rigidity of outlook or an inability to let go.

### Try a herbal remedy

There are several herbal remedies available that have a good track record at easing pain and inflammation. **Pilex** (tablets and cream), a combination of ayurvedic (traditional Indian) plant extracts, is well worth trying. Other useful remedies include **bilberry, horse chestnut** and **witch hazel**.

▶ **Witch hazel** (*Hamamelis virginiana*) has been used for centuries by Native Americans to treat a number of conditions including haemorrhoids, varicose veins, ulcerated or broken skin, insect bites and skin rashes. Traditionally, a poultice was made with the bark and leaves of the plant and applied to the troubled area. Witch hazel is still regarded as one of the most useful applications for skin disorders; a clear example of an old and trusted botanical remedy becoming an accepted part of mainstream medical advice.

   Scientists now know the active ingredients that make witch hazel such an effective skin treatment. Tannins and volatile oils provide a strong astringent effect and help to take down inflammation. Flavonoids are vitamin-like substances that improve circulation and strengthen blood vessels, in particular, the fragile capillaries near the surface of the skin. They also have important anti-thrombotic and anti-inflammatory properties. The active flavonoids in witch hazel are called proanthocyanadins, which also turn up in dark fruits such as bilberries, cranberries and black grapes. The deep tonic effect of this herb can relieve that awful dragging heaviness and tiredness of the legs so frequently associated with varicose veins. It is also sometimes recommended for the treatment of venous oedema (fluid retention). Witch hazel is available as capsules, cream, ointment or clear liquid. Always follow the pack instructions.

▶ **Horse chestnut** (*Aesculus hippocastanum*) is well known as a remedy for poor circulation – a frequent factor in haemorrhoids and varicose veins – and is sometimes recommended by herbalists to be taken in conjunction with witch hazel. For internal use, I would choose aesculus tincture (liquid herbal extract) or horse chestnut capsules. For external use, try a gel that contains extract of witch hazel perhaps with bilberry leaf and horse chestnut. Your health store should be able to advise you.

▶ Another great circulation booster that may also help relieve the symptoms of piles and varicose veins are the essential fatty acids found in **starflower oil, blackcurrant seed oil** or **evening prim-rose oil**.

▶ **Californian poppy** (*Eschscholzia california*) is probably best known as a sleep-inducing herbal remedy; a useful non-addictive alterna-tive to the opium poppy as it does not contain the morphine-codeine alkaloids. Californian poppy capsules could be helpful if you are very anxious and find that you are having difficulty sleeping or are being disturbed by nightmares. A less well-known talent of Cali-fornian poppy is its ability to ease the intestinal spasms so common of irritable bowel syndrome and the muscle tightness associated with piles.

The Native Americans harvested the stalk, leaves and flowers dur-ing peak flowering time between early summer and early autumn, air-dried them in the shade, and made a tincture which was used to treat colic pain. Although they had no scientific knowledge as to why the medicine worked, we now know that the benefits come from the plant's active ingredients – alkaloids, flavones and glycosides.

Alkaloids are potent plant constituents that have a physiological effect on a number of body systems including the nerves and the digestion. Glycosides include some of the most effective plant drugs; these particular glycosides may exert their beneficial effect on the intestinal muscles. Flavones are one of the most common groups of plant substances and have a wide range of activities; in particular an anti-spasmodic action which may be of benefit to IBS and other forms of bowel discomfort.

# What Can You Do to Improve Your Digestion?

## Nutrition Advice is Always Changing

Scientists and doctors don't always get it right. Since Dr Denis Burkitt's famous research in the 1970s into regularity and roughage, advice to eat more of it has become engraved in the stone of official health recommendations. Bran was the thing, and only a heretic would have dared question the benefits of a high-fibre diet. However, as a promoter of bowel health, too much *cereal* fibre may not be so helpful. Recent research emanating from an important long-term study of nearly 90,000 nurses, carried out by a team at Harvard Medical School, suggests that the insoluble fibre (such as bran) so favoured by Dr Burkitt may not, after all, provide the protection against bowel cancer that everyone had been led to expect. A follow-up study of 47,000 male health professionals came to a similar conclusion. But that doesn't mean we should all dump every kind of dietary fibre.

Fibre helps prevent constipation by increasing the volume of the stools and making evacuation much easier. In addition, it seems likely that the soluble kind of fibre found in beans, seeds, nuts, salads and vegetables, which is already known to be helpful in keeping blood glucose balanced, may also improve the balance of beneficial microflora in the gut and could help protect us against coronary heart disease too.

Just as interesting is the suggestion that a diet rich in complex starches, antioxidant nutrients and healthy gut flora could offer more protection against bowel cancer than the familiar string and sawdust roughage. (By the way, if you see the term 'non-starch polysaccharides' – 'NSPs' for short – turning up in health articles or medical advice, don't dismay. This is nothing more than the new nutrition-speak for dietary fibre).

If you're feeling confused, the following advice will set you straight.

## MY TRIED AND TESTED TIPS FOR IMPROVING DIGESTION AND REGULARITY

### Always have breakfast

A fruit meal makes a refreshing start to the day and is a light alternative if you're not up to facing food first thing in the morning. The extra fluid provided by fresh fruit can sometimes be enough to kick-start your bowel into gear without the need for medication or fibre supplements.

### Don't get over-hungry

Don't allow yourself to get so hungry that your stomach feels sore. If you can't take a decent break from the task in hand, at least stop for ten minutes and have a light snack.

### Don't eat on the run

However pushed for time you are, never eat on the run. When the stomach is tense, it can't digest properly. Sit down to meals. Don't just say you'll do it. Do it.

### Give your digestion a chance

Don't rush off as soon as you've finished a meal. Sitting, relaxed – chatting, reading or contemplating – for five or ten minutes after eating gives digestion a head start.

### Promise yourself you'll eat more slowly

Chew your liquids and drink your solids. Puzzled? Think about it. Moving liquids around your mouth before swallowing mixes them with saliva and so helps digestion along. Chewing solid food until it becomes semi-liquid before swallowing not only adds in valuable digestive enzymes from saliva (especially important if you are eating something sweet or starchy), it breaks food down so that the stomach juices can reach a larger surface area. Taking time over each mouthful also encourages you to relax and not rush.

### Don't allow your own mealtimes to be interrupted

It's all too easy to be disturbed by the telephone or to get up from the table to fetch something for someone else. Your nourishment is just as important as theirs.

### Avoid very hot and very cold food

If you have any kind of digestive or bowel discomfort, avoid very hot (hot temperature and hot spicy) and very cold foods. The stomach isn't designed for them and the liver doesn't like them. If curries or other spicy dishes are part of your culture, could you make them milder?

## Cut down on tea and coffee

Too much tea or coffee disturbs digestion and can also rob your body of some nutrients. There is no need to avoid these beverages entirely. Apart from anything else, they're enjoyable – and that means they are bound to be of benefit. A cup of tea can be wonderfully relaxing and a cup of coffee is known to increase our attention span when we're flagging. But don't overdo it. Two or three cups per day is about right. Enjoy tea and coffee between meals, not with a meal or straight afterwards.

## Eat little and often

This takes the strain off a tired digestive system and can also be valuable if you have high cholesterol or are trying to lose weight. Smaller, more frequent meals can help to normalise cholesterol levels and encourage balanced bodyweight.

## Don't eat late at night

Eating late in the evening is sometimes unavoidable but there is no doubt that food swallowed late will go to bed with you. Could you have your main meal at lunchtime or adjust your routine a little and try to eat earlier in the evening? It really is best to leave three hours between consuming dinner and going to sleep to give food a reasonable chance of digestion. There is also some evidence to suggest that late meals are more likely to encourage weight problems.

## Pace yourself

Allow a few minutes between courses. Better still, go for a one-course meal.

## Don't eat a large meal if you are stressed or anxious

The digestion won't be working properly if you are wound up like a coiled spring. Enjoy something that is easier to digest such as fresh fruit, a light salad or soup.

## Try to food combine when eating out

If you eat out a lot, it isn't that complicated to food combine a restaurant meal. For example, if you have ordered a chicken or fish dish, say no to potatoes or rice and ask for extra vegetables or a green salad. If it's pasta, choose a non-cheese sauce and wave away the Parmesan. Ask for fruit salad as a starter and refuse the dessert. If the recipe is particularly involved and you're not sure about the ingredients, just enjoy the meal and forget about combining it this time.

## Cut back on sugar

Better still, train yourself to manage without it. Use cold-pressed raw honey (available from health stores) as an alternative sweetener. Check the **Swap Sheet** (pages 80–1) for other options. Avoid the use of sweeteners such as sorbitol, saccharin and aspartame. If you're unsure what's in a product, check the label.

## Steer clear of foods that can be hard to digest

These include red meat, bread, wheat cereals, corn, spicy foods, puddings and desserts, anything deep-fried, rich sauces, pastry, pies, quiches, packaged orange juice, and foods containing artificial preservatives such as the flavour enhancer monosodium glutamate and sodium nitrite preservative.

## Keep fruit separate

Eat fruit and drink fruit juice separately from concentrated proteins and starches. Pages 22–33 explain why this is important.

## Go organic whenever and wherever possible

Most supermarkets and grocery stores in the UK now stock a good range of organic alternatives including onions, mushrooms, potatoes, carrots, bananas, apples, milk, soya milk, cheese, yoghurt, cream, eggs, chicken, breakfast cereals, biscuits, crackers, bread, fruit juices, soups and canned pulses. About 80 per cent of my weekly shop is organic now and I believe the small extra cost is worth it. If you're not sure where to find organic produce, pages 438–44 have details.

## Wash fresh produce

Wash all fruit, vegetables and salads really thoroughly before use. We usually remember to do this for vegetables and salad, but will eat an apple or a bunch of grapes without giving a second thought to the stomach-churning bacteria that they may have on their skins. There have been several reports of serious cases of food poisoning from imported fruit. Washing won't remove systemic pesticides, but will help reduce the load.

## Keep cow's milk to a minimum

Cow's milk is a common cause of discomfort, bloating, nausea, cramps, diarrhoea and gas. Unless you are very sensitive to dairy foods, small amounts of milk in tea or coffee are more likely to be tolerated but large quantities (such as by the glass, or on cereal) may not be. Several patients tell me that organic milk, now available in all major supermarkets, causes less disturbance than non-organic. If you can't manage your tea without a tiny splash of milk, going organic may be the answer.

## Include plenty of variety in your diet

Sticking with a limited number of foods limits your nutrient intake and increases your risk of food allergies.

## Choose food that is as close to its normal, natural, unrefined state as possible

This doesn't mean you have to plough your way through piles of roughage or a load of lettuce and lentils to be healthy. But every time you buy food that is packaged or pre-prepared in some way, check to see if there is a fresher, less-processed equivalent available instead. Preparing meals from basic ingredients means that they are likely to be more nourishing and, just as important, you know what goes into them.

## Take regular exercise

If nothing else, try to take a brisk walk for 15–20 minutes every day – or 30–40 minutes three times each week. Don't go jogging on a full stomach. Any kind of really vigorous exercise immediately after a meal can cause indigestion. But a walk after dinner is said to be good for the digestion.

## Relax your insides

Even if you are the world's worst worrier, always stressed, always rushing, always hyper and never still, a few minutes' quiet time each day can do wonders for your digestion, your bowels and your general health. Five minutes, that's all I'm asking. Regular deep breathing is one way to 'open up' all those tubes and improve digestive and bowel 'motility' (the word doctors use when talking about the transit and movement of food through the gut).

Sit down or lie down in a warm and comfortable place where you can be still and quiet:

▶ Let all the tension go out of your body. Make sure you have relaxed your jaw and your shoulders.

▶ Breathe in slowly and deliberately, allowing the abdomen to rise on breathing in and settle on breathing out.

▶ Repeat for ten in-breaths and ten out-breaths.

▶ Remain relaxed, and keeping your eyes closed, return to breathing normally for a further three to four minutes.

Don't do more deep breathing than this. Short sessions are very beneficial but too much, unless you are breathing deeply during aerobic exercise, could encourage over-alkalinity. You might be interested to know that in Chinese medical philosophy, anxiety and distress can lead to dysfunction of the lungs and the large intestine. Improving the quality of the breathing can increase the energy flow between these organs.

## Massage your abdomen

In case you skipped the section earlier on in the chapter about irritable bowel syndrome and piles, another helpful way to 'exercise' and relax the digestive system is to massage your abdomen.

Take a small amount of good-quality natural oil such as almond, olive, grapeseed or linseed (that's nutritional-grade linseed oil, not the stuff you treat wood with). About half a teaspoon is usually enough. Warm it between your hands and then, lying down on a bed or couch, massage the oil into your abdomen. Use the pads of your fingers or the heel of your hand and make small, firm circular movements, working from left to right until you have covered the whole area from your waist to the tops of your legs.

This should take about four or five minutes. Any abdominal gurgling, farting or burping is a good sign that the massage is having a beneficial effect. Repeat the massage whenever you remember – once a week is fine, twice a week is better. This is a very soothing exercise if you are stressed or have a stomach upset.

## Wear comfortable clothes

Avoid tight-fitting clothing, belts, corsets and skin-gripping elastic. Anything that restricts the chest, waist or abdomen can disturb the digestion and aggravate conditions such as IBS and diverticulitis.

## Check your posture

Constantly leaning forwards over a desk, or sitting or standing in a stooped or crouched position, can cause chest and stomach cramps and heartburn, and can aggravate conditions such as hiatus hernia. Think 'shoulders' several times a day and remind yourself to relax them. Lift your arms out to the sides so that your hands are level with your shoulders. Take a few deep breaths (this helps to open up the chest area and relieve cramps), and then let go.

## Let your bowel rule your brain

By ignoring the call to go to the toilet, you increase the risk of poisons in the large intestine being reabsorbed into the body. Constipation also puts pressure on the rest of the gut, increasing the likelihood of bloating, distension, heartburn and hiatus hernia. Experts advise that once you get the urge to empty, don't put it off. Don't strain. Breathe deeply and slowly. Massage the abdomen while sitting on the toilet. If you are tense, try putting your feet up on a book or low footstool. This puts the body into a natural semi-squatting position and relaxes the colon. Another 'trick' that some people find helpful is to stretch the arms up above the head and then to rest the palms on top of the head, breathing slowly and steadily all the time.

## Keep aluminium out of your life

It can disturb the balance of nutritional minerals in the body. Even though it is found in many indigestion remedies, aluminium can upset digestion and cause flatulence in some people. Don't cook with aluminium pans, pressure cookers or cooking utensils. Check packet labels, too. Aluminium is sometimes added to dried food to stop powder sticking together.

## Use a natural indigestion remedy

If you need an indigestion remedy, use something chemical-free and natural such as the herb meadowsweet or slippery elm – both from health stores.

## Choose fibre carefully

If you've been advised to eat more fibre, think again before using wheat-bran cereals. Plain coarse wheat bran can cause severe irritation and, for some people, makes diverticulitis and irritable bowel syndrome worse. Some bran cereals are also very high in sugar (check the label) although they may not taste overly sweet. The fibre found in oats, brown rice, seeds, vegetables and pulses is usually far more soothing.

---

**Vegetables, fruits, beans and nuts provide excellent fibre scores**

These are some of the best:

| | | |
|---|---|---|
| Almonds | Cauliflower | Peaches |
| Apples | Courgettes (zucchini) | Peas |
| Bananas | Dried apricots | Potatoes with skins |
| Beans (all kinds) | Dried figs | Prunes |
| Blackberries | Grapefruit | Pumpkin seeds |
| Broccoli | Hummus | Raisins |
| Brown rice | Lentils | Sweetcorn |
| Brussels sprouts | Nectarines | Walnuts |
| Cabbage | Oats | Whole rye |
| Carrots | Onions | Wholewheat pasta |

---

## Take organic linseeds or psyllium fibre

If you have problems with regularity, suffer constipation, piles, diverticulitis or irritable bowel syndrome, take a daily supplement either of organic linseeds or psyllium fibre. Health stores are the place to find them. Both are very gentle forms of roughage that help not only regularity but also encourage the bowel to let go of some of its compacted waste. They also seem to be just as helpful at soothing and slowing up a loose bowel as speeding up a reluctant one. Linseeds and psyllium must be taken with a good-sized glass of water.

## Drink plenty of water between meals

Sometimes, constipation can be caused not by too little dietary fibre but by lack of fluid. To work effectively, fibrous foods need to be hydrated with water to enable them to pass safely, comfortably and effectively through the gut.

## Don't drink too much liquid with your food

A small glass of water or wine is about right.

## Take supplements during meals

If you take supplements, it helps absorption and reduces the risk of indigestion if you swallow them in the middle of the meal. Eat half the meal, take your tablets or capsules with a little water and then finish the food. Take your supplements at a different time of day to any prescribed or over-the-counter medication.

## Don't let the dog or cat lick your face

Animal saliva can carry bacteria which increases the risk of dyspepsia, ulcers and intestinal parasites.

## Take a course of probiotics

Once a year, and especially if you have had to take antibiotics, follow them with a course of probiotics – concentrated friendly flora usually supplied in capsule or powder form – that repopulate the bowel. Probiotics have a number of important functions. They curb the population of bad bacteria and discourage pathogenic organisms from taking up residence. They also help the contraction and relaxation of the muscles in the gut wall, improve the consistency of bowel motions, reduce inflammation, reduce flatulence and increase absorption of vital nutrients. I have found only a handful of products to be consistently helpful. Page 443 has details.

## Follow a detox programme

Take the strain off the digestion by following the detox programme described on pages 231–46.

# CHAPTER 11

# Food Combining and Food Allergies

'Nouns of multitude: a pair of spectacles, a gaggle of geese, a pack of wolves, a pride of lions.

Nouns of medical multitude: a rash of dermatologists, a flood of urologists, an eyeful of opthalmologists, a retina of orthoptists, a mouthful of dentists, a pile of proctologists, a whiff of anaesthetists, a muscle of rheumatologists, a traction of physiotherapists, a mindful of psychologists, a cast of orthopaedists, a hive of allergists.'

How are you feeling right at this moment? How did you feel after breakfast or after lunch, yesterday or today? Think about it. Energetic, alert and alive or lethargic, bloated and completely devoid of brain power?

Food affects not only the way we feel but also how efficiently we function – both physically and emotionally. It can determine whether we are happy, ratty or depressed and will influence attitude, concentration and recall. Most of us recognise the importance of eating healthily and know that what we put in our bodies has a direct bearing on our well-being. To maintain peak performance, it's vital that the goodness in our food gets to where it's needed; that means through our digestive systems and into our blood. For a seemingly increasing number of people, though, that doesn't appear to be happening. One of the reasons, some nutrition experts believe, could be the growing problem of food allergies or, more correctly, food sensitivity.

One of the most successful ways I've found of dealing with food sensitivity is to make sure the digestion is working really efficiently. Probably the best way of achieving this is to food combine for a whole month. If you feel better, this could be a clue that your digestive system was not working too well and was aggravating your symptoms. Before we look in more detail at how we can alleviate problems, let's see exactly what the problems are and what causes them.

## Allergy, Intolerance or Sensitivity?

Confusingly, the words 'allergy', 'intolerance' and 'sensitivity' tend to be used interchangeably but there is a clear difference in meaning.

### What is An Allergy?

An allergy is defined as an abnormal response to a normal substance. When an allergen – such as pollen, pet dander or a potentially troublesome food – enters the body, the immune system shouts for help. In someone who is not allergic, antibodies are produced that deal with the troublemaker quietly and without fuss. Indeed, there may be no obvious symptoms at all. But in someone who is allergic, large quantities of sensitising antibodies are produced which attach themselves to cell membranes, causing them to rupture and release a number of chemicals including histamine, and toxins called leukotrienes. Such a reaction can cause a good deal of havoc. Blood vessels dilate. Nasal and sinus cavities block up. Muscles go into spasm. There may be sneezing, a runny nose, watery eyes, skin rashes, and, in more severe cases, vomiting or diarrhoea, migraine and restricted breathing. The severity and kind of response depends on which part of the body and which type of tissue is affected by which particular allergen.

## Fixed food allergies

True allergic reactions to food, sometimes referred to as fixed allergies, always involve the immune system. Although, thankfully, these are relatively rare, for some sufferers they can be life-threatening. Examples are peanut or seafood allergies where even the tiniest amount can cause symptoms scary enough to require emergency treatment. Strawberries, eggs and some food additives can also trigger very unpleasant symptoms. Allergies of this nature are very often genetic in origin and therefore a lifelong hazard and, if you have one, chances are you will already be very much aware of it. The effect of the allergen on the body can be severe. Large amounts of histamine are produced. The throat and tongue swell up, cutting off the flow of oxygen to the lungs, resulting in wheezing and chest pain. Blood vessels dilate and fluids are lost from the circulation, creating a dramatic fall in blood pressure. Toxins are released that send the muscles of the bronchioles (breathing tubes) into spasm, causing an asthma-like attack and suffocation. The resulting shock, known as anaphylaxis, can occur within seconds, minutes or a few hours of coming into contact with the allergen, very often an offending food. Sufferers usually carry special shots of adrenalin for use in emergencies. Adrenalin counteracts the effects of the histamine by opening up the airways and recovering the breathing. Even a moment's hesitation and it could be too late. Other less threatening reactions, such as migraine, asthma, skin rashes, vomiting or diarrhoea, can also be the result of food allergy.

## What is Food Intolerance?

The term 'food intolerance' usually indicates that someone has lost the ability to digest a particular food because of an enzyme deficiency. A good example is lactose intolerance, where there is a deficiency of the enzyme lactase needed to digest the natural sugar in milk. Enzyme supplements are available that help to 'pre-digest' the milk sugar and, so, remove the symptoms. Lactase tablets or drops can be particular helpful if a sufferer is eating away from home and has no way of knowing whether a particular food might contain lactose. However, one of the simplest ways of dealing with lactose intolerance is to avoid milk products altogether. The immune system is not involved in food intolerance.

## What is Food Sensitivity?

Whilst true allergies may be rare, food sensitivities definitely appear to be on the increase. In the majority of cases, if what you eat gives you digestive grief, bloats you up and makes you feel tired or spaced-out, then you are far more likely to be experiencing food sensitivity than allergy. Reactions are linked, primarily, to the digestive system. More recently, some allergy specialists have suggested that the immune system may also be involved, although the type of reaction is clearly not as severe as the life-threatening anaphylaxis described above. A growing number of today's complementary health practitioners believe that a whole range of conditions, including weight problems, loss of energy and even some types of arthritis, can be linked to food sensitivity.

## Not All in the Mind

Complaints of food sensitivity are very often dismissed as a passing fad or fashion. But adverse reactions to 'something you ate' are nothing new, nor is it likely to be a figment of the imagination. Dr Herbert Shelton took a particular interest in the problem throughout his medical career. He observed that an amazing number of food sensitivities clear up completely when supposedly allergic individuals eat their foods in digestible combinations. What they suffered from, said Shelton, was not allergy but indigestion. Although this is not a theory that finds favour with many in the medical profession, it may be premature to dismiss it. A number of the signs of food sensitivity are very similar to those of long-term poor digestion and malabsorption. If it's true that 20 per cent of the population think it suffers from sensitivity to certain foods and yet only 1–2 per cent are truly affected, something must be upsetting the other 18 per cent who experience symptoms that seem suspiciously like food sensitivity but aren't – if you get my drift.

### Symptoms of food sensitivity or poor digestion

| | | |
|---|---|---|
| Bloating | Fluid retention | Nausea |
| Catarrh | Indigestion | Non-descript headache |
| Chest pain | Insomnia | Palpitations |
| Circles under the eyes | Irritable bowel | PMS |
| Confusion | Hives | Puffiness |
| Constipation | Hyperactivity | Runny nose |
| Cravings | Joint pain | Scaly, itchy scalp |
| Depression | Joint swelling | Skin flare-ups |
| Diarrhoea | Leaded limbs | Sneezing |
| Dizziness | Lethargy | Sore, itchy eyes |
| Eczema | Migraine | Sore mouth or tongue |
| Flaky scalp | Muscle spasm | Weight fluctuations |
| Flatulence | | |

### Author's note

I have found from my own experience with patients that a combination of dull, woolly headache, bloating, joint pain, lethargy, energy loss, and either diarrhoea or irritable bowel symptoms, are reasonably reliable indications that food could be at fault, and are worth investigating.

## What Causes Food Sensitivity?

Experts can't agree on what causes someone to be suddenly sensitive to a food that, at one time, didn't appear to be a problem. It seems unlikely that one single cause will be found but there are several possible triggers, including:

▶ A restricted diet

▶ An imbalance of friendly gut flora

▶ Disturbed acid-alkali balance

▶ Insufficient digestive enzymes

▶ Intestinal parasites

▶ Leaky gut syndrome

▶ Low immunity

▶ Poor protein digestion

▶ Over-exposure to potential allergens

▶ Too few vitamins and minerals

▶ Weaning too early

## Not enough nourishment?

A restricted or unimaginative diet might increase our risk of sensitivity. If our diet is limited in variety, there may simply be too few vitamins, minerals and other nutrients to support the immune system or to help in the manufacture of vital enzymes and natural antihistamines. Although no one knows why, the body seems much more likely to over-react if the diet lacks variety and contains too many similar foods – for example, lots of dairy or wheat-based products.

## Weaning too early?

Some practitioners are concerned that early weaning, or the use of cow's milk formula instead of breast milk, may expose an infant's immature digestive system to concentrated animal protein before they can cope with the change, and could go some way to explaining the massive increase in childhood allergies. Over the years I've observed that children who are formula-fed or weaned early demonstrate far more problems with food sensitivity and conditions such as asthma, eczema, hay fever, and digestive and bowel complaints than those who are breast fed. This doesn't mean that all breast-fed babies are immune from allergies or food sensitivities but that those who take formula might be less well protected.

## Leaky gut?

An explanation supported by a number of leading therapists and allergy specialists is that allergies and sensitivities are more likely to occur if the gut wall is too porous. If the wall becomes damaged, allowing bigger or partially digested particles to wheedle their way into the bloodstream, this is known as leaky gut syndrome (or intestinal permeability). In a healthy, undamaged gut, the special absorptive surface between the tubes of the small intestine and the bloodstream acts like a security fence. The barrier is designed to keep out unwanted substances but will allow things with a special pass to get through. If the gut wall is injured or damaged, the fence can be breached by large protein particles and other debris that would not normally be allowed in. Instead of accepting that these particles are just a whole load of food bits and pieces that didn't get broken down properly, the body sees them as invaders, reacting a bit like it does when it encounters pollen or house-dust mites.

The immune system over-reacts. Chemicals and toxins find their way into the bloodstream which, in the ensuing chaos, can cause symptoms such as fluid retention, bloating, digestive and bowel discomfort, headaches, muscle spasm and joint swelling.

The first stage of treatment is to identify and then stop eating the offending foods. However, long-term improvements are only likely if the gut wall is healed, using dietary therapy and specialised supplementation. Repopulating the gut with friendly intestinal flora is also an important part of the process. I have seen this type of treatment bring about dramatic improvements in the health of an allergy sufferer.

## Poor acid-alkali balance

Some writers have suggested that disturbed body chemistry in the form of an over-acid system may leave the body more susceptible to food sensitivity. Clinical evidence suggests that increasing the amount of alkaline-forming food in the diet can help to reduce the number of adverse reactions to food. Alkalising vegetables and fruits are important for strengthening the immune system to resist allergens.

It is also the case that acid-forming foods are generally far more difficult to digest than alkaline-forming foods, increasing the risk of partially digested proteins being taken into the bloodstream. There is a good deal of clinical evidence to suggest that inadequate digestion of proteins could be a key factor in the investigation of food sensitivity. Improving digestion, healing a leaky gut and boosting immunity are three important steps to relieving symptoms. I have treated many allergic patients very successfully by improving digestive function using nothing more than food combining and specialised supplements.

## The system can't cope

Another possible reason for our reduced resistance to common foodstuffs is that our digestive systems haven't yet learned to cope with so many unnaturally produced, hybridised or otherwise modified or altered foods, or the many different manufactured chemicals and other additives that are allegedly necessary in the modern diet.

### Poor immunity plus over-exposure = overload

Some experts think that the lower the immune strength and the higher the number of potential allergens to which someone is exposed, the more likely they are to be a candidate for food sensitivity. This is what is known as the 'System Overload Theory' or 'Total Load Concept'. That is, the probability that someone will react to a food, inhalant, chemical, airborne dust or pollen increases in direct proportion to the number of allergens to which they are exposed. The more potential allergens, the greater the risk of unpleasant reactions. I call it the 'Camel Loading Theory'. Each additional allergen is another straw on the camel's back. You can keep piling them on until the last straw, however lightweight it might appear to be, breaks the back of the body's resistance.

### Immune-boosting nourishment

A properly nourished person with a strong immunity should be well able to deal with potential allergens. However, someone who is, say, under a lot of stress, missing meals, not digesting properly or not getting enough sleep, may be more prone to allergic responses than someone who is taking care of themselves. Other risk points might include too much sugar in the diet, daily exposure to heavy traffic fumes or other environmental pollutants. And as we have seen above, someone who has a family history of allergies or who already suffers from conditions such as asthma or hayfever may also be more prone to food sensitivities – and vice versa.

## Weight problems?

The idea that sensitivity or allergy to certain foods might be responsible for weight problems is still controversial. However, some practitioners are convinced that reactions to common allergens are a major reason why so many of us suffer poor general health and may also experience difficulty in losing weight. As explained above, many cases of allergy are believed to be related to partially digested foods wriggling their way into the bloodstream through a porous gut wall. Once there, they cause irritation and inflammation. In trying to 'flood out' the irritants, the body accumulates extra fluid which, in turn, can lead to unwanted 'water weight'. In addition, some of the chemicals that are released during this process actually increase the appetite. As a result, we eat more and put on more weight. The same chemicals may also slow up the metabolism, releasing hormone-like messengers that reduce the body's ability to burn fat.

For a long time it has been theorised that, even if we muster up huge helpings of willpower and overcome our desire to overeat, the presence of food allergies will still cause us to gain weight. This could explain why some people put on weight despite the fact that they don't consume excess calories.

## Finding the Answers to Food Allergies

So what should be your first move? You may think you are already doing all the diet-wise things and yet are still waking up tired, feeling jaded after lunch and running out of steam before the nine o'clock news. The suggestions I make here are those that I've collected over ten years of clinic work and found to be the most helpful.

## TOP TIPS FOR FIGHTING FOOD ALLERGIES

### Eliminate problem foods

▶ As a first step, avoid the five most common problem groups:

1. Wheat bran and wheat-based breakfast cereals

2. Bread, cakes, pastry and biscuits

3. Food additives such as flavour enhancer E621 monosodium glutamate, preservative E250 sodium nitrite, and colourings E110 sunset yellow and E102 tartrazine

4. Cow's milk and cow's milk cheese

5. Sugar and sugary foods

These items cause symptoms in so many people that it really is worth trying to manage without them. You may get an early and effective improvement and have no need to take your food sleuthing any further.

▶ If you feel no better after two weeks, continue to stay off the first group and begin to eliminate the second five culprits:

6. Eggs

7. Tomatoes, bell peppers, aubergines and potatoes

8. Coffee, chocolate, tea and cola

9. Soya beans and anything made from them

10. Shellfish

▶ If you feel better after two weeks of avoiding all ten food groups listed above, then you could be on to something. My advice is always to stay off the 'Big Five', *wheat cereals, bread, food additives, cow's milk and sugar*, whether they turn out to be problem foods or not. The next thing to do is to reintroduce the other five groups –

but only one group at a time each week. Do this carefully and be absolutely specific as you note the results. Eat the reintroduced food every day for seven days. Symptoms should soon show up once you consume the problem food again. If nothing happens, move to the next food and follow the same pattern. When you locate the problem food, the best way of dealing with it is simply not to eat it again or to eat it only very occasionally.

▶ If you still get no result, it can be worth playing around with combinations. I have met several food sensitive people who didn't react to any individual groups in the list but found certain combinations produced symptoms. For example, one lady was upset by cheese only if she ate it with bread. A cheese salad caused her no discomfort. Another patient complained that tomatoes only caused a problem when they were cooked, not when they were raw. And a third patient said he could eat boiled or scrambled eggs perfectly happily on their own, but found they produced gas and nausea if he ate them with toast, bread or with a cup of coffee or tea.

▶ Always try to find suitable replacements for the foods you are giving up. This is very important. The chapter **Eating for Better Health** (pages 60–81) gives plenty of additional information on where to begin. The section on how to reduce chemical overload (pages 248–57) is also essential reading. And for instant information, turn to pages 80–1 for my **Swap Sheet**.

If you are not improving as a result of these suggestions, you will need to get down to some more detailed investigations (see below).

## Keep a food diary

For four weeks keep a diary of everything you eat. Be really diligent about this. Write down any symptoms and see if you come up with a common denominator. Reactions don't usually occur straightaway and may not happen for several hours or until next day – or even a couple of days later. You need to be able to look back over at least the previous 48 hours and check your menus.

**Author's note**

The reason I don't suggest keeping a food diary at the very beginning is because most of the ten foods in the list above appear so frequently in most people's diets that you would probably find it almost impossible to identify the culprit.

## Identify favourite foods

Is there a particularly favourite food that you eat all the time? Be aware that 'favourite' foods – or those you have most cravings for – are often the ones to watch for, even if there are no apparent or immediate symptoms. An additional difficulty can be that a problem food might not present any clues simply because you feel better, not worse, when you have eaten it. The 'lift' it gives you can last for several hours, by which time you may have eaten the offending food again, giving yourself another temporary 'high'. The result of this hidden or masked reaction is that you are, unwittingly, concealing the real symptoms.

To recap, if you suspect a particular food, avoid it for seven days and then reintroduce it. If it still upsets you, think about avoiding it altogether – or try reducing the quantity. Sometimes the body will tolerate small amounts but be thrown off balance by a larger portion of something.

## Do some research

Ask your parents or brothers and sisters about foods you or they were allergic to as children. Allergies and intolerances can affect anyone at any age and they can develop during childhood or adulthood. Sometimes, childhood allergies can return in adulthood and can also be passed from parent to offspring. To make detection more difficult, symptoms may vary between childhood and adulthood even though the food culprit may be the same. I know one particular case where cow's milk was found to be the cause of childhood eczema and, several years later in that same person, triggered asthma-like breathing problems. Similarly, someone who suffered a severe rash as a child every time he ate tomatoes, found that, as an adult, tomatoes no longer caused a rash but aggravated his arthritis instead.

## Consider the possibility of candida

Although not everyone with allergies or sensitivities will have candidiasis, I can't ever remember seeing a candida patient who didn't have difficulty dealing with at least some food substances. *Candida albicans* is a yeast fungus, a natural inhabitant of everybody's gut, which is kept in check by healthy intestinal flora. Unfortunately, if the normal ecology of the digestive system is disturbed, the yeast becomes prolific. Its structure changes from a simple cell to a fungus (like a bread mould) that can invade the whole digestive system. The condition is then known as candidiasis.

---

**Some of the most likely causes or triggers for candida overgrowth include:**

- Adrenal exhaustion
- Antibiotics
- Extended negative stress
- Frequent dieting
- High alcohol consumption
- High sugar intake
- Hormone replacement therapy
- Illness
- Leaky gut syndrome
- Low intake of nutrients
- Poor immunity
- Poor liver function
- Sensitivity to environmental pollution
- The contraceptive pill
- Toxicity

---

There are so many symptoms relating to candidiasis that diagnosis without professional help can be very difficult. Many are similar to those of leaky gut syndrome and food sensitivity, making it almost impossible to know which came first. The presence of candida can also cause or aggravate a number of other conditions.

If any of the following symptoms sound like you, I would very strongly recommend a consultation with a qualified therapist who is familiar with the condition and who has a good track record of successful treatment.

- ▶ Bad breath or sour taste in the mouth
- ▶ Bloating
- ▶ Bowel problems
- ▶ Catarrh
- ▶ Cravings, especially for sweet foods
- ▶ Depression or anxiety
- ▶ Difficulty losing weight
- ▶ Digestive discomfort
- ▶ Feeling 'spaced-out'
- ▶ Feeling tired all the time
- ▶ Flatulence
- ▶ Headaches or migraine
- ▶ Hypoglycaemia (low blood sugar)
- ▶ Itchy skin or scalp
- ▶ Menstrual problems
- ▶ Noisy or rumbling stomach other than when hungry
- ▶ Persistent infections
- ▶ Poor concentration
- ▶ Recurring cystitis
- ▶ Recurring thrush
- ▶ Running out of energy quickly or suddenly

▶ Sensitivity to several foods

▶ Unable to tolerate even a small amount of alcohol

▶ Unexplained muscle or joint pain

## Don't restrict your diet

No matter how keen you are to find the culprit, don't be tempted to give up a long list of foods all at once. A restricted diet can lead to serious malnourishment without you realising the dangers. There is also a risk that, by giving up too many foods and limiting your diet even further, your body could then become sensitive to other foods that were previously not a problem.

## Food combine

I've said it earlier, but I'll say it again. Try food combining for a month and, if you feel an improvement, you'll know that your digestion has been under par.

## Get professional help

If your symptoms persist, seek help from a practitioner who specialises in diet therapy and is qualified to carry out tests for allergies, leaky gut syndrome and, as I mentioned above, candidiasis.

## ! TECHNICAL STUFF

### Tips on Testing

**ELISA** The conventional way of detecting food allergies is to undergo an enzyme linked immuno-sorbent assay (ELISA). This is a blood test which measures the antibody reaction to common foods. It is a relatively painless procedure and can be done at home. However, I would strongly recommend that it is carried out by a qualified allergist who has direct access to a recognised laboratory. The blood sample will be analysed and the results reported to you or to your practitioner. I have found this test helpful for some patients but not for others. It can be useful for detecting allergies but may not be able to pick up food sensitivities that do not involve the immune system.

**Vega** Another way of detecting problem foods is by using applied kinesiology (muscle testing), with or without a machine called a Vega. These methods rely very much on the skill of the practitioner, so it is imperative to locate not only a qualified therapist but also one who has recognised expertise in this field. Beware of Vega testing offered by healthfood outlets. However good the practitioner or the equipment in these circumstances, results are likely to be much less reliable if the tests are carried out on a limited timescale in a busy or noisy environment.

**Pulse test** The pulse test is something that you can try at home. It is often (although not always) the case that allergies and sensitivities can cause a significant increase in pulse rate. Here's how.

▶ Sit down quietly for five minutes. Don't watch television or involve yourself in any other activity. Don't wear your watch while you are doing this test; take it off and put it down alongside you where you can see it.

▶ Locate your pulse on the thumb side of your wrist. Count how many times it beats in 30 seconds and then double the answer. For example, if it beats 36 times in half a minute, then your resting pulse rate will be 72.

▶ Then eat a normal portion of the food you suspect is causing symptoms.

▶ Fifteen minutes after you have eaten, take your pulse just as you did before. Note the result.

▶ Then take it again after half an hour, one hour and two hours, each time noting the result. Try not to do anything exertive during this time.

If the results show an increase in pulse rate of anything over 5 beats per minute, this could indicate that you are sensitive to the food you are challenging.

For information on where to find clinics specialising in testing procedures, see page 445.

## IMPORTANT NOTE

**All these tests are capable of producing false positives, indicating certain foods to be a problem when they are not, and false negatives, telling you that there is no problem when, in reality, you may be genuinely sensitive or allergic. For this reason, it's wise to use testing as a back-up to other methods of diagnosis, not as a fool-proof diagnosis on its own.**

## ESSENTIAL READING

Get hold of a copy of *Allergies – Disease in Disguise* by Carolee Bateson-Koch (Alive Books). If you'd like more information on candida, read *The Practical Guide to Candida* by Jane McWhirter (Green Library).

# CHAPTER 12

# Food Combining Detox

## Including the Benefits of Skin Cleansing and Better Breathing

'The good news is that the European Union is drawing up a positive list of pesticides. So far it has taken eight years to give three pesticides the all clear and take seven off the market. The bad news is that there are a further 850 to go. At the current rate of progress, it should take another 680 years to consider the rest.'

From *The Food Magazine*, July/September issue, 1999

The principle of detoxification is rooted in the foundations and traditions of naturopathic medicine. Fasting and the avoidance of solid food also have strong associations with medical and religious practices the world over. Nature-cure practitioners believe that removing toxic materials and waste products from the system opens up the pathway to natural self-healing, and some groups see fasting and cleansing as part of the journey to spiritual enlightenment.

Dr Shelton observed that all mental powers, including memory and attention span, are improved, senses are heightened and 'intellectual and emotional qualities are infused with new vigour and meaning'.

On a purely practical level, detoxification takes the strain off our physical bodies, helping slowly to reduce the overload. This isn't a cure for pollution. Like the old line about painting the Sydney Harbour Bridge in Australia or the Forth Bridge in Scotland, by the time you finish the job, the rust has already set in at the other end and you need to begin again. When you dust or vacuum your home, you don't expect the dirt and grime to stop. But you clean so that bacteria don't take over and so you don't disappear under layers of dust.

Regular dietary cleansing is a bit the same. It can't prevent further exposure – but it does help to protect your health by preventing a build-up of excess waste and keeping toxicity at manageable levels. And, especially valuable when used in conjunction with food combining, it can lift away lethargy, increase your energy levels, kick-start stubborn weight into gear, lighten your body and take a load off your mind. Towards the end of this chapter you'll also find information on skin cleansing and breathing techniques – both of these have an important part to play in detoxification.

## A Toxic World

Every day our systems need to get rid of large quantities of naturally produced debris including the by-products of digestion and metabolism, dead cells and other unwanted waste products.

In an ideal world, a healthy body will see to this ongoing clean-up automatically. So sophisticated are the mechanisms for dealing with metabolic rubbish that we wouldn't even notice it was happening.

But is it an ideal world? There have been many mind-blowing advances in technology, communication systems no one would have thought possible half a century ago, vehicles that travel at incredible speeds and satellites that beam information around the globe. We have fast food, fast cars, faster aircraft, mobile telephones, digital TV and spare-part surgery. Homes are filled with microwave ovens, washing machines, dishwashers and Dysons™. Offices bulge with computers, scanners, photocopiers and fax machines, and almost anything can be connected to virtually anything else in any other office or home anywhere in the world, via a modem and a www dot com.

It certainly sounds ideal. But in amongst all these amazing advances, one thing hasn't changed.

Us.

You and me.

The human body is an intricate organism with a brain so advanced that it is still light years ahead of the most complex computer. And yet, according to paleopathological data, recorded by osteologists (who study skeletons), archaeologists (who examine history by digging for remains) and anthropological historians (who are interested in the study of humankind and its societies and customs), it seems likely that the workings of our liver, kidneys, intestines, lungs, lymphatic system and skin are little changed in the past 10,000 years. Some experts suggest that our basic genetic make-up is much the same as it was as long as 40,000 years ago.

From skeletal – and occasionally from mummified – remains, osteologists can pick up surprisingly detailed information, including general health, disease patterns, degenerative changes and even the amount of stress suffered by our primordial predecessors. The results are surprising.

Our perception of human progress relies heavily on stereotypes we have created about being 'primitive' or 'civilised'. As a result, it's easy to assume that our prehistoric ancestors were poor, ill, ignorant and malnourished. In reality, investigations show that hunter-gatherers were well organised socially, well nourished and had surprisingly good health records. Anthropologists studying the few remaining hunter-gatherer tribes, such as the Kalahari San, the Hadza of Tanzania and tribes of South America, New Guinea, and South and Southeast Asia, have concluded that, since these nomads have no coronary heart disease, no excess cholesterol, no high blood pressure, no angina, no anaemia, no diabetes and no sudden death associated with illness, it is extremely likely that their ancestors had similar health profiles. These nomadic peoples live in relatively unpolluted areas of the world. They have none of the trappings of so-called developed countries. There are no shops or supermarkets. They have no gas or electricity, and no petroleum products – so no agrichemicals, food additives or cleaning fluids and no need of the internal combustion engine. Their diet focuses on simple meals of vegetables and lean meat from wild animals and yet there is no evidence of vitamin or mineral deficiency or malnutrition.

Our modern civilisation is almost identical in its anatomical and physiological development, and yet is exposed to a completely different lifestyle of sudden changes, new inventions, and masses of synthetic chemicals, the health legacy of which will remain, for many years to come, an unknown quantity.

The evidence is already there to show that exposure to pesticide residues and a long list of other pollutants (which have been part of our lives for only a relatively short period of time) are playing havoc with our health and our environment.

Despite pronouncements by agrichemical companies that their products are safe, investigations have already linked farm chemicals to nervous system damage and the slow death of brain cells. Worry has also been expressed that pesticide and other toxic residues might be responsible for an increase in Parkinson's disease, Chronic Fatigue Syndrome (ME) and osteoporosis (brittle bones).

## Insecticides

Used to kill crawling and flying insects, insecticides work in a similar way to nerve gases, by attacking the central nervous system of the bugs they aim to eradicate. Some types of organochlorine sprays are particularly attracted to fatty substances and can build up to high concentrations in such foods as cow's milk, meat, cheese and human breast milk. Apart from concerns about potential damage to the nervous system and the possibility that some of these chemicals may turn out to be carcinogenic (cancer forming), it is a long-held theory of some practitioners that the build up of toxicity in human fat tissue could make it more difficult to lose weight.

## Herbicides

These are used to get rid of weeds either by exhausting the plant through unnaturally rapid growth or by killing them off altogether. Some herbicides work systemically and are absorbed right into the plant so that washing the chemical out becomes impossible. Because most tests for chemical sprays check only the peel on vegetables and fruit, it's easy to underestimate the actual amounts of chemicals being consumed. Peeling the produce might reduce the quantity of chemicals you swallow but won't necessarily protect you from contamination.

## Fungicides

Designed to destroy the fungus that can attack fruit, vegetables and grain crops, fungicides have been linked to tumours and birth defects in laboratory animals. One class of fungicides is said to be used on 70 per cent of potatoes, 40 per cent of apples, and 10 per cent of wheat grown in the UK.

## No Need to Worry?

Fears about the potentially damaging effects of farm chemicals are far from irrational and are supported by much evidence. Tests have shown that agrichemicals do accumulate in foods, sometimes to what officialdom terms 'unacceptable levels'. If they are found there at all, to me that's unacceptable.

Some samplings have revealed that one-third of basic staples such as bread, potatoes and milk, and approximately one-third of all vegetables and fruit were found to contain contaminants in excess of the government's safe limits. And I'm sure you don't need me to tell you – these figures don't mean that the rest of foods tested were pesticide-free, only that they were within the maximum limits allowed!

Everyone agrees that large quantities of pesticides, herbicides or fungicides are potentially hazardous but no one seems to have addressed the possibility that small doses could kill people, animals and birdlife just as effectively, although perhaps not so easy to trace, over a longer period of time. As Graham Harvey points out in his book *The Killing of the Countryside*, written in 1997, science knows virtually nothing about the dangers of prolonged exposure.

And that's only the tip of the toxic iceberg. There are many hundreds more pollutants, other than farm chemicals, that we expect our bodies to detoxify, without complaint, every day of our lives. Most of them are new. Few of them are properly tested for long-term exposure. No wonder that today's *Homo sapiens* may be experiencing some difficulty dealing with the consequences of so many discoveries and contrivances that have occurred in only the past couple of hundred years. We are a wonderfully resourceful species, but there are limits.

## Long-term Dangers

How are we *really* being affected by such close acquaintance with vehicle exhaust emissions, artificial preservatives, food colourings made from coal tar, vapours from aerosols and household cleaning products, solvents, industrial smog, plastic packaging, food processing, refined sugar, hydrogenated fats, artificial hormones, over-use of antibiotics, steroids, and the residues from a myriad of other twentieth century leftovers? No one really knows. It's all sort of OK, isn't it? We don't seem to have come to any direct or immediate harm. Or have we?

How are you today? How are you *really*? There is growing concern that the many artificial chemical substances and pollutants in today's modern world could be one of the reasons why hardly anyone can say they feel *really well*.

## Recycling the Twentieth Century

Saving and separating glass, cans and paper, buying products made from recycled materials, walking to work or to school, composting and tree planting all make small ripples in the bigger pond. But the twenty-first century has inherited a massive pollution problem from the twentieth century that isn't going to go away. Even if we manage to eat only organic produce, drink truly chemical-free water, live in ecologically sound dwellings and suffer from absolutely no stress, we still breathe the air and come into contact with potentially toxic materials in our own and other people's everyday lives. Just one example is the estimate that, from the pollution levels in an average traffic queue or city centre, even a non-smoker could breathe in the equivalent of two packs of cigarettes per day.

## Time to Take Notice

The world is, at last – perhaps too late, perhaps not – beginning to pay serious attention to how pollution is affecting our external environment. However, little attention is paid to the effect of externally produced toxicity on our inner environment, *the inside of us*, and even less on taking steps to protect it from further damage. Regular detoxification could provide at least some vital support.

# Detoxification

Almost as important as the detoxification itself, is the need for it to fit comfortably with our usually hectic lifestyles. Some detox programmes expect a lot in the beginning, even if they say they don't. Cold showers, Epsom salt baths, skin brushing, exercise, relaxation, affirmations, meditations. All these things are undeniably beneficial in the right circumstances, but can also cause a great deal of stress if the person trying to do them is trying to do them all at once and fast at the same time. We know that, in an ideal world, we should slow right down and pay ourselves a great deal more attention, but it isn't always workable for those of us who have families to care for, homes to run or other full-time jobs. Few of us are in a position to be able to take days or weeks away from our responsibilities to follow a strict regime and to cope with all that it entails. But we can gain a number of benefits by following a far less stringent detox.

---

**Fasting and detoxing – what's the difference?**

It's easy to confuse fasting with a simple detox but they are not the same thing. People sometimes talk in terms of juice 'fasts' or fruit 'fasts' but although taking juices or fruit entirely on their own are stringent methods of detoxification, they are, in fact, juice or fruit 'cures' or 'diets', not fasts. A true fast means eating no solid foods, and surviving on water only, for a period of several days or weeks. Unless you are very experienced and know exactly what you are doing, fasting should only be carried out under medical supervision.

---

# Understanding the Body's Elimination Systems

Regular spring-cleaning sessions are designed to give the body's major elimination systems, the skin, the lungs, the lymphatic system, the kidneys, the liver and the bowel, a helping hand. All these areas of the body are hard-working performers in the detox story, ridding it of naturally accumulated waste via sweat, faeces, gases and urine. Persuade them to work more efficiently and it should be possible to improve digestion and absorption of nourishment, stir a sluggish bowel into life and get rid of the garbage, ease bloating and gas, reduce allergies, enhance the health of the skin, hair and nails, increase resistance to colds and infections, and improve energy levels.

According to feedback from a number of patients, detoxification could also cast off a couple of pounds or so of unwanted weight.

## The skin

This is the body's largest organ, covering between 15–20 square feet (1.5–2 square metres). It's washable, waterproof and self-repairing, but is also a major route for the elimination of wastes. Each day, through many hundreds of thousands of skin pores, the average human secretes over 1½ pints (850ml) of fluid; primarily, sweat from the sweat glands keeps us cool and a waxy secretion, sebum, from the sebaceous glands, gives the skin lubrication and protection. But those same glands are also an essential route for the elimination of toxins collected via the blood and lymphatic system. Apart from discharging wastes, the sweat that results from aerobic exercise might also speed up the removal of cancer-forming chemicals from the body.

Because of its ability to rid the body of unwanted substances, the skin is sometimes referred to as the third kidney. Toxins that aren't removed via the kidneys, the bowel or the lungs may find their way out through the skin. In addition, if one or other elimination route is blocked, if you are constipated or perhaps your kidneys or liver are under par, your skin will try to take over some of the work. Naturopathic medicine has it that skin diseases, such as eczema and psoriasis, are signs that the skin is trying to correct imbalances deep within the body. Blocking the skin could chase the wastes back inside the system.

Dampen down the effects of eczema with steroid creams, say some practitioners, and you may see other problems such as asthma or bowel disorders starting up in its place.

---

**Signs of skin under strain can include:**
Excessive oiliness, flaking, blotchy patches, cellulite, roughness, spots and pimples. White skins may show red blotchy patches and a greyish pallor. Dark skins can become dull and take on a greyish tone. Healthy skin, whatever its colour, has an obvious glow.

---

## The lymphatic system

This is the body's garbage collector; an elaborate network of capillaries, not unlike tiny blood vessels, that removes excess fluid, cellular debris and other unwanted material from the tissues. The average adult human has just over 8 pints (4.5 litres) of blood pumping through veins and arteries. Around four times this amount of lymph fluid is being pushed though the lymphatic system at any one time. Most of the lymph fluid is propelled towards collection channels in the chest area before being emptied back into the veins. On the way, lymph fluid passes through lymph nodes which latch on to and destroy bacteria. Once the rubbish is discharged into the blood, it is transported to other exits via the liver and the kidneys.

Lymph channels are not only routes for rubbish, they are also a major pathway for nutrients absorbed from the digestive tract. Maintaining good lymph circulation is vital if the body is going to be able to transport nourishment and deal with wastes. The lymphatic system has valves and collecting vessels into which the lymphatic capillaries empty. But the body doesn't 'pump' lymph fluid like the heart pumps blood through arteries and veins. Rather it is moved along by the contraction and propulsion of the lymphatic capillaries which are helped by the general movement of the body and contraction of muscles. Just as the blood circulation can become sluggish, so, too, can the circulation of lymph. Keeping it moving is essential for effective lymph drainage. During exercise, the lymphatic pump becomes very active and can increase lymph flow as much as tenfold to thirtyfold. Full body massage and deep breathing also improve lymph drainage. (For more on the benefits of deep breathing, see pages 262–72.)

---

**Signs of a sluggish lymphatic system can include:**
Puffy ankles or fingers, tender breasts, spotty skin, poor resistance to infection, puffy eyes, dark circles under the eyes, weariness, lethargy and cellulite.

---

## The lungs

To say that good-quality breathing is essential to health is self-evident. But breathing well is not something most of us are too good at. For one thing, we tend to take it for granted. In fact, the only time we really become aware of our lungs at all is if we are out of breath, or if we get a cold or chest infection that causes tightening, pain, wheezing or coughing.

The obvious goal of the lungs is to take oxygen into the body and to remove carbon dioxide from the body. The breathing in is called inspiration and the breathing out is known as expiration. At the same time that blood picks up oxygen in the lungs, carbon dioxide is released from the blood into the lung spaces and breathed out into the atmosphere. This doesn't mean that oxygen is all good and carbon dioxide is all bad. It is the continuous exchange and balance of gases that is important to healthy breathing and a healthy body.

Intertwined with all the supportive tissues of each lung are the lymph drainage channels which work to remove unwanted particles and fluids from the lung area. If we don't breathe properly, the movement of the lungs is affected and the lymph channels can become sluggish.

---

**Signs of poor lung function can include:**
Congested mucus, chest cramps, general fatigue, allergies, headaches, poor circulation, cold extremities.

---

## The kidneys

These are responsible for filtering the blood, recycling and saving any good stuff that the body wants to keep and use again (such as some nutrients, salts, water and glucose), and removing waste products to be excreted in the urine.

> **Signs of sluggish kidney function can include:**
> Strong-smelling urine, dark-coloured urine, cloudy urine, passing water less than four times per day and persistent tiredness. These signs may also suggest dehydration, so, if this is happening to you, ask yourself if you are drinking enough fluid.

## The intestines

Food is broken down in the small intestine and nutrients and fluid are absorbed from there into the bloodstream. Solid matter that can't be absorbed (such as plant fibre) passes into the large intestine. Other toxins are taken up by the liver which processes them ready for elimination. Unfortunately, highly refined foods, lack of fibre and/or too little fluid can lead to constipation and compaction of waste, allowing toxins that should be excreted to be reabsorbed into the body.

> **Signs of sluggish intestines can include:**
> Bloating, flatulence, indigestion, constipation.

## The liver

A complex organ, the liver carries out a mind-blowing number of different tasks. One of its major jobs is to keep the bloodstream clear of anything that might be poisonous to the body, for example, pesticide residues or the leftovers from drug medications. Because the liver has so much hard work to do, it can become overloaded and exhausted, and unable to cope. Keeping the liver healthy is therefore a key factor in keeping the body healthy too.

The liver is arguably the hardest working of all the organs. It picks up the processing tab for the majority of undesirable substances that we take into our systems from food, water, medication and environmental factors – and as a result of internal body activity.

It acts as a store cupboard for energy-producing foods such as starches, sugars and fats and for some vitamins and minerals. It recycles hormones and keeps cholesterol levels in check. Every 60 seconds, this amazing little factory filters, cleans and recycles around two pints (1 litre) of blood.

The liver is an absolutely vital part of the detoxification process. It acts as a huge cleansing plant, sifting and deactivating toxic substances, metabolic leftovers, foreign poisonous matter and infective organisms. It produces bile, which – apart from being used to break down fats – helps to carry unwanted residues of hormones, drug medicines and pesticides away from the body via the bowel. When bile is not flowing freely, toxins build up and the liver cannot function efficiently. Wastes in the form of poisons, dead cells and micro-organisms build up in the bloodstream. The strain that this puts on the immune system may lead to chronic fatigue, aching muscles and joints, repeated infections, elevated cholesterol, high blood fats and an increased risk of allergies. An overworked, undernourished liver can also result in a slower metabolism, increasing the possibility of weight gain. It's easy to understand why there is concern that toxic overload could damage liver cells, congest the lymph system and affect our immunity to viruses and bacteria. When the liver isn't in peak condition, bile production can be affected. Bile, made by the liver and stored in the gallbladder, helps to stabilise the pH of the gut. It acts a bit like a natural disinfectant and encourages the accumulation of 'good bugs'.

In Traditional Chinese Medicine, an overheated liver manifests as irritability and bad temper. Liver imbalances are also believed to be linked to reproductive and menstrual disorders. There is even research evidence to suggest that sluggish liver detoxification can increase the risk of lung cancer. Part of the detox process requires certain enzymes, known as GSTM1 and GSTT1 (glutathione S-transferase M1 and T1), that are produced from the amino acid glutathione. Researchers have found that there was a greater incidence of lung cancer in people who had consistently low levels of these enzymes. In addition to its importance in the detoxification of a whole range of undesirable substances, including heavy metals, glutathione is also used by the body as a free-radical scavenger and to enhance the immune protective status of certain cells, including liver cells.

---

**Signs of a sluggish liver can include:**
Allergies, dry skin patches, headaches, high cholesterol, lethargy, nausea, skin problems, poor skin tone, repeated colds, coated tongue.

---

**IMPORTANT NOTE**
If stools change colour, or if the whites of the eyes, the nails or the tongue are tinged yellow, this could be sign of more serious liver problems requiring an immediate appointment with a medical practitioner.

---

# The Two-day Detox Programme

If you are suffering from any of the symptoms listed above, you might like to try a simple two-day detox and see how you feel afterwards. As you give your digestive system a break, toxins will begin to be turned out from various sites around the body.

## Last In – First Out

The law of detoxification states that any *dis*-ease will retrace itself as the remedial process begins deep within the system, and then work its way to the surface. Healing is also believed to happen from the head down or in the reverse order to the way symptoms developed in the first place. As the rubbish is collected up and passed to one or more routes of elimination, it is possible that unwanted debris may, at one or more stages, spread through all of the circulatory system, causing transient symptoms such as headaches, catarrh, slight nausea, a more heavily coated tongue, strong-smelling urine and stools, bad breath, body odour and tiredness. Sometimes, the body reacts by becoming constipated for a couple of days. Such profound changes can also bring about unexpected emotional releases such as depression, tearfulness, irritability, remembered dreams or disturbed sleep. These symptoms, referred to by naturopaths as a healing crisis, are an indication that the detox is working.

If you are affected by any of the above, here's how to deal with them.

▶ Rest as much as possible.

▶ Walk in the fresh air but don't do any vigorous exercise on detox days.

▶ Chew half-a-dozen sweet dried figs. They are an excellent remedy for constipation and one of the best alkaline-forming foods.

▶ Drink plenty of water to keep the toxins moving and persuade a sluggish bowel to get going. Add 6 drops of the Bach flower remedy, **crab apple**, to each glass. Dr Bach's crab apple is a traditional cleansing remedy for mind and body.

▶ Relax in a warm bath. Add 3 drops each of **juniper**, **geranium** and **lavender** essential oils to help you wind down.

▶ Take 2 grams of **vitamin C complex** with a glass of water. This is a useful remedy for a headache.

▶ Take plenty of deep, slow breaths.

▶ Rinse out your mouth and gargle with **tea-tree** or **propolis** mouthwash.

▶ Skin brush regularly – see page 259.

▶ Use an exfoliating scrub on your face, neck and upper chest areas.

## Don't Overdo it

The number of symptoms you experience can be related to the level of toxicity in your body. Or, sometimes, there may be no symptoms at all. However, if your system is very sluggish and your liver and lymph are overloaded, you could feel a little worse before you feel better. If you decide, at this stage, that two days is too much all at once, go for a one-day cleanse, once a week or once a fortnight to begin with, and work your way gently towards the two-day detox. Look upon the cleansing process as a slow unwinding of waste products out of your system.

There is no need to go to any kind of extreme. In someone who is very toxic, detoxing quickly can cause those toxins to be released much too fast for comfort. One of the places that toxins like living is in our fat cells. During detoxification, fat is broken down and mobilised into the bloodstream. Along with it go a whole heap of stored chemicals, whoosh, straight into the bloodstream – just like pouring undiluted poisons into the body all at once. While they are being carried to various exits, they can, not surprisingly, cause some extremely unpleasant symptoms.

In addition, going without food can cause massive swings in blood glucose levels, encouraging hypoglycaemic symptoms such as poor co-ordination, lack of concentration, a fall in body temperature, hot or cold sweats, stomach pains and dizziness.

Two days of detox can't cleanse a very toxic body all at one time but regular detox can, as long as it's in conjunction with healthy diet. The information in the chapter **Eating for Better Health** (pages 60–81) and the section on **Long-term Protection** (starting on page 247) should also lighten the pollution load.

## HERE'S A RECAP

Although regular short-term sessions take longer to despatch debris, they are less of a shock to the body and so are less likely to produce unpleasant symptoms. However, don't underestimate the ability of this short two-day session. It can have a really beneficial deep-cleansing action. Extended detoxification is not, in my view, either practical or safe for most people.

## Abdominal Massage

This is a really valuable form of exercise and helps the detox process by encourage improved bowel movement. I've mentioned it elsewhere in *The Complete Book of Food Combining* and it's something that anyone can try. As well as aiding detox by improving bowel function, it is great for relieving constipation and may help to reduce the symptoms of candidiasis, diverticulitis and irritable bowel syndrome.

Here's how to do it:

▶ Lie down on the bed with a towel spread out underneath your lower back (this is to prevent any oil getting on to bed linen).

▶ Lubricate the belly area with a little olive oil or vitamin E oil.

▶ Using the pads of your fingers, massage the whole area for four to five minutes.

▶ Begin at the lower right side, just inside the right hip bone and work your way upwards towards the waist, then across and down the left side.

▶ You should hear some gurgling and you may pass trapped wind. This is a good sign and to be encouraged.

▶ If you find the massage action hard work on your hands, try using a pressing movement, working over the abdomen in the same clockwise direction. Or find a willing partner to do the massage for you.

▶ Rub any excess oil into your hands, chest and thighs.

## How Often Should I Detox?

Introduce the two-day detox programme any time you have time. Once or twice a month is about right. It doesn't matter whether you choose weekdays or weekends, but try to organise your personal routine so that you have a little less stress around you and not so much pressure from other people. If you have tried lots of different diets and had little or no success in losing weight over the years, please do try this. I have talked with so many patients who had more or less given up trying to shed excess pounds but who succeeded by using this system.

## WHEN NOT TO DETOX

▶ If you are pregnant or breastfeeding.

▶ If you are waiting for – or are just recovering from – an operation.

▶ If you are diabetic or have a blood glucose disorder.

▶ If you are taking any prescribed medication or are undergoing any kind of treatment, talk to your doctor or specialist before undertaking any dietary changes including detox.

## Preparing for the Two-day Detox

For best results, to improve body function, speed elimination of wastes and boost energy levels, introduce two detox days into your regular routine every two to four weeks.

Alternatively, use any of the days, singly or together, as a 'refresher' any time you are feeling sluggish, stressed, exhausted, need to recharge your batteries, are suffering the effects of too many late nights or, indeed, any kind of excess. Read the whole of this section right through before you begin and make a shopping list of the items you are going to include for your first detox session. Before you shop for the items you've listed, read the section on **Long-term Protection** (pages 247–8). To maintain progress, follow the simple food combining guidelines given on pages 46–7. If you haven't food combined before, it could be helpful, now, to turn to page 15 and remind yourself of those foods that combine well and those that do not. You'll also find food combining guidelines alongside the main meal recipes below.

By all means use the programme on workdays if that suits you. However, it's much better if you can find 48 hours when you're at home and under less pressure. At a weekend or during the week – it doesn't matter just as long as you give yourself priority.

## Short Cut

If you're too pushed for time to do the full two-day detox, then give your system a treat by simply changing your diet for a day. Stock up on fresh fruit, fresh vegetables and salads. Make a big fruit salad for breakfast, a king-sized green salad or large bowl of vegetable soup at lunchtime, and a delicious vegetable stir-fry for supper. Make sure that portion sizes are generous. If a hunger pang hits you, reach for some fresh fruit or snack on a few dried figs. For this one day, avoid all meat, poultry, eggs, cheese, fish, fatty foods, crisps, alcohol, coffee, tea, sugar, ready meals, take-aways, packaged and processed foods. Keep fluid intake high by drinking plenty of filtered or bottled water and herbal teas throughout the day.

---

**IMPORTANT NOTE**

On detox days, ignore your usual set meal breaks during the detox. If you feel hungry anytime between the recommended meals, then it's absolutely fine to tuck into any kind of fresh fruit, a vegetable or fruit juice, soup or herbal tea. It's important that you never let yourself become over-hungry.

Above all, keep your fluid intake high. Drink plenty of filtered water. For hot summer days, keep bottles of organic vegetable and fruit juice in the refrigerator; health stores stock them. Or have fresh produce on hand so that you can make your own using a juicing machine. They provide tasty, nutritious and satisfying drinks, especially when the weather is warm, or your energy is flagging, or you're simply not all that hungry. In the winter, warming and sustaining home-made vegetable soup makes a terrific pit-stop and adds healthily to your daily fluid intake.

See pages 31–3 and 244 for more information on juicing.

## The Two-day Detox Menu Plan

# DAY ONE

## Day one – first thing in the morning

### Lemon and honey refresher drink

juice of 1 lemon (organic if possible and remember that pre-packed lemon
juice contains preservative)
2 teaspoons cold-pressed raw honey, preferably New Zealand Manuka or similar
250ml (approx ¼ pint) just-boiled filtered water

Squeeze the lemon juice into a tumbler or large mug, add the honey
and pour on the boiled water. Stir until the honey has dissolved. Sip
slowly – don't gulp. If you are short on time, take the drink with you
while you wash and dress.

## Day one – breakfast

### Fresh melon

Buy a small ripe melon – cantaloupe or galia are the best. Wash it really
well and cut it in half. Scoop out the seeds and discard them. Eat one
half now and wrap the other half and refrigerate it for tomorrow.

## Day one – mid-morning

### Cleansing juice

I've recommended this cleansing juice for many years. The recipe has
been handed to patients, students and visitors to my seminars. It's an
excellent detox drink but also a tasty aperitif while you are preparing
your evening meal, or a refreshing drink between meals any time. If
you are away from home during the day and can't prepare this juice

mid-morning, enjoy a glass of fresh fruit juice or a couple of pieces of fresh fruit instead. Make the healing juice to drink while you are preparing your evening meal instead.

2 organic carrots, well scrubbed
1 or 2 apples, peeled
a couple of dozen grapes, any colour
1 raw beetroot, peeled
a few sprigs of parsley (see tip on herbs, page 334)
a few sprigs of watercress or baby spinach
4 'feathers' of fennel, about 7.5cm (3in) each

Try to find as many organic products as possible. Wash everything really thoroughly and discard any peel. Then chop all of the ingredients and push them through your juicer or blender. Drink the results immediately but slowly, holding each sip in your mouth for a few seconds before swallowing. If you can't obtain all the ingredients, at least include the carrots, apples and grapes. Grow fennel in your garden or in a tub or windowbox. It is the most rewarding herb, very decorative and incredibly forgiving of neglectful treatment.

---

**Servings**

All the recipes in this section serve one. Simply double the quantities if two of you are doing the programme together.

---

**Organic carrots**

I've suggested throughout the book to buy organic produce whenever possible. That way you'll not only avoid unnecessary pesticides, you'll probably get a better flavour too. This applies especially to carrots. There's much concern over the levels of pesticides in some commercially grown carrots and, for this reason alone, I think it's worth avoiding carrots unless they are organic.

# Day one – lunch

## Hearty vegetable soup or big fresh salad

Choose from the list of vegetable ideas on page 43 or the salad suggestions on 365. For a tasty salad dressing, add a tablespoon of balsamic vinegar to a tablespoon of extra-virgin olive oil. Mix with a little bit of black pepper and pour over the salad.

# Day one – mid-afternoon

## Organic golden linseeds

1 dessertspoon organic golden linseeds (available from health stores)
a tumbler of filtered water

Linseeds provide the body with soluble and insoluble fibre and vitamin-like substances called essential fatty acids. The nutrients they contain are very easily damaged by exposure to heat, light and air. To ensure the best quality, choose only organic linseeds that are sold in sealed opaque tubs, boxes or bags (not in loose or see-through wrapping). Reseal the bag carefully after each opening or pour contents into an airtight storage jar and keep carefully in the refrigerator. The fibre in linseeds is very gentle and easily dealt with by the body. A daily dessertspoon with a large tumbler of water will coax a sluggish or irritable bowel to life and help remove wastes and poisons from the system. Don't forget to drink plenty of water with your seeds. To work properly and safely, fibre needs fluid.

---

**Avoid . . .**
Try to avoid very cold food and chilled drinks. They can disturb the digestion and liver function.

---

# Day one – before supper

## Vegetable or fruit juice

If you haven't had your cleansing juice today, now would be a good time. Otherwise, enjoy a glass of vegetable or fruit juice while you are preparing your meal. Whenever possible, prepare your own juices from fresh organic ingredients. If you buy cartoned or bottled juices, make every effort to seek out products that are, preferably, organic and at least additive-free. Health stores may hold a wider range than supermarkets.

# Day one – supper

## Colourful rice

This recipe follows food combining guidelines by mixing the rice (a complex starch) with vegetables. There is no concentrated protein (i.e. meat, eggs or fish) served at this meal. Try to use as many organic ingredients as possible.

1 good portion basmati rice, cooked
1 onion, chopped
1 clove fresh garlic, crushed
½ teaspoon of freshly grated root ginger
2 tablespoons extra-virgin olive oil
½ small bell pepper, any colour, finely grated
2 small tomatoes, chopped
1 organic carrot, finely grated
2 tablespoons frozen peas
1 tablespoon sunflower seeds and/or pumpkin seeds (mixed or separate)

First, cook your rice according to the packet instructions. Then in a wok or large pan suitable for stir-fry, sauté the onion, crushed garlic and ginger in the olive oil until the onion is just tender. Add the cooked rice, bell pepper, tomatoes, carrot, peas and seeds and keep the mixture moving over a hot ring for 5 minutes.

Serve with any kind of salad from the list on page 365. Any leftovers can be served cold with salad tomorrow if you wish.

---

### Rice

Rice is a great detoxifier and an excellent source of dietary fibre. It's also a very useful food for settling a sore stomach or calming an irritated digestive system. Also worth remembering is the fact that freshly cooked brown rice in its bland, plain and unflavoured state can be sustaining and soothing following a bout of nausea or food poisoning. However, cooked rice does not keep well. Always store leftovers in the coldest part of the refrigerator and use up within 24 hours.

---

## Day one – 1 hour before bed

### A medium tub (approx 200g/7oz) sheep's milk yoghurt

# DAY TWO

## Day two – first thing in the morning

**Lemon and honey refresher drink, as yesterday**

## Day two – breakfast

### Fresh fruit yoghurt

1 medium tub (200g/7oz) sheep's or goat's yoghurt, plain
1 ripe kiwi fruit, washed, peeled and sliced
1 apple, washed, peeled and sliced
1 teaspoon cold-pressed raw honey
1 tablespoon organic spirulina flakes or green barley powder
(available from health stores)

Put all the ingredients into a blender and mix into a smooth liquid.
Drink at once.

## Day two – mid-morning

**Cleansing juice, as yesterday**

## Day two – lunch

**Vegetable soup or salad, as yesterday**

---

**Snacks**
If you are hungry at any time during your detox days, snack on
either fresh or dried fruit, or a glass of fruit or vegetable juice.

# Day two – mid-afternoon

## Apples

For your mid-afternoon snack, have two apples – washed well, peeled and sliced – and a cup of herb or fruit tea if desired.

# Day two – before supper

## Cleansing juice or 1 dessertspoon of linseeds with a tumbler of filtered water, as yesterday

# Day two – supper

## Half an avocado pear filled with hummus, followed by a jacket potato served with green salad

This supper follows food combining guidelines by serving a starch (the potato) with vegetables or salad. There is no concentrated protein at this meal. Avocado pear combines well with either proteins or starches. Hummus is made from chickpeas which are quite starchy.

½ ripe avocado pear
enough hummus to fill half an avocado (see recipe on page 368)
1 good-sized potato, scrubbed
extra-virgin olive oil
cider vinegar
a selection of green salad items (see page 365) or cooked vegetables
(see page 43)

Prepare your avocado at the last minute to avoid it going brown. Spoon in enough hummus to fill the centre.

If you have an oven timer, why not prepare the potato in the morning and set the cooker to switch on automatically? That way, your main course is ready when you need it. Drizzle your baked potato with extra-virgin olive oil and cider vinegar and serve with a green salad or with cooked vegetables. And, remember, only eat the potato skin if it's organic.

*Or*

If you are really pushed for time, any rice and vegetables left over from yesterday, served with a big green salad.

# Day two – 1 hour before bed

## A medium tub (approx 200g/7oz) sheep's milk yoghurt

---

**Remember to drink water**

I've said it before, but I'll say it again. Make sure you drink plenty of filtered or bottled water during the two-day detox. It's vital for helping to flush the toxins from your system.

---

# Juicing for Detoxification

I would recommend anyone to take up juicing. Freshly prepared juice is a wonderful way to start the day. Invigorating, energising and an excellent way to get your inner workings working! If you have your own juicing machine (available from hardware and electrical stores) you can make a delicious variety of nourishing juices. Make your juice first thing before you disappear to the bathroom and then eat breakfast when you are dressed. Remember that you can enjoy fresh juices at any time of day, to drink before meals as a healthy aperitif, between meals as an energy booster or simply as a refreshing alternative to tea and coffee.

It's worth knowing that home-made juices deteriorate (oxidise) extremely rapidly once they are extracted from the fruit or vegetable, so it's important to consume them as soon as they are ready. All the goodness will be lost even if you leave them to stand for only a minute or two.

## Try a Juice Day

Taking nothing more than fruit and vegetable juices, or plain vegetable broth, gives the digestive system a complete rest, allowing detoxification to take place without hindrance and pushing the body's energy into boosting the immune system. These kinds of fluids on their own contain relatively little in the way of dietary fibre. Something not to be recommended, you might think. However, the digestive system has to work much harder when it is dealing with roughage, especially the insoluble cereals. Juices, on the other hand, provide easily absorbed vitamins and minerals without the need for extensive digestion. Just the thing if you're suffering from a cold or have really pushed alcohol or rich food to excess!

If you are feeling liverish or bloated, are getting over a virus, trying to get back into gear after a late night or are generally under par and need a lift, try my emergency rescue juice.

## Emergency rescue juice

2 organic carrots, well scrubbed and sliced

2 apples, washed, peeled and sliced

a handful of black grapes

1.5cm ($\frac{1}{2}$in) piece of fresh root ginger, peeled

2 teaspoons organic spirulina flakes or powder (available from health stores)

Scrub the organic carrots and peel the apples. Slice them so they fit the juicing machine. Wash the grapes. Cut and peel the ginger. Blend everything well and stir the spirulina flakes or powder into the juice before serving. Remember to use as much organic produce as you can.

> ### Cleaning tip
> Juicing machines are easier to clean if emptied and rinsed straightaway after using.

## Anything Goes

Almost anything goes when it comes to juicing. You can add fresh culinary herbs, green leaves such as spinach or watercress; in fact, any fruit or vegetable that takes your fancy.

---

**These are some of my favourite mixes:**

Apple and carrot

Apple, grape and beetroot

Apple, grape and cucumber

Apple and celery

Pineapple, mango and papaya

Blackcurrant and pineapple

Orange and grapefruit

Banana, raw honey and yoghurt

Fresh figs with black grapes and kiwi

Kiwi and mango

---

If you don't have a juicer, then buy bottled non-carbonated, additive-free juices (organic if possible) and keep them refrigerated. If you're thinking of buying a juicer, see pages 31–2.

## ESSENTIAL READING

▶ Juicing is one of the healthiest habits to get hooked on to. If you want to broaden your horizons, do get hold of a copy of a wonderful book called *Super Juice* by Michael Van Straten (Mitchell Beazley). This is a beautifully presented and colourful collection of the best juice recipes around. Great fun. I highly recommend it.

▶ Or go for Friedrich Bohlmann's handbook, *Energy Drinks* (Gaia). Not as comprehensive as Van Straten's book but a useful starting point for those new to juicing.

# Long-term Protection – Reducing Your Exposure to Toxins

Just as important as a regular internal spring-clean, is the need to reduce exposure to the pollutants and chemicals that contribute to toxicity in the first place. This means being a little more vigilant about the food and household products that we buy.

**Did You Know?**

▶ Organophosphates are neurotoxic chemicals originally developed as nerve gases.

▶ Farmers who use organophosphates suffer from more psychiatric and nervous-system disorders and loss of mental skills than those who are not exposed.

▶ Pregnant women who work with farm chemicals are nearly three times as likely to miscarry than others who have no direct contact.

▶ It has been suggested that chemical residues in breast tissue may be linked to an increased risk of breast cancer.

▶ There may be a connection between organophosphate contamination and osteoporosis (brittle bone disease).

▶ Figures suggest that there may be as many as three million severe cases of pesticide poisoning and over 200,000 deaths worldwide each year.

▶ Researchers who discovered a connection between organophosphates and Chronic Fatigue Syndrome (ME) have also found that there is a long delay between the actual exposure to the pesticide and the onset of the illness.

▶ Biologists have linked a number of pesticides and hormone residues in the environment to feminisation and infertility of male birds, alligators, fish and turtles. Animal studies show that even the minutest exposure to these chemicals, far less than are known to cause cancer, is sufficient to damage reproduction. Researchers are concerned that similar changes may affect humans.

▶ The annual US production of synthetic pesticides exceeds 600,000 tonnes. This figure *does not include* herbicides, fungicides, fertilisers and other crop chemicals.

▶ Out of 426 commonly used chemicals listed in one toxological survey, 68 were found to be carcinogenic, 61 could mutate human genes, 35 were found to adversely effect reproduction and 93 caused skin irritations.

▶ We may choose to buy perfect looking, blemish-free produce because it looks healthy. But it's worth knowing that to obtain the perfect look, most fresh produce will be heavily sprayed, in some cases as many as 25 times during a growing cycle. If you find a slug or insect inside your cabbage or lettuce, be thankful that it lived long enough to get that far. You can remove a slug or a greenfly from your cabbage but you can't 'pick off' systemic agrichemicals.

▶ Organic farmers have higher sperm counts.

▶ Organically managed farmland supports more wildlife (including birds) than chemically managed land.

## MY TIPS FOR REDUCING YOUR CHEMICAL OVERLOAD

### Go organic

▶ Whenever possible, choose organic produce over commercially grown foods. Some areas operate a 'veggie box' scheme. Run by local growers of organic produce, the service aims to make ecologically acceptable food available at affordable prices. Although not so geared-up in isolated and rural areas, doorstep deliveries of locally produced organic fruit and vegetables are increasing nationwide. Contact The Soil Association (see page 441) who can advise you of your nearest supplier in the UK.

▶ Even if local organic farm supplies or organic home deliveries are not available in your area, you can still go the organic route for quite a lot of shopping. Good supermarkets, grocery stores and healthfood shops now sell a wide range of organics including bread, brown rice, breakfast cereals, cheese, meat, poultry, rice cakes, soya milk, yoghurt, flour, eggs, pasta, stock cubes, olive oil, honey, apples, avocado pears, carrots, mushrooms, onions, oranges, potatoes, even chocolate. You may not find all the items under one roof and have to shop around, but it is worth the effort to be able to reduce your intake of unnecessary chemicals.

▶ If you're concerned about the cost of going organic, don't be. It's true that organic produce can be a little more expensive but that depends where you shop. With careful planning, food bills don't need to be higher. We all tend to eat too much protein but there really is no need to eat expensive meat products every day. If you're a vegetarian, you'll know that already. By preparing vegetarian dishes using cheaper ingredients such as beans, brown rice, couscous and fresh organic vegetables on three or four days of the week, you'll still be well nourished and you'll stay within your budget.

▶ If organic options are not available to you at all or you still really feel that they are beyond your budget, don't give up on fruit and vegetables. It's true that pesticide residues cannot be totally removed by washing – or even by peeling. However, the benefits may still outweigh the disadvantages. Some wise mathematician once estimated that it's 15 times better to eat the commercially-grown non-organic produce than it is to avoid fruit and vegetables just because they've been sprayed.

## Wash fruit, vegetables and salad foods thoroughly

Whatever your source of supply, and whether organic or not, wash all fruit, vegetables and salad foods thoroughly. It's not well publicised but bacteria and moulds, just as deadly as those implicated in food poisoning caused by poultry, meats and soft cheeses, are also found on other produce including melons, tomatoes, mushrooms and lettuces. Even if you intend to remove the peel or outer leaves on any vegetable or fruit, *wash it thoroughly first.*

## Don't buy foods from roadside stalls

They are not always locally grown or organic. Even if they are not contaminated with pesticide, herbicide or fungicide residues, they could be laced with the fall-out from vehicle exhaust emissions.

## Eat the following foods

Try to include the following foods regularly in your diet. The nutrients they contain are all believed to be beneficial to the liver, kidneys or colon. Fresh grapefruit, fresh lemon juice, apples, bananas, green salads, fresh beetroot, cabbage, celery, carrots, artichokes, onions, leeks, shallots, garlic, fresh root ginger and fresh culinary herbs. (Avoid pre-packed lemon juice or packed pre-cooked beetroot which usually contain preservative.)

## Cut down on . . .

Artificial sweeteners, foods containing artificial colours or preservatives, coffee, battery-farmed eggs and poultry, deep-fried and fatty foods, non-organic red meat, ready meals, soft drinks, sugar, sugary foods and take-aways.

## Eat lots of fibrous foods

Try to include porridge, oat bran, brown rice, dried figs, jacket potatoes, sweet potatoes, linseeds, pulses and a wide variety of green and root vegetables in your diet.

## Drinks lots of water, preferably filtered

Aim for four glasses of water (about 2 pints/1 litre) per day in addition to teas and juices.

## Try to avoid chemicals

As far as possible, avoid cow's milk and meat products unless they are organic. Apart from the inevitable concerns about BSE, these foods are also common sources of dioxin residues. Dioxins, recently at the centre of another health scare, are toxic by-products of the chlorine bleach and paper pulp industries and are given off during chemical reprocessing and medical waste incineration. They then 'fall out' from the atmosphere and settle on grass land which is then eaten by farm animals and wildlife. Dioxins are known to cause cancer, infertility and birth defects. Apart from household bleach, chlorine is used in the production of disposable nappies, tissues and cleansing pads, loo rolls, sanitary protection and even some teabags. The remains of other toxic chemicals such as DDT and lindane, that have been found in some milk supplies, are believed to contribute to a wide range of health problems but are said by government sources to be at 'safe levels'. High dioxin levels in fish have also been reported.

As dioxins are most concentrated in animal fats, humans are more likely to consume them by eating meat or dairy products from animals fed on foods that are themselves contaminated. Cow's milk, in particular, is an accurate guide to past and present levels of environmental pollution because animals grazing in polluted areas pick up pollutants and pass them down the food chain via their milk.

Dioxins have also been implicated in toxic shock syndrome (TSS) an extremely serious and potentially fatal infection caused by a toxin known as TSST-1, produced in the warm environment of the vagina by the bacteria *Staphylococcus aureus*. Women using barrier contraceptives are at increased risk from TSS but the greatest danger of all comes from the use of tampons, which allow bacteria to creep into the bloodstream by drying and ulcerating the vaginal wall. Dioxins have also been implicated as a major cause of endometriosis.

---

**Endometriosis**

This is a condition where tissue, known as the endometrium, normally only present in the lining of the uterus (womb), also occurs in other sites around the body, such as the abdomen. These tissue fragments behave in just the same way as the uterus lining, responding to the menstrual cycle and bleeding each month. Unfortunately, the blood cannot escape, resulting in – sometimes extremely large – cysts, which can cause pressure and pain.

---

## Reduce your milk quota

Cut right back on milk intake or give it up altogether. Or drink only small quantities of organic milk (now available in all major supermarkets).

## Cut back on cuppas

Limit your intake of tea, especially if it is made with bleached teabags. Go for good-quality loose black tea and green tea.

## Buy bleach-free products

Avoid tampons totally and use the older type of bleach-free cotton sanitary pads. If you feel that you can't manage without tampons, then make sure that you change them even more frequently than you do at present. And always buy bleach-free products. See page 439 for stockist information.

## Avoid meat unless it is truly organic

Get your first-class proteins from organic poultry, free-range eggs from birds fed organically, sheep's and goat's milk yoghurt and cheeses, fresh oily fish, organic soya milk and other organic soya products or a combination of pulses, grains and vegetables.

## Filter your tap water

Reduce chemical exposure further by filtering all your tap water. If you can't afford the much more expensive 'reverse osmosis' plumbed-in systems, go for an inexpensive jug filter. Most filters will take out a significant proportion of aluminium, nitrates and chlorine, improving the taste and the quality of tap water. Do remember to change the cartridge regularly; at the very least once a month. Wash the jug out thoroughly between each change. Don't use water that has been standing for long periods or stored for more than a day either in or out of the fridge. Old cartridges and stale water breed bacteria. If you are away from home during the day, either take freshly filtered water with you or buy reputable bottled water. On holiday, I use a small portable water filter unit.

## Reduce indoor air pollution

Household products such as cleaning materials, air fresheners, building materials, carpets, furnishings, wood and bedding may all contain chemicals and undesirable pollutants. It can be difficult to avoid them all, but when you get to the stage of needing to replace bedding, floor coverings, paints or other finishes, you may be able to reduce chemical sensitivity and potential allergies by going for natural materials. You might take other precautions too, such as installing air purifiers and ionisers in your home and workplace. Special air filters are available for cars which fit over the air intake on the fan or air-conditioning unit. These prevent pollens and other airborne pollutants, as well as the exhaust emissions from other vehicles, from entering the passenger compartment. Read *Your Healthy House*, a special report in the journal *What Doctors Don't Tell You*, available from Satellite House, 2 Salisbury Road, London SW19 4EZ. (Cost £3.95, including postage.) For suppliers of filters, see page 439.

## Reduce exposure to house-dust mites

Introduce dust-mite-proof bedding to your home. Most large department stores now stock linen designed to protect against dust-mite allergy. Barrier cases and non-toxic sprays for mattresses, duvets and pillows are also available from a number of mail-order catalogues. More information in the **Resource** section on page 401.

## Keep aluminium out of your life

Not only can aluminium disturb digestion, it's yet another toxin that the body has to deal with. It has also been reported that the relatively small amounts of aluminium to which we are exposed every day are enough to upset the liver and mimic symptoms similar to those asso-ciated with alcohol-induced cirrhosis. You'll find aluminium lurking in dried foods such as baking powder, milks and dried soups (as an anti-caking agent), in regular brand toothpastes, dental amalgam, antacid medications, some deodorants and in tap water in some areas of the country. If your cooking pots and pans are light in weight, the chances are they could be aluminium. Stainless steel or glass are healthier options.

## Try to ease up on as many household chemicals as possible

And try not to breathe in too deeply or directly when using them. Whenever possible, choose biodegradable cleaning products, natural soaps and shampoos. Use non-chlorine cleaning products.

## Use a chemical-free herbal/mineral toothpaste

Health stores stock a good range. Apart from the aforementioned aluminium, many ordinary toothpastes contain a whole array of chemicals which, although not directly or immediately harmful, may contribute to the build-up of toxicity. There is also some evidence that the foaming agents and detergents (such as sodium laurel sulphate), used in a number of ordinary toothpastes, are not re-moved by mouth rinsing as they actually bind to gum tissue. Formaldehyde, bromchlorophen and chlorhexidin are designed to kill bacteria but they also destroy friendly and helpful flora, upset-ting the natural balance. It has been suggested that more dangerous bacteria may remain untouched and unharmed. In addition, there is increasing concern about the effects of fluoride toothpaste and fluoridated water on our long-term health and that of our children. And if that were not enough, the membranes of the mouth are a short-cut route to the bloodstream. That's great for vital substances (sub-lingual drugs for angina are administered this way; so, too, are some vitamin preparations) but not when it comes to potentially harmful chemicals.

## Change to a non-chemical deodorant

I find most anti-perspirants/deodorants, especially aerosols, make my skin sore – I suspect it might be the aluminium chlorohydrate. So, I've changed to using only those products, such as Pitrok or Crystal Spring, that contain natural ingredients. These look like chunks of clear quartz, but are compressed mineral salts which work by killing the bacteria that cause odour. After washing, wet the crystal and wipe it under the arms, over the soles of the feet, in the groin and between the breasts. One pack usually lasts a year or more, and although they are deodorants not anti-perspirants, I have found them to be effective in the hottest of climates. Good health stores stock a wide range of deodorant products that are free from artificial chemicals.

## Avoid chemicals in the garden

If you are a gardener, avoid the use of weed-killers and other chemicals. It isn't difficult. I'm a very keen gardener but even distant contact with most garden chemicals makes me feel nauseous. Ever noticed the odour given off by the packaged weed-killers and pesticide products when they are stacked side-by-side in the garden centre? Even this apparently mild exposure can cause queasiness, smarting eyes or sneezing in some sensitive people. If you're convinced that chemicals are absolutely necessary, take the greatest care when applying them. Read the instructions carefully (you'd be surprised how many people don't) and use only the smallest amount required for the job. Store chemicals carefully and safely with caps secured, away from heat, sunlight, food, pets and children.

## Lobby retailers and politicians

Write to the head office of the supermarkets you shop at most regularly and ask to see local managers too. Tell them you want more pesticide-free food and accurate labelling on those foods that are sprayed, to give you freedom of choice when buying. Complain about unnecessary additives and ask for more organic produce. Supermarkets come in for a lot of stick for being too commercial and not caring enough, but I have to say that visits to my local Tesco and Waitrose supermarkets have brought some surprises. They have taken an amazingly impressive stand against genetically modified foods. Tesco couldn't have been more helpful when I asked why there were relatively few organic foods in my local store. Within a matter of weeks the situation was remedied to the point where, if I chose to do 100 per cent of my weekly shop at the supermarket, three-quarters of it would be organic. Write to your MP and MEP, Senator and Congressman and tell them your concerns. Politicians and retailers do respond to public pressure.

## Subscribe to *The Food Magazine*

Take out that subscription I was talking about to *The Food Magazine*. Published by The Food Commission (UK), an independent, non-profit-making organisation that campaigns tirelessly for safer, healthier food. They receive no government subsidies, and are not supported by advertising or by the food industry. Very highly recommended (see page 79).

## Avoid petrol fumes

When filling your car up with petrol, try to avoid breathing deeply and, particularly, breathing directly over the nozzle of the pump. Apart from exhaust emissions spewed out of incoming and outgoing vehicles, fuel vapours give off volatile compounds that are considered by scientists to be potential carcinogens. Unleaded petrol maybe no safer than leaded in this respect.

## Wherever possible, avoid cigarette smoke

This is well known as a class A carcinogen and supplier of toxic by-products! There are, for those who don't know, 100,000,000,000,000 (that's one hundred million million) free radicals in every puff which is why heavy smokers have been found to have five times as many wrinkles as non-smokers. (The havoc created by free radicals suppresses production of new tissue and causes old tissue to degenerate, encouraging premature ageing and wrinkles.) It is estimated that only a few lungs full of cigarette smoke, or similarly polluted air, uses up 25 milligrams of vitamin C. This vital vitamin is just one of many very important antioxidant nutrients that help protect cells against oxidation (cell degeneration) and free-radical damage and, according to studies, could be a major factor in reducing our risk of cancer and heart disease.

## Take a daily antioxidant supplement

Low levels of antioxidants have been implicated in a number of diseases. Studies show that supplementing nutrients such as vitamin E and selenium can be protective, *even if there is enough in your food supply*. Go for a capsule or tablet that contains more than the basic vitamins A, C and E. Choose a product that includes those three, plus the B group (especially B1, B3, B5 and B6) and minerals manganese, selenium and zinc. See the **Resources Section** (page 438) for details of where to find the best quality supplements.

### ESSENTIAL READING

▶ For more detailed information on detoxification, read *The Detox Plan* by Jane Alexander (Gaia) or *Detox Yourself* by Jane Scrivner (Piatkus).

▶ For a scary read about how pollution and pesticides are affecting wildlife and the countryside, read *The Killing of the Countryside* by Graham Harvey (Jonathan Cape).

▶ Get hold of a copy of the book I was telling you about, back in **Eating for Better Health** (See page 76). *The Food We Eat*, by award-winning author Joanna Blythman, tells it how it is in the food industry and recommends how to buy food that you can trust.

## Skin-cleansing Programme

*'Foolish the doctor who despises the knowledge acquired by the ancients.'*

Hippocrates, Greek physician, c.460–c.377 BC

We've already talked about how important a part the skin plays in healthy detox and how, along with the lungs, lymphatic system, kidneys, liver and large intestine, the skin is an important route of elimination. One of the ways of enhancing the cleansing process is to 'skin brush'. If you've not heard about skin brushing, you could be forgiven for thinking that I'm talking nonsense.

It does sound strange, doesn't it, until you realise what very good sense it makes. It's really not a lot different to brushing our hair, which we do so that the strands stay smooth, impurities and loose hairs are removed, and the circulation of the scalp is improved.

When we talk about cleaning the skin, we tend to think about cleansing lotions or soap and water. But there is more that we can do to prevent those pores from becoming clogged and congested. Regular brushing off of dead skin cells helps to eliminate impurities and allows our skin to breathe. Most importantly, by stimulating the lymphatic system, it speeds up the elimination of toxins from inside our bodies. And a nice little bonus is that, done regularly, it can also improve circulation and smooth out the dreaded orange peel at the same time.

There are many different approaches to skin brushing. This is the method that I have always recommended to patients and have found to be most beneficial for myself.

## HOW TO SKIN BRUSH

▶ Use a special natural-bristle skin brush with a long handle, specially designed for the purpose. They are usually available from health stores. If you can't find one, buy a long-handled, soft-bristle bathing brush from the chemist. For sensitive skin, use a very soft nylon brush or loofah or towelling mitt.

▶ Brush regularly (once or twice a week) while the skin is still dry – before bathing or showering.

▶ It's very important that you – and your muscles and skin – are warm, so do make sure the bathroom isn't chilly.

▶ First, brush the tops and soles of your feet. If your feet are extra sensitive or ticklish, begin brushing at the ankles instead. Remember that while light strokes may be ticklish, firm strokes are usually not. If you have particularly 'touchy' feet, you might find it more comfortable to use an exfoliating paste just for this area.

▶ Next, brush up the backs and fronts of your lower legs, over the knees and up the thighs. Avoid the genitals but brush inside the thighs around the groin area where there are lots of lymph nodes.

▶ Then move over the buttocks, lower back and hips. Don't twist to reach inaccessible areas.

▶ Use circular movements over and across the tummy in any direction.

▶ Then brush up the arms and across the shoulders and chest, avoiding the nipples.

▶ Don't strain to reach your back and, it's worth repeating, don't twist. If you have stiff joints or other limited movement, just brush the parts of the body that you can reach and don't worry about the rest.

▶ Brush firmly but not fiercely, until your skin feels tingly and glowing (two to three minutes for the whole body is usually enough). There is no need to brush roughly or to make your skin sore.

▶ When you have finished, rinse the brush and put it to dry.

▶ For the face and neck, use a gentle skin-scrub (exfoliating paste or lotion). See page 440 for stockists details or check your chemist or health store for a wide range of products.

▶ Then bathe or shower as usual or, if you are incapacitated in any way or have mobility problems and cannot bathe easily without help, wipe the brushed areas with a warm flannel or face cloth, rinsing it out between each wipe.

▶ Finally, after bathing or wiping, apply a body lotion or moisturiser made from natural ingredients.

## OTHER SKIN-CLEANSING TREATMENTS

### Try a home-made oil and salt scrape

This is based on a method used by Olympic athletes preparing to take part in the ancient games at Olympia. The Greek writer Lucian (*c.* AD 120–200) observed that, before training, the athletes covered themselves in olive oil and then sprinkled on sand to protect themselves from heat and cold. After the exercise, they used strigils or scrapers to remove the layers of dirt before bathing in a vessel of water.

Happily, we don't have to go to such extremes.

You will need about two tablespoons of warmed extra-virgin olive oil, two tablespoons of ordinary salt, and two large, clean, preferably old, towels.

▶ Run a hot bath (comfortable, not scalding).

▶ Put down one of your towels to protect floor coverings.

▶ Rub the arms, torso, legs and buttocks with the olive oil, just as you would if you were applying a body lotion.

▶ Next, pour a little ordinary salt into the palm of your hand and then rub it over all the oiled areas, massaging with slow circular movements.

▶ Then get into the bath (very carefully because the oil will make everything slippery), and soak for about ten minutes.

▶ Don't use any soap or bath bubbles.

▶ When you get out, dry yourself vigorously with the clean spare towel. Take care, you will still be slippery.

▶ As you rub yourself dry, not only will you remove excess oil but you should also get rid of skin grime and other impurities.

## Or you could use an Epsom salt or mineral salt bath

This is an excellent method of detoxification and is sometimes recommended for relieving joint stiffness, aching muscles, or for easing the symptoms of a cold. Epsom salts are usually available from pharmacies. If you can't find Epsom salts, use prepared mineral salts such as Dead Sea salts (sold in chemists and health stores) and follow the pack instructions as to quantity.

▶ Dissolve about half a pound (8oz/225g) of Epsom salts, or the recommended amount of mineral salts, in a warm bath.

▶ Relax for ten minutes.

▶ Take care as you get out of the bath.

▶ Instead of drying off, wrap your body in a warm towelling robe and your feet and legs in a large, dry bath-towel and go to bed either for an hour's complete rest or for the night.

▶ When you get up, shower off and rub yourself dry.

▶ If your skin feels tight or dry, apply a natural, fragrance-free body oil or lotion.

---

**IMPORTANT NOTE**

Go very gently with any kind of exfoliating scrub. Vigorous rubbing is not only unnecessary but can scratch the skin and damage the living layer.

Don't use salt baths if you have a heart condition, a blood pressure problem, are diabetic, pregnant or suffering from chronic fatigue.

---

# Better Breathing Techniques

'The space between heaven and earth is like a bellows; the shape changes but not the form; the more it moves, the more it yields; more words count less.'

Lao Tzu, *Tao Te Ching*

The breath also has a key part to play in detoxification. The lungs are an important organ of elimination and deep breathing can improve lymph drainage. But it goes much further than that. Before we look at ways of protecting ourselves from pollution in the air that we breathe and how we can help ourselves to expel toxicity, let's look in general terms at the benefits of better breathing.

Ask anyone what he or she thinks is the most important nutrient needed by the body and they may tell you the name of a vitamin, a mineral or a food perhaps. Few will think of oxygen. Breathing is so automatic that hardly anyone gives a second thought to this most vital nourishment. We can survive for very long periods of time – weeks or months – without food. We can manage for a few days without water. But starve us of oxygen and we die in seconds.

Deep breathing has major benefits and should be a fundamental part of any fitness programme. It is generally cleansing, alkalises the blood, calms an over-active mind, enhances efficient cell turnover, improves the transport of oxygen and nutrients throughout the bloodstream, reduces anxiety and strengthens the lungs. Deep breathing also improves circulation and is a useful exercise for warming you up if you're chilled.

## Breathing is Life-Giving

And yet most of us don't breathe properly. Watch anyone breathing and, if you see any movement at all, it is often only the upper chest that rises and falls. The diaphragm and abdomen rarely move, except when someone sighs or breathes in sharply because of anxiety or fear.

Ask anyone to indicate where in the body their lungs are positioned and they will usually point to the upper chest. It's easy to forget that these most important air bags take up most of the space inside the rib-cage. They fill the beehive-shaped area from just below the shoulders, all the way down to the diaphragm, the dome-shaped partition that sits above the waist, separating the chest from the abdomen.

## Breathing isn't Initiated by the Lungs

Breathing begins in the brain, in a 'control centre' known as the medulla oblongata, which sends nerve impulses to the intercostal muscles, telling them to alternately contract and relax. As we breathe in, the intercostals open up the rib-cage and the diaphragm descends, creating space for the lungs to draw in oxygen. When we breathe out, the intercostals and the diaphragm relax, deflating the lungs and pushing out air containing carbon-dioxide waste. The brain monitors the levels of carbon dioxide and oxygen in the bloodstream and, under normal circumstances, adjusts the nerve impulses so that there is always enough oxygen and never too much carbon dioxide.

Unfortunately, there are lots of things that can disturb this delicate balance. Crying, laughing, singing and running all make us breathe in and out less rhythmically. We may appear to be breathing more deeply, but may not always exhale fully enough. Even going from a warm room to cold outside air can lead to short, sudden, shallow and accelerated breathing. Our posture also cramps our breathing. We are told that to achieve good posture we must hold in our stomach muscles. If, like me, your father had a military background, the 'chest out, shoulders back, stand up straight' orders were probably issued with the best of intentions, but unfortunately can have the effect of severely restricting the breathing. Restrictive clothing, tight waistbands, corsets, belts or bras can all limit lung capacity.

## Breathing and the Emotions

Our mental and emotional state has a profound effect on the oxygen/carbon-dioxide exchange, too. A sudden shock, anxiety, anger, frustration, fear or nervous tension – all akin to the 'fight or flight' stress response – cause breathing to become faster and more shallow. When the body is tense and the breathing restricted, the movement of blood is also affected, reducing the supply of oxygen and nutrients to all parts of the body. People who are under persistent and unrelenting stress may 'overbreathe' habitually, to the point where their general health and well-being is affected.

There are specialists who believe that the way we breathe can have a greater influence on our long-term mental, emotional and physical health than on how much sleep we get, how much exercise we take, or even the type of food we eat. My view is that sleep, exercise, diet and breathing are all parts of the whole and are as important as each other.

## Ancient Philosophy

The breath nourishes us. It feeds the body and the brain. The Eastern concept of health and disease is that the qi or chi (the life force) is obstructed not only by an inadequate diet, not enough rest and relaxation, too much work, too little exercise, an over-active mind, negative stress and disturbed emotions, but also by poor-quality breathing. Many ancient traditions teach that it is air, not food, that sustains energy. In Indian philosophy, life force is *prana*, a Sanskrit word meaning the underlying energy that pervades the universe, flowing to and from heaven and earth. Anyone familiar with yoga will understand *pranayama* or control of the breath, one of eight yogic steps to enlightenment. It is this same energy that flows through the meridians or channels of a healthy body. Hatha yoga, qi gong, tai chi, and the meditation disciplines of Buddhism, Zen (a form of Buddhism), and

Taoism all recognise the importance of the breath in healing the body and the mind.

## Holding on Tight

To the Western world, unfamiliar with Eastern philosophy, relaxing and resting the physical body is difficult enough; unwinding the mind doesn't come easily at all. Some people are too afraid to let go. Staying in control seems like the simpler option. Even in the most peaceful of surroundings, many of us find that worry wanders in and out of tranquillity and over-active thoughts seem impossible to eradicate. We set into rigid postures. Shoulders are hunched, jaws are clenched and throats are tight. Our mouths turn down at the corners and our toes grip, claw-like, inside our shoes. All this puts a huge physical strain on the skeleton, especially the spine, and on internal organs, including the chest cavity. The lungs are tense, and we become physically unable to breathe as nature intended. We inhale and exhale enough to stay mobile, but we do so in a jerky, stilted kind of way, hardly moving the lungs at all. To compensate, we overbreathe or hyperventilate.

## A Common Cause of Illness

A disordered breathing pattern is recognised as being responsible for a whole range of diseases that, at one time, might have been branded as 'all in the mind'. Overbreathers tend to suffer with a lot of vague symptoms and numerous health problems that can't be defined. When no medical explanation can be found for their headaches, heartburn, irritability, panic attacks, palpitations, extreme fatigue, disturbed sleep and depression, they may be labelled as neurotic or as hypochondriacs, and their complaints not taken seriously. But symptoms aren't imagined.

It's interesting that overbreathers seem to belong to a particular personality type. They are usually meticulously tidy perfectionists who worry a lot about seemingly insignificant details. Men who overbreathe are usually competitive and ambitious, easily irritated by delays or inefficiency. I found female patients, especially, to be outwardly gentle and quiet, but internally in turmoil, having difficulty explaining how they felt about a particular issue and reluctant, at least at first, to show emotion. Questions about their childhood often revealed a lack of attention and affection from parents. I have to say that these are personal observations, but I've talked with a number of other practitioners who find similar traits.

## Getting a Rhythm

The best-quality breathing should be steady, relaxed and rhythmical. Breathing *too* deeply or *too* slowly is just as unhelpful as very rapid shallow breathing. A natural response to stress is to hold our breath or to breathe so shallowly that we then need to take a big breath (usually sounding like a sigh) to make-up for not breathing properly. Or the body may respond by overbreathing; instead of an average of 12–15 breaths per minute, hyperventilators can take anything from 20–30 breaths every 60 seconds.

---

### O2 & CO2

It would be easy to imagine that overbreathing pushed up the levels of oxygen ($O_2$). In fact, what actually happens is that carbon dioxide ($CO_2$) levels fall, causing a range of symptoms including dizziness, extreme tiredness, lack of concentration, palpitations and unexplained anxiety.

---

## MY TIPS FOR RE-EDUCATING THE BREATH AND DETOXING THE BODY

No one taught us to breathe. Nevertheless, breathing lessons can eradicate bad breathing habits. There are many different types of breathing exercise available. Those that follow here are the ones I have used most successfully with patients. My own first lessons, many years ago, were given to me by Joy Burling at the Bristol Cancer Help Centre. I have never forgotten her sound advice and excellent tuition.

If you identify with any of the symptoms mentioned in this chapter, or if you want to discover the detox benefits of deep breathing and learn how to protect yourself from pollution, give the following a go.

## Discover if you're a chest breather or a belly breather

This is an important first step. To do this, lie down on a couch or bed, or if it's comfortable enough for you, on the floor – anywhere where you can stretch out fully and flat is fine. Place the right hand on your chest and the left hand on your abdomen. Breathe normally and make a mental note of which hand moves the most. If the right hand moves more than the left hand, then it's likely that you are a chest breather, only taking air into the upper parts of the lungs. If the left hand moves more than the right hand, you are extending your abdomen, an indication that you are probably breathing more deeply than a chest breather.

Air doesn't actually fill the abdomen because it cannot pass through the diaphragm, the muscular floor of the chest. When you breathe out, the diaphragm rises in the chest and air is expelled through the nostrils. Then, as you breathe in, the rib-cage expands, drawing air into the lungs and pulling the diaphragm downwards, causing the abdominal area to expand as if air was moving directly into it. This only happens if you breathe fully and deeply – so checking up on whether your abdomen moves when you breathe is a good indication of how effective your breathing really is.

## Try this first basic breathing exercise

Do the following exercise twice a day, just before you get up in the morning and again last thing at night while you are waiting to go to sleep. The room should be warm, quiet and well ventilated. If you can open a window to let in fresh air, without intrusion from noise or traffic fumes, then so much the better.

▸ Lie on your back and make sure that you are completely comfortable. Check your body, from your toes to the top of your head, to make sure there are no tight, tense muscles.

▶ Close your eyes.

▶ Let your tongue fall naturally behind your teeth.

▶ Relax your jaw.

▶ Breathe in and, as you breathe out, pull the abdomen deliberately in as if you are trying to squeeze all the air out of your belly.

▶ Then breathe in, making as much room as possible by pushing your belly up and out. As you continue to breathe in, your chest should open up so that the whole of the front of your torso is 'lifted'.

▶ Relax and let go.

▶ Then repeat this exaggerated breathing twice more. This should help you to get the feel of how the body responds to full, deep breathing.

▶ Now breathe in and out normally and steadily, paying particular attention to the lower chest and the abdomen.

▶ On the high point of each inhalation, hold the breath for one second before exhaling. Do this for ten in-breaths and ten out-breaths.

▶ Don't push yourself and don't strain. Breathe to comfortable limits. If you are used to breathing only into the upper part of the chest, moving the abdomen can seem strange and sometimes difficult to begin with. But the change will come with practice.

### Try this second breathing exercise

The benefit of this particular exercise is that it is not only calming but also warming.

▶ Lie down flat on a comfortable surface. Make sure that you are warm enough and unlikely to be disturbed.

▶ Concentrate on your abdomen and begin with a long slow out-breath.

▶ Breathe in again, slowly and fully, counting as you inhale. If you are unused to deep breathing, you will probably only count comfortably to five or six.

▶ When you breathe out, continue to count but slow down so that the air is expelled much more slowly than it was inhaled. For example, if you counted six as you inhaled, try to regulate breathing out to a count of eight. The idea is simply to breathe out more slowly than you breathed in.

▶ Repeat this action another eight times.

▶ Then breathe normally for a few minutes before getting up.

## Use this basic relaxation technique

This simple exercise can be carried out sitting or lying down. The room should be warm, quiet and well ventilated. If you are sitting, choose a chair that has good back support and is high enough off the ground so that your thighs are parallel with the floor. If you knees are higher than your hips, then the chair is too low and the abdominal area won't be relaxed. If you lie down, make sure your neck and your lower back are well supported. If you find it more comfortable to lie on your side, then that's fine. Just make sure that your chest isn't cramped.

▶ Close your eyes.

▶ Position the tongue so that the tip touches – gently – the roof of the mouth.

▶ Breathe steadily through the nose, in and out, counting 'one' for each complete inhale and exhale. Do this for ten in-breaths and ten out-breaths.

▶ Stop counting, let the tongue relax behind the lower teeth and keep breathing normally.

▶ Then think through your body, being aware of any tight or tense muscles, relaxing as you go. Work from the toes and feet, up the legs to the hips, buttocks, lower back, chest, arms, fingers, shoulders, neck, jaw, face and brow.

▶ Then repeat the ten in-breaths and ten out-breaths.

▶ As you count, concentrate on the breath itself, becoming aware of the coolness of the air in the nostrils.

▶ Each time you breathe out, imagine that you are pushing away all anger, impatience, irritability, resentment and tension. As you breathe in, draw comfort, peace, warmth, tranquillity and love into your body.

▶ When you have completed the exercise, before getting up, lie quietly for ten minutes and allow your mind to wander.

## Quieten your mind

▶ Lie down in a warm, quiet and well-ventilated room.

▶ Loosen any tight clothing, belts, corsets, or restricting elastic.

▶ Close your eyes and relax.

▶ Do the first basic breathing exercise as above.

▶ Then make a picture in your mind of a hamster running round inside a wheel. Just like your racing thoughts, he can't stop running.

▶ Watch him for a while. See how tired he gets and how his running is getting him nowhere. Notice that you can't even see the rungs of his ladder wheel because the movement is so fast.

▶ Then see the wheel slowing down to a walking pace. Slower and slower still he walks until the wheel stops going round. You can see each rung of the ladder in detail now.

▶ The hamster is still there but he has turned over on to his back, closed his eyes and is using his wheel as a hammock, rocking gently backwards and forwards.

▶ Each time an outside thought intrudes into your head, bring your attention back to the gentle rocking of the wheel.

▶ After a while, the rocking stops and the hamster is asleep.

## Protect yourself from pollution

We can't give up breathing and, although many of us do our bit to reduce damage to the environment, we can't do a great deal to improve the quality of the outside air. But there are a number of protective measures we can take to reduce the effect of pollution on our delicate lungs.

▶ If you enjoy walking or running, don't do it alongside heavy traffic. If possible, get away to a less polluted park or street.

▶ If you have to take your exercise where the air is polluted, why not think about using a mask? Bikers wear them; why not pedestrians? The answer may be that they are not considered a fashion accessory. Perhaps, one day, they will be as bright and as sought-after as helmets or trainers. Or maybe the air will be so clean that we won't need them? (For more information on masks, see page 443.)

▶ If you drive regularly in heavy traffic, consider having a filter unit fitted to your car that cleans incoming air and absorbs toxic chemicals and pollens, preventing them from reaching the passenger compartment. In the meantime, get into the habit of shutting off incoming air when you are following vehicles with heavy exhaust emissions. Better to breathe your own carbon dioxide for a minute or two than someone else's deadly carbon monoxide. The in-cab air in most vehicles can be a dangerously concentrated form of the smoke and smog outside. (For more information on filters, see page 443.)

▶ Steer clear of cigarette smoke as much as possible.

▶ Always ask for seats in non-smoking areas.

▶ Fill your home and workplace with anti-polluting green plants such as the peace lily or spider plant.

▶ Make sure your diet contains plenty of fresh fruit, vegetables and salads, rich in protective antioxidant nutrients.

▶ Take a daily antioxidant supplement – it should contain vitamins A, C, E, B6, manganese, selenium and zinc. If you live or work in a polluted area, or live or work with smokers, take an extra one gram of vitamin C complex together with your antioxidant every day.

▶ Make your home a safer place by reducing the number of chemicals. Read *Your Healthy House,* a special report in the journal *What Doctors Don't Tell You* (see page 447).

# CHAPTER 13

# Food Combining and Eating Disorders

'From early childhood many had felt they were expected to be perfect but didn't feel they had a right to express their true feelings to those around them . . . creating in them a compulsion to "dissolve like a Disprin" and disappear.'

Diana, Princess of Wales, 1993

During my years in nutrition practice, I was involved in the treatment of a number of patients with eating disorders and have seen, at first hand, the distress and unhappiness caused to sufferers and to their families. It's one of the saddest things to observe. The sufferer is suffering and the family is suffering and yet they can't understand each other's pain. Increasing knowledge and understanding of eating disorders, as well as clearing any stigma and blame, is essential in reducing the incidence of these potentially life-threatening illnesses. Research has shown that recognising an eating disorder at an early stage, followed by appropriate treatment and support, will result in a much better chance of recovery. While food combining doesn't cure eating disorders, I have sometimes recommended its basics as part of the nutritional support given to people receiving treatment. One of the nicest, most fulfilling moments of my whole career was given to me by a former anorexic who told me that food combining had been such an important part of her recovery. Because there were no calories to count, she wasn't afraid of it. 'When I was first anorexic, I didn't want to get well, but I didn't want to die either. A girlfriend told me she was food combining and how much better she felt and I reasoned that it could help me too.' Another former sufferer told me she was surprised to find how 'ordinary and completely unintimidating' food combining was.

In a debate about diet five or so years ago, I remember facing a fairly grumpy and disgruntled professor-type who accused me of 'causing eating disorders by promoting silly diets like food combining'. I asked him what he thought food combining was about. His answer? 'Yet another extreme that gets people obsessed about food.'

Unfair, as well as inaccurate. Anyone who knows my work also knows that everything I have ever written about food highlights the need for common sense and moderation. And I am absolutely against any kind of extreme. Food combining certainly isn't extreme. But because of its success in helping overweight people to lose weight, it is sometimes, mistakenly, lumped under the same heading as low-calorie weight-loss regimes, some of which probably could be considered severe and intense. The difference between extreme diets and food combining is that, if followed correctly, food combining encourages balanced and steady weight control, not dramatic or dangerous weight loss.

To the best of my own knowledge and research, I can find not a scrap of evidence that food combining ever caused any kind of eating disorder. Nor is it a cure. So you may be wondering why I have included a chapter on eating disorders in this book. I've always thought that anorexia, bulimia and binge eating don't get nearly enough publicity or support and I hope that by discussing them openly in these pages, at least some sufferers and their families might be encouraged to seek help.

Nutritional advice can play an important part in the treatment of eating disorders but, on its own, is very unlikely to be the answer to anorexia or bulimia or binge eating. Those suffering eating disorders already have an abhorrence of calories and a fear of loss of control. If stress, exhaustion, boredom, habit, lack of self-esteem, self-disgust or other psychological trauma is causing someone to be afraid of food or the effects of food, or to use food as a way of dealing with emotional pain, the last thing they want to hear is how food can help them get better. No new eating plan, however nutritious in its own right, is going to offer any kind of complete answer to someone who is suffering from unresolved and ongoing emotional tumult or seems set on self-destruction.

# The Background to Eating Disorders

It is almost impossible to estimate, with any accuracy, the extent of anorexia nervosa, bulimia nervosa and binge eating because of the reluctance of so many sufferers to admit to any problem. The number of reported cases appears to be on the up but it's extremely difficult to say if this results from greater awareness and willingness of sufferers to ask for help or simply that the problem is, genuinely, getting worse. The results of a survey carried out in the UK in 1999 suggest that anorexia and psychological problems associated with body-image may be on the increase in boys and young men.

The Royal College of Psychiatrists' best guess is that around 60,000 people may have anorexia nervosa or bulimia nervosa at any one time in the UK. However, because of the concealment and stealth surrounding both conditions, the Eating Disorders Association believes there could be as much as 1 per cent of the population suffering from anorexia and 3 per cent affected by bulimia. That doesn't sound too serious until you work-out that 1 per cent and 3 per cent of just the UK population translates into 600,000 anorexic and 1,800,000 bulimic lives being ruled by food. I have read other reports suggesting that as many as 7 per cent may be affected by eating disorders.

Anorexia may eventually give itself away as a sufferer loses weight and looks unwell, but in its early stages may be just as hampered by secrecy and denial as its binge eating and bulimic bedfellows. There are believed to be more than five million Americans suffering from eating disorders with an estimated 1000 women each year dying from the effects of the disease.

## Who Gets an Eating Disorder?

Anyone can develop an eating disorder, regardless of age, race, sex or background. However, young women are most vulnerable. The age group at greatest risk for developing anorexia is 10 to 19 years old, although some say the gap is wider – between 15 and 25. It is the third most prevalent chronic illness in teenagers, although there is a worrying trend of anorexics aged as young as six, seven or eight years. Bulimia can affect teenagers too but is more common in the twenties and thirties age groups. Eating disorders are said to last an average of six years but can persist throughout life. Sufferers may also fluctuate between anorexia and bulimia nervosa. And the condition can repeat itself over and over. For example, an anorexic might be persuaded to accept hospital treatment or controlled feeding until they reach a normal weight, only to be discharged and start the undereating, overexercising regime all over again.

## Nothing New

Surprising as it may seem, anorexia is not a modern illness confined only to the youth population of the Western world. Young people from all countries have been afflicted over the centuries. However, eating disorders were not common where heavier women were prized and admired. This remains so today, suggesting that the incidence of anorexia and bulimia appear to be strongly influenced by culture.

## Doing What Friends Do

Anorexia or bulimia may develop simply as a result of joining in with friends at school and then the situation getting out of hand. Copying one's peers and being 'in the gang' is a part of growing up. The fact that there is no need to lose weight is no deterrent. As the situation spirals out of control, there may be a complete denial of being underweight. This point was illustrated starkly by a study of adolescents in Finland (reported at the Eighth European Nutrition Conference in Lillehammer in June 1999). One in every three girls of normal weight thought they were too heavy, and more than half of underweight girls believed themselves to be overweight. One in five underweight boys were convinced they also needed to lose weight. I talked to one former anorexic who told me that she only started crash dieting because she thought no one at school liked her. 'I didn't need to lose weight but I told myself that if I was thinner, they would stop pointing at me and let me in. I didn't do it because I wanted to be a model or anything; I just wanted them to like me.'

'You have a situation where girls of eight want to lose weight and at 12 they can tell you the fat content of an avocado . . . but they don't know what constitutes a healthy meal.'

Mary Evans Young, Chairwoman of Dietbreakers, *The Observer*, 1 May 1994

## Peer Pressure

We live in an era when our image and how we are seen by family, friends and colleagues can seem to dominate daily life. Alongside this is a national preoccupation with food and diet. Almost every magazine or newspaper bombards us with advice on how to be slim and trim, planting the idea firmly in many people's minds that, unless we all achieve this 'perfect shape', we have somehow failed ourselves and others. As a consequence, eating disorders are in the public eye to an extent that would have been unimaginable 20 years ago.

## Media to Blame?

'Unnecessary dieting is because everything from television and fashion ads have made it seem wicked to cast a shadow. This wild, emaciated look appeals to some women, though not to many men, who are seldom seen pinning up a *Vogue* illustration in a machine shop.'

Peg Bracken, US writer and humourist

It has often been said that eating disorders are caused by the continual publicity given to weight-loss diets or stick-thin catwalkers. There is, in fact, no direct evidence that the media obsession with dieting – or with fashion designers and their models – *causes* eating disorders. However, in the same way that violent films and television are known to influence the behaviour of some susceptible individuals in everyday life, the persistent use of underweight models to advertise the fashions of the day presents a powerful and influential image to an age group that is easily swayed by media mentors.

It is certainly likely that the massive interest in dieting and body-weight has created an image that being thin is somehow desirable. Since lack of self-esteem and the desire to please others are major handicaps for those with eating disorders, anything that suggests desirability is likely to be seen as helpful or beneficial. It is also the case that people with eating disorders may be influenced by someone close to them, say, a colleague at work or a member of their family. If that influential source is always counting calories or going on a diet, then it's possible that the message that food is fattening (and therefore undesirable) could rub off on to someone more vulnerable or impressionable.

## Likely Causes and Triggers

Eating disorders are believed to develop as outward signs of inner emotional or psychological problems. They become the way that people cope with difficulties in their life. Overeating, or not eating, is used to help block out painful feelings.

### All in the genes?

Research suggests that a person's genetic make-up may make them more likely to develop an eating disorder. It can run in families. Identical twins are more likely both to have anorexia than are non-identical twins. However, genes alone are unlikely to provide the whole answer. There are many other reasons too. The interaction between genes, the environment and developmental factors may hold some clues. For example, low stress tolerance could be an important trigger for anorexia.

## Adverse influence

A key person in someone's life – perhaps a parent or relative – may adversely influence other family members through his or her attitude to food.

## Pressure

In situations where there are high academic expectations or social pressures, a person may focus on food and eating as a way of coping with these stresses.

## Trauma

Traumatic events can activate anorexia or bulimia nervosa. Bereavement, being bullied or abused, – physically, sexually or mentally – upheaval in the family (such as divorce) or concerns over being gay or lesbian are all possible triggers.

## Long-term illness

Someone with another long-term illness or disability – for instance, diabetes, manic depression or deafness – may also experience eating problems.

## The zinc link

If someone doesn't eat enough, or eats and then vomits, it's pretty obvious that they are likely to become deficient in a number of nutrients. Although zinc deficiency is very unlikely to be a direct cause of anorexia, there is good evidence that at least some cases could be helped by the introduction of zinc supplementation. There are also similarities between symptoms. Anorexia and low zinc both lead to changes in appetite and taste, weight loss, yellowing skin, loss of periods and mood changes. It is also interesting that some anorexics appear to absorb zinc less efficiently than normal subjects. Anorexics who receive zinc supplements as part of their treatment have been shown to gain weight faster than those taking a placebo.

## Low serotonin levels

Imbalances of the hormone serotonin – involved in the regulation of mood – have been implicated in bulimia. I've also seen several bulimics and anorexics who suffered symptoms suggestive of winter depression or seasonal affective disorder (SAD). Serotonin levels vary in everyone throughout the year and are lowest during the winter months. In SAD sufferers, serotonin levels are believed to be much lower than normal. Perhaps this explains why treatments including the use of light boxes, plus additional time spent out of doors, have helped some sufferers of bulimia. The use of light therapy (the use of a special type of bright indoor lighting) is now a recognised treatment for SAD.

A symptom of SAD that affects some – but not all – sufferers is food cravings which can trigger binge eating and winter weight gain. If you know you have a problem with binge eating but also suffer from depression, especially during the winter, you could ask your doctor to refer you to a specialist who treats seasonal affective disorder.

### SOME USEFUL SELF-HELP MOVES

### Eat small meals

Small, nutrient-dense meals using ingredients chosen by the sufferer may be less of a threat and of greater value than larger controlled meals.

### Try amino-acid supplements

Broad-range amino-acid supplements are an additional non-calorific way of introducing essential nourishment into a malnourished body. Amino acids are the building blocks of protein, needed for almost every single body function. They are particularly valuable where there have been long periods of low-calorie intake, dramatic loss of weight, poor digestion and malabsorption.

## Supplement vitamins and minerals

Supplementation of magnesium, chromium, zinc and vitamins B3 and B6 have helped to improve mood in bulimics, anorexics and binge eaters, resulting in more balanced eating habits. Vitamin B3 is part of the nutrient pathway essential for serotonin production. Chromium may help reduce cravings and regulate appetite by balancing blood glucose. Zinc is, as explained above, often found lacking in anorexics. A plus point for the use of nutrient supplements in the treatment of anorexia and bulimia is that they contain only negligible calories and so are more likely to be perceived as non-threatening.

## Take probiotics

Experience suggests that people with eating disorders may have an imbalance of friendly gut flora. A three-month course of probiotics could be helpful.

The **Resources** section on page 438 has details of supplement suppliers.

# Long-term Dangers of Eating Disorders

In addition to a range of serious health complications, including heart, kidney and digestive disorders, cessation of periods and loss of fertility are two of the earliest complications to manifest themselves in eating disorders. Later in life, thinning bones (osteoporosis) and the consequent increased risk of fractures can be a major problem.

## Hormonal imbalances

Pre-existing hormonal imbalances seem to be common in anorexia and bulimia. It is certainly the case that loss of periods (amenorrhoea) occurs in some anorexics long before there is any evidence of significant weight loss. In all cases of anorexia – but particularly where there is a family history either of eating disorders or hormone-related health problems such as endometriosis, PMS or period problems – it is always worth asking for tests to be carried out to check for any hormone imbalances.

Researchers have noted a connection between ovarian cysts and bulimia. Polycystic ovarian disease (PCOS) is a common cause of infertility and may also be linked to obesity. In one study, only around 15 in every 100 bulimics had normal ovaries. Indeed, the association between bulimia and PCOS hormones is so strong that it has been suggested gynaecologists screen all patients for abnormal eating patterns and, where appropriate, provide counselling and other support.

I highly recommend you read PCOS: *A Woman's Guide to Dealing with Polycystic Ovary Syndrome* by Colette Harris with Dr Adam Carey (Thorsons), or visit www.pcosupport.org, www.soulcyster.com or www.verity-pcos.org.

---

**Polycystic ovarian disease (PCOS)**

In this condition, numerous small cysts occur under the surface of the ovaries. This not only causes the ovaries to enlarge, but also affects oestrogen production. Sufferers may experience infrequent or absent periods, infertility, abnormal hair growth and obesity.

---

## Understanding the Sufferer's Pain

Worryingly, an opinion poll carried out in 1999 demonstrated a sad lack of understanding of eating disorders. Although three-quarters of those taking part believed that anorexics and bulimics suffered low self-esteem, there were several serious misconceptions. Results showed that one in every four people believed that anorexics and bulimics were vain. More than a third of those interviewed thought that anorexics and bulimics were attention seekers. And well over half of those questioned thought that having an eating disorder meant someone was mentally ill.

One of the most poignant ways to bring home the desperation associated with eating disorders is to hear the pain directly from a sufferer.

'Eating disorders, whether it be anorexia or bulimia, show how individuals can turn the nourishment of the body into a painful attack on themselves and they have at the core a far deeper problem than mere vanity,'

said Diana, Princess of Wales.

Speaking at the Eating Disorders International Conference in 1993, Diana expressed what so many sufferers already felt but that most non-sufferers could not comprehend:

'From early childhood many had felt they were expected to be perfect but didn't feel they had a right to express their true feelings to those around them – feelings of guilt, of self-revulsion and low personal esteem, creating in them a compulsion to "dissolve like a Disprin" and disappear. The illness they developed became their shameful friend . . .'

## Anorexia Nervosa – Specifics

The term 'anorexia nervosa' – meaning 'loss of appetite for nervous reasons' – can be misleading because there is far more to this condition than merely 'nerves'. In addition, most people assume that anorexics have no appetite when the truth is that they are often struggling with raging hunger through every waking moment. What the person has lost is the ability to *allow* themselves to satisfy their appetite, but this doesn't mean they don't feel hungry. They restrict the amount they eat and drink, sometimes to a dangerous level, focusing on food in an attempt to cope with life, rather than to starve to death. It is a way of demonstrating that they are in control of their bodyweight and shape.

Ultimately, however, the illness itself takes control. Loss of proper nourishment leads to malnutrition, resulting in chemical changes that distort thinking to the point where a person can no longer make rational decisions about food. As the illness progresses, many people will suffer from the exhaustion of starvation. The risk of dying from the effects of anorexia are 'occasional' or could be as many as one in every ten sufferers, according to different researchers. It is certainly the case that anorexia nervosa has one of the highest death rates for any psychiatric disorder.

## Signs of anorexia

### Physical symptoms of anorexia may include:

▶ In children and teenagers – poor or inadequate weight gain in relation to their growth

▶ In adults – extreme weight loss

▶ In men – loss of libido

### Other signs are:

▶ Abdominal pains

▶ Absent periods

▶ Cold hands and feet

▶ Constipation

▶ Depression

▶ Disrupted menstrual cycles

▶ Dizzy spells

▶ Downy hair on the body; loss of hair on the head when recovering

▶ Dry, rough, discoloured skin

▶ Fainting

▶ Loss of bone mass and, eventually, osteoporosis (brittle bones)

- Loss of taste and smell

- Poor circulation

- Shivering

- Swollen stomach, face and ankles

- Yellowing skin pigmentation

## Psychological signs:

- Changes in personality and mood swings

- Denial of the existence of a problem

- Distorted perception of bodyweight or shape

- Intense fear of gaining weight, even within the normal weight range according to height

## Behavioural signs:

- Obsessive interest in taking exercise

- Restlessness and hyperactivity

- Rituals attached to eating, such as cutting food into tiny pieces

- Secrecy

- Taking laxatives

- Vomiting

- Wearing big baggy clothes

## Long-term Effects of Anorexia

The long-term effects of anorexia on the body and mind can be alarming and severe. Fortunately, many of these effects can be reversed once the body receives proper and regular nourishment, although it can take some weeks or months for the body and mind to readjust.

Eating and drinking regularly after so long without proper nourishment can cause temporary bloating. Personality and mood swings may also take a while to settle, depending on the emotional difficulties associated with anorexia.

## Anorexia and the Family

Anorexia not only overwhelms the person with the disorder – the whole family is affected. Each family is different but some common trends have been identified.

People who develop anorexia may have been compliant and obedient children. They would be less likely to become angry than their brothers or sisters and more willing to be the doormat. Inner feelings and anxieties can be hidden by an outwardly pleasant and genuinely kind personality, coupled to an overwhelming desire to please and care for others. They are committed to achieving high standards that have been set – or that they assume have been set – by parents or teachers. Their fear of failure – of not making the grade – or not matching up to a brother or sister who is held as brighter or more successful in some way, may commit the sufferer to strive constantly to be the best. Often the high standards are self-imposed but can also be the result of badgering to succeed, or the belief or constant reminder that 'you could do better'.

Some families are so close and loving that the child finds it difficult to become independent. Some parents can be almost suffocating in their concern. The sufferer becomes afraid that they cannot manage on their own away from the family and uses anorexia in an attempt to demonstrate independence through control over food and eating.

The father of one patient talked about his daughter constantly, to everyone, wherever he went, whether they wanted to listen or not. His desperation was clear. He had no answers and was trying to find them. But his daughter was stifled by this concern. She felt that her father controlled her life completely and never allowed her any kind of free reign. 'I know he's worried,' she told me, 'but he never lets me forget my illness. I'm 22 years old but I've never been me,' she said. 'I'm like a puppet dominated by the puppeteer.' She began to recover once she had left home. Back to her normal weight, she is now married and expecting her first child.

Sufferers often blame themselves for their predicament. A teenage male anorexic pulled himself out of the disease because his complementary medicine practitioner, who used nutritional therapy and plenty of 'good listening', helped the young man 'to stop blaming myself and to take responsibility'. 'I liked the diet because there were no calories to count and I liked the therapist because he was completely non-judgemental.'

## Bulimia Nervosa – Specifics

It is only in the last 30 years that bulimia nervosa has been recognised by doctors as an eating disorder in its own right. The term 'bulimia nervosa' means literally 'the hunger of an ox'. The hunger, however, is often an emotional need that cannot be satisfied by food alone. After binge eating a large quantity of food to fill the hunger gap, the person will immediately rid themselves of the food they have consumed by vomiting or taking laxatives (or both), or they will work off the calories with exercise – all in an attempt to purge the guilt and prevent weight gain.

A person is most likely to develop bulimia in their late teens to early twenties and may have already suffered from – or go on to develop – anorexia.

Bulimia is more difficult to detect than anorexia as the person often will not lose weight so dramatically. In fact, even people close to them at home or work may not recognise the illness and so it can persist for many years undetected. 'I used to get up and disappear to the bathroom between courses,' one bulimic told me. 'I did it for years but no one ever guessed I was going out to vomit.' The sufferer's chronic lack of self-confidence is often hidden. For example, people with bulimia may have high-powered jobs that often demand them to be outgoing and self-assured. As with anorexia, those who develop bulimia rely on the control of food and eating as a way of coping with emotional difficulties in their life.

A 40-year-old woman who talked to me about her bulimia said that the big difference in her life was learning to touch. She had never been cuddled or hugged by her parents or encouraged to express her own opinion. Her reluctance to touch in adulthood had eventually resulted in divorce from her first husband. Finally, she consulted a practitioner who also happened to believe that hugging was an important part of healing. 'She recommended all kinds of different things for me to do but one thing will always stay in my mind,' she told me. 'It was the sign on her consulting-room wall reminding all visitors that arms are for hugging. I must have stared at it or something and she just got up from her chair and hugged me. I cried for nearly an hour. It was a real break-through.'

## Purging Shame and Guilt

Whilst some bulimics are binge eaters, others don't overeat. They may simply choose to vomit to get rid of a normal-sized meal. Whatever they've eaten, as the sufferer starts to feel full, feelings of guilt, shame or self-disgust come into their mind. For some sufferers, feeling full may equate with feeling dirty or out of control. In desperation, they vomit or take laxatives to purge themselves of everything they have consumed.

At this point, some people describe feeling emotionally relieved and physically light-headed. This cycle can keep inner pain and unhappiness at bay – but only for a short time.

The frequency of the binge-vomit cycle will vary from person to person. Some will suffer from an episode every few months whilst others, who are more severely ill, may binge and purge several times a day. So ingrained does the habit become that sometimes sufferers will vomit automatically after they have eaten any food without any need to force themselves to be sick. Others will appear to eat socially without problems but may be bulimic in private.

Some people accept their eating disorder as a kind of normality, whilst others despise and fear the vicious and uncontrollable cycle they are in.

# Signs of bulimia

## Physical signs of bulimia may include:

▶ Frequent weight changes

▶ Hormonal imbalances

▶ Lethargy and tiredness

▶ Poor skin condition

▶ Sore throat and tooth decay caused by excessive vomiting

▶ Swollen salivary glands making the face more round

## Psychological signs:

▶ An obsession with food

▶ Anxiety and depression; low self-esteem, shame and guilt

▶ Distorted perception of bodyweight and shape

▶ Emotional behaviour and mood swings

▶ Isolation – feeling helpless and lonely

▶ Uncontrollable urges to eat vast amounts of food

## Behavioural signs:

▶ At mealtimes, disappearing to the bathroom/toilet between courses

▶ Bingeing and vomiting

▶ Excessive exercise

▶ Excessive use of laxatives, diuretics or enemas

▶ Food disappearing unexpectedly

▶ Periods of fasting

▶ Secrecy and reluctance to socialise

▶ Shoplifting for food

▶ Spending abnormal amounts of money on food

## Long-term Effects of Bulimia

In a similar way to anorexia, bulimia can take over the life of the person with the disorder, making them feel trapped and desperate. Chaotic eating and dramatic loss of fluids can cause a number of health problems. Encouragingly, most can usually be corrected once the body is nourished in an even and moderate way.

Although the dangers of anorexia are more apparent because of a person's substantial weight loss or very low weight, bulimia can, in extreme cases, be fatal due to, for instance, a heart attack. An imbalance, or dangerously low levels of the essential minerals in the body, can significantly or fatally affect the workings of vital internal organs. Other dangers of bulimia include rupture of the stomach, sore gullet, choking, and erosion of tooth enamel caused by the regurgitation of stomach acid.

# Binge Eating

Like bulimia, binge eating has only recently been recognised as a definite condition. There is a difference, however, between bingeing and bulimia. Binge eaters may eat to uncontrollable excess, but do not purge themselves. Many more people suffer from binge-eating disorder than either anorexia or bulimia nervosa, and it's estimated that approximately ten per cent of people with binge eating disorder are obese.

A person may begin to binge in an attempt to cope with emotional difficulties or to ease tension, but may find the situation running rapidly out of control. The foods they eat are generally high calorie, high carbohydrate and high fat. Bingeing is eating for the sake of eating, when you aren't hungry, because you are upset, distressed about your body-image or simply feeling low. If you can work your way systematically through excessive amounts of food to the point of being sick but do not deliberately vomit (as in bulimia), this is bingeing.

## Signs of binge eating

▶ Cravings, especially for sweet and starchy foods (seasonal cravings may be linked to SAD, winter depression)

▶ Eating alone because of embarrassment at the quantities of food consumed

▶ Eating in a 'trance'

▶ Eating large amounts of food when not physically hungry

▶ Eating much more rapidly than usual

▶ Eating until feeling uncomfortably full

▶ Feeling ashamed, depressed or guilty after bingeing

▶ Horror of vomiting

## Some comments made by sufferers of binge eating:

▶ 'I just feel awful about myself.'

▶ 'I hate my body.'

▶ 'I'm useless at everything.'

▶ 'I'm not good enough for anything.'

▶ 'I'm trying to forget how bad things are.'

▶ 'I'm trying to convince myself that it doesn't matter what people think about me even though I care very much what they think.'

▶ 'Food? Well it's like mountains. It's there.'

▶ 'Stress.'

▶ 'Boredom.'

▶ 'Poor self-image.'

▶ 'Habit.'

▶ 'I'm ugly anyway. Who's going to notice the fat.'

## Identify Your Triggers

The following list of questions may help you to identify what drives you to bingeing. Answer the questions honestly.

### Section one

*Do you eat:*

▶ When you're depressed?

▶ When you're anxious or nervous?

▶ When you're stressed?

▶ When you've had a row with someone?

▶ When you're overwhelmed by circumstances?

▶ When you're trying to cope with a crisis?

▶ When you're watching television?

▶ When you're tired?

▶ When you've had a bad day?

▶ When you're irritable?

▶ When you have money worries?

▶ When you're overworked?

Questions in **Section 1** relate to stressful situations. If you thought 'yes, that sounds like me' to any of these, then you may be under too much stress or not coping well with the effects of stress. When you're overtired, worried or under pressure, your perspective goes and you don't see things rationally. Food is a way of diverting attention from the problems at hand. Stress responses to food may be more than psychological, too. Levels of serotonin (that all-important brain chemical which helps to keep us calm and is also involved in regulating hunger), fall when we are stressed. There is a chapter in this book especially for you (from page 329) on how to help your body cope safely with the effects of stress.

## Section two

*Do you eat:*

▶ When you feel intimidated?

▶ When someone hurts your feelings?

▶ When someone makes you angry, irritable, annoyed or frustrated?

▶ When you're criticised?

▶ When you feel unwelcome?

▶ When you think no one cares about you?

▶ When you think people don't understand you?

▶ When you hate yourself?

▶ When you're put upon or taken for granted?

▶ When you're telling yourself you couldn't care less about what anyone thinks?

▶ When you think you're undeserving?

▶ When someone says 'you could have done better'?

If you ticked any of the questions in **Section 2**, it could be that your self-esteem has taken a bashing and you are having difficulty in your relationships with other people. It's usually the people closest to you that do such a good job of destroying your self-esteem. Because you love them or trust them, you believe what they tell you. If you hear 'you're useless' often enough, you'll convince yourself that it's true. From this inevitable lack of confidence, it's easy to form a persecution complex that says nobody likes you or everyone is whispering behind your back. Don't believe it. It is very unlikely to be true. No one is useless. Most people have a huge contribution to make if only given the chance. If people really are making silly remarks or criticisms, don't forget the old adage that when a finger is pointing at someone, there are three other fingers pointing back. Point with your finger now and you'll see what I mean. Generally, people accuse others only of what they themselves are guilty.

## Section three

### *Do you eat:*

▶ When you have nothing else to do?

▶ When you see cakes on display or food on someone else's plate?

▶ When you see other people eating?

▶ When you're bored?

▶ When you're watching television?

**Section 3** is all about boredom, habit and lack of interest in things around you. No wonder you want to fill the void with food. Boredom begets boredom and, soon, the link with food becomes a habit. But it is a breakable habit. Read My Hot Hints for Healthy Weight Loss on page 139.

## Section four

▶ Do you suffer from depression?

▶ Is your depression worse in the winter?

▶ Do you suffer from mood swings?

▶ Do you have problems sleeping?

▶ Do you suffer from frequent colds or recurring infections?

▶ Do you crave particular foods?

▶ Do you have favourite foods that you eat every day?

▶ Do you crave sweet and starchy foods?

▶ Do you suffer from twitchy limbs or nervousness?

▶ Do you suffer from joint pain, muscle cramps or spasms?

▶ Do you have a history of pre-menstrual tension?

▶ Do any particular foods upset or disagree with you?

▶ Are you tired all the time?

▶ Do you suffer from frequent headaches or migraine?

▶ Do you suffer from fluid retention or bloating?

▶ Do you have any kind of bowel or digestive discomfort?

**Section 4** relates to nutritional deficiencies and food sensitivities. If you think any of these symptoms apply to you, you could be low in some nutrients or may be suffering from sensitivity to certain foods. Very little research has been carried out in this area in relation to eating disorders, but it is one worth exploring. Symptoms of sensitivity can include joint pain, constant fatigue, mood swings, migraine, headaches, irritability, fluid retention, bloating or any kind of ongoing digestive discomfort or irritable bowel. Or there may be no symptoms at all. The roots of food sensitivity or allergy may be in childhood. If you suffered as a child from colic, hyperactive behaviour, asthma, eczema, ear infections or glue ear, were not breast-fed, were weaned early or showed an intolerance to cow's milk – even if you no longer have any symptoms as an adult – your eating disorder still might be related to, or caused by, an allergic reaction. Don't try to self-diagnose or self-medicate. I would strongly recommend that you ask to be referred to a naturopathic physician, homoeopath or nutrition-oriented practitioner who specialises in the treatment of eating disorders and allergies.

## Other Eating Disorders

Conditions as complex as eating disorders inevitably mean that there are many variations in the typical signs described in this chapter. Not all of the symptoms will apply to all sufferers. Some people may cut their food intake dramatically only for a few weeks or may binge only when they are under particular pressure or stress. Instead of swallowing large amounts of food and then vomiting, another action is to chew and spit. Appalling to a non-sufferer as it may sound, yet another example is re-chewing food that has already been swallowed and then regurgitated. Some people have become so concerned about the effect that calories might have on their weight that they choose to eat non-foods, such as paper tissues, to fill themselves up.

# Finding Support and Help for Eating Disorders

## FIRST STEPS

Eating disorders are complex illnesses and although the recovery rates are said to be encouraging, the relapse rates, especially for anorexia, are not so cheery. Specialist medical and nutritional care is vital, not only to assess and treat the physical problems and to restore a nutritious eating pattern but also for the psychological difficulties that cause such unhappiness and trauma. Helping someone come to terms with the underlying emotional issues enables them to cope with difficulties in a way that is not harmful to them.

However, with illnesses like anorexia, bulimia or binge eating, the person must themselves want to get better before help can be really effective. People with eating disorders often have mixed feelings about 'giving up' their illness. This is because their eating habits have become a way of coping with their profound emotional difficulties.

There are a variety of ways in which people can be treated. Recovery is not easy but it is certainly possible. A patient may be offered a combination of different forms of therapy, such as:

▶ Counselling

▶ Self-help and support groups

▶ Psychotherapy; drama or arts therapy

▶ Therapy sessions that involve the family or small groups of patients

▶ Diet and nutritional advice

► Treatment for food sensitivities

► Light therapy

If medication is required for illnesses that occur as a result of the eating disorder, this could be provided by a doctor or specialist out-patient clinic. In-patient hospital or clinic care might be necessary for the patient who is severely ill.

## What To Do Next

### Contact the Eating Disorders Association

This is a good first port of call. The Eating Disorders Association is there to talk to anyone with any kind of eating disorder. It also runs a telephone counselling programme for people with bulimia. Feedback from some of those who have attended their self-help and support groups confirm that they have proven to be highly beneficial.

The adult Helpline is manned five days each week from 9.00 am to 6.30 pm. The Youthline is supported by trained counsellors and has a callback facility so that youngsters don't have to worry about anyone finding out that they have used a telephone at home or at work. The Association is there to help partners, parents, concerned friends and families as well as sufferers and can put any one in touch with local support groups.

If you are living or working with someone who you think may be suffering from an eating disorder, look for the signs listed above. If you are sure there's a problem, call the Eating Disorders Association helpline for further advice or talk to your own doctor.

If you are a sufferer, whatever your age or circumstances, the Eating Disorders Association is there to help you too. All calls are completely confidential and you don't have to do anything you don't want to do. But do talk to them. Their telephone lines are supported by trained counsellors and experienced volunteers, many of whom have been through what you are going through now.

If you think you have a problem but are not sure, still talk to someone. If emotional upset, stress, exhaustion, boredom, habit or lack of self-esteem are causing you to eat for comfort, then dealing with the reasons why this is happening to you should be a priority. Impulse eating can develop into more serious eating disorders.

Adult Helpline: 01603 621414     9.00 am–6.30 pm, Monday to Friday
Youthline: 01603 765050     4.00 pm–6.00 pm, Monday to Friday

## Contact Priory Healthcare

Another point of contact is Priory Healthcare. Sufferers and families can get in touch by e-mailing *eatingdisorders@prioryhealthcare.co.uk* and can also write for an information pack to Eating Disorders, PO Box 195, Uxbridge, Middlesex UB9 5QE. Please send a large s.a.e. All letters are completely confidential.

## In the US

Call the American Anorexia Bulimia Association on 212 575 6200. Again, all calls are confidential.

## Use the internet

For more information on books, videos, where to turn for support, how to get involved in self-help groups, how to choose the best therapist and how family and friends can help, the internet is an excellent resource. The websites listed below are well worth visiting.

▶ **The Mirror Mirror Eating Disorders** website can be found at *www.mirror-mirror.org* When you arrive, just click on Eating Disorders at the top of their first page.

▶ The **Anorexia Nervosa and Related Eating Disorders** organisation is at *www.anred.com*

▶ A useful site known as **Cath's Links to Eating Disorders Resources** is *www.nvg.org/~cath/ed*

## ESSENTIAL READING

▶ *Fear of Food* by Genevieve Blais (Bloomsbury)

▶ *Eating Your Heart Out* by Julia Buckroyd (Vermilion)

▶ *Transforming Body Image* by Marcia Germaine Hutchinson (Crossing Press)

▶ *You Can Heal Your Life* by Louise Hay (Eden Grove)

### Author's note

My grateful thanks to the **Eating Disorders Association** for their help in supplying some of the statistics and research for this chapter.

# CHAPTER 14

# Food Combining and Blood Glucose

**M**ost of us are familiar with that slightly unpleasant sensation of feeling empty and slightly spaced-out because we've gone too long without food. But, if, only a couple of hours after a fairly decent-sized meal, you're experiencing hunger pangs, loss of concentration, unexplained irritability, shivering, or a complete and sudden drop in energy – and if it happens regularly – then you could be suffering from a condition known as reactive hypoglycaemia.

If you haven't heard of it before, don't panic.

If you have heard about it, you'll probably know that hypoglycaemia simply means low blood glucose or sugar, sometimes just called 'the hypo'. If you diet regularly for weight loss, for example, you are almost certainly going to be very familiar with the hypo. The cravings that are so often associated with low-calorie weight-loss programmes are one of the most common reasons for not sticking to a diet plan. And that's where food combining comes in.

Food combining has become famed for its ability to help people achieve permanent weight loss. One of the reasons it works so well to stabilise bodyweight is because, if it's followed correctly, it can also be very effective at keeping blood sugar on an even keel. Cravings associated with PMS (pre-menstrual tension) should also respond well to the advice in this chapter.

# The Background to Hypoglycaemia

Perhaps a more accurate description of the reactive hypo is that blood glucose doesn't just fall, it fluctuates quickly and wildly between high and low levels. In fact, there is a growing conviction that hypoglycaemic symptoms are not only triggered when glucose levels plummet, but by how often and how quickly they fall. Low blood sugar is certainly a major symptom of the condition we know as hypoglycaemia – but the wildly fluctuating see-saw pattern of glucose in the blood from high levels to low and back again could make the description *erratic* or *unstable* blood sugar more accurate of its true nature.

## No Obvious Symptoms

The tendency to hypoglycaemia can creep up on us almost unnoticed. We may have a few unpleasant symptoms but dismiss them as nothing more than hunger. Eat something, fix it and you'll be fine. But let's look at what happens when the mechanisms for balancing blood glucose get out of control:

Your blood sugar levels are falling and you're beginning to yawn.

You feel dizzy, drowsy, light-headed, sweaty or shaky.

Your brain fogs up, too. Because the brain takes priority over the rest of the body when it comes to being fed and because the only fuel the brain can use is glucose, a major symptom of hypoglycaemia is a sudden inability to concentrate.

Sometimes, when a hypo hits you, you'll reach for the nearest and easiest sustenance – a bar of chocolate, a packet of biscuits or a can of cola. This 'safety net' is your own internal messenger service calling up instant sugar supplies. That's why, when a hypo happens, we so often crave sweet foods; because the body knows that they'll release their energy quickly into the system and stave off the emergency.

But the effect is short-lived.

Insulin shoots out from the pancreas to mop up the excess sugar but, because there is too much insulin and not enough truly sustaining food, blood glucose falls again and you're back where you started.

Running on empty.

The next meal seems like miles away.

## The most common signs of low blood sugar

These symptoms are more likely to occur when your body has been without food for anything from 90 minutes to three or four hours. Symptoms tend to come on suddenly, and resolve quickly after eating.

▶ Blurred vision or difficulty focusing

▶ Clamminess

▶ Cravings

▶ Dizziness

▶ Drowsiness

▶ Excessive thirst

▶ Fast, shallow breathing

▶ Feeling light-headed or shaky

▶ Feeling spaced-out

▶ Feeling the cold

▶ Fluid retention

▶ Headache

▶ Hollow, gurgling stomach

▶ Irritability

▶ Insomnia

▶ Loss of energy

▶ Loss of libido

▶ Mood swings

▶ Muscle cramps

▶ Night sweats

▶ Palpitations

▶ Poor concentration

▶ Poor co-ordination

▶ Shivering

▶ Waking hungry during the night

▶ Yawning

Well, never mind. It's worth putting up with the symptoms just to avoid the calories, isn't it?

Your body doesn't agree.

You must eat something fast.

Your hand reaches out for more chocolate.

You munch through the whole bar.

Ah! That's better.

Blood sugar rises rapidly and you feel fine again, but usually only for a half an hour, or even less.

More insulin is produced to deal with the sudden influx of sugar but then, once again, there is too much insulin circulating in the blood so the glucose falls dramatically and the vicious circle is completed.

## Wide-Ranging or Rare?

The popular view is that hypoglycaemia has reached epidemic proportions. Some authorities say that as many as one in two people may be affected. But other, equally highly qualified, experts are sure that the hypo is nothing more than hype. A major problem is that, although doctors acknowledge the existence of organic hypoglycaemia, in conditions such as alcoholism or chronic liver disease, most do not accept the possibility of reactive hypoglycaemia.

Misdiagnosis is common.

I have met a number of patients who were dismissed as stressed, confused, mistaken and, in several cases, as having a psychological disorder only, eventually, to be diagnosed with reactive hypoglycaemia. None was diabetic or had any other serious illness.

## So, What Exactly Does Hypoglycaemia Mean?

Well, the word, when you split it up, simply translates as 'not enough glucose in the blood'. *Hypo = under or low; glykis = sweet; aemia = in the blood.* Many people assume that the condition of low blood sugar is the opposite of diabetes which, of course, is a condition of high blood sugar. But hypoglycaemia and diabetes can be just two different stages in the same disease process. A growing number of nutrition experts believe that if reactive hypoglycaemia is allowed to go unchecked, there is a risk of it leading to full-blown diabetes.

In between the two – and linked to both – is hyperinsulinaemia (say *hyper-insu-lin-eemier*), which simply means over-production of insulin, a major hormone in the glucose balancing act. If insulin is persistently over-produced, it can result in a condition known as insulin resistance. I've talked about this in more detail on page 307 but, briefly, the problem has to do with the levels of glucose in the bloodstream and how effectively insulin deals with that glucose.

## Body Fuel

Glucose is a major body fuel, a simple sugar that is produced when food is digested and absorbed. As glucose is absorbed and levels in the bloodstream rise, insulin is squirted out of a gland called the pancreas, latching on to glucose and moving it into cells, where it is either burned as an energy source or stored as fat. This is a normal and continuous process. Unfortunately, our diets and lifestyles have changed so dramatically in the past 100 years or so that the body's glucose- and insulin-balancing mechanisms are finding it hard to cope.

## Could Diet Be to Blame?

For hundreds of thousands of years, our ancestors existed on a diet of lean protein, vegetables, seeds and fruit. These foods are digested very slowly, resulting in a gradual rise in glucose levels and in normal insulin production.

In the past century, the average Western diet has altered almost beyond recognition. One of the worst 'hazards' is that grains are often stripped and processed to produce white flour, white bread, rolls, cakes, biscuits, pastries and all manner of baked and packaged goods that are high in refined sugars. These foods are broken down extremely rapidly by the digestive system so that the simple sugars from them are absorbed at great speed. Glucose levels rocket upwards, triggering insulin which, in these circumstances, is usually produced in too large a quantity, leaving unused amounts floating unchecked in the blood-stream.

This situation can continue unnoticed for years, usually without any obvious symptoms. Eventually, though, the cells that normally respond to insulin become 'resistant'. The pancreas tries to compensate by producing even more insulin but, by this time, the cells are reluctant to respond. As a result of this imbalance, both glucose and insulin levels in the blood remain high, generating large numbers of destructive molecules known as free radicals that have been linked to degeneration and age-related diseases including Alzheimer's, heart disease and cancer. Over-production of insulin and poor management of glucose can create a pre-diabetic state, increasing the risk of diabetes in later life.

And because insulin promotes the storage of fat, it makes weight problems more likely, too.

Now this doesn't mean that everyone who suffers occasional symptoms of low blood sugar is going to become insulin resistant, obese or diabetic. But it does mean that if symptoms are persistent and there are other risk factors involved (see pages 312–16), then some action should be taken sooner rather than later to reduce that risk. It is also the case that nearly everyone who diets regularly for weight loss is likely to have an underlying problem with blood sugar control and balance.

## But Why Does Blood Sugar Get Out of Control?

First of all, let's look in a bit more detail at how the body keeps blood sugar levels in check and why erratic blood sugar levels can make us feel so dreadful.

Just as a car is propelled by petrol or diesel and a building is heated by gas or oil, the body is fuelled by glucose, which is converted from the carbohydrates (starchy and sugary foods) in our diet. When the carbohydrates reach the small intestine, enzymes break them down into simple sugars, the majority of which is glucose. The glucose then passes across the gut wall into the bloodstream and, in doing so, it raises the level of blood glucose.

Some glucose will be used right away to keep the body supplied with energy. As it is absorbed, a message is sent to the pancreas to produce insulin, which converts any glucose that isn't needed into glycogen, another kind of fuel that is stored in the muscles and the liver. Then, between meals when food isn't available and blood glucose concentration begins to fall, other hormones – glucagon from the pancreas and adrenalin from the adrenal glands – are called up. They work in the opposite way to insulin, pulling glycogen back out of the liver and muscle stores and turning it back into glucose, so that blood levels remain normal. If glycogen stores are full, any glucose still left over will be converted into a fatty substance known as triglyceride and sent to a different storage area – our body fat. It's not difficult to see that, if this keeps on happening, we could put on weight.

## Diet Right

Controlling blood sugar is all about eating the right foods. Proteins, fats and vegetables don't trigger insulin as carbohydrates do. And some carbohydrates stimulate insulin production far more readily than others.

If you have just eaten some refined food such as white bread, sugar-coated or low-fibre breakfast cereal, chocolate, buns, doughnuts or a sugary drink, glucose is usually pushed very quickly into your bloodstream. This kind of speedy absorption provides instant energy but also demands extra insulin. The result is a bit like burning paper. Unless other slower burning fuel is added, the fire fizzles out. On the other hand, complex starches such as wholemeal pasta, oats, rye, beans, peas and lentils take longer to be broken down and release their natural sugars more slowly; like a log stove that burns gradually and steadily. Glucose doesn't rush so quickly into the blood and less insulin is needed.

---

### Mood and attitude

A side-effect of low blood sugar that is not often considered is mood and attitude. When glucose levels in the blood swing frequently from high to low and back again, periods of irritability and bad temper may alternate with lack of concentration, lethargy and drowsiness. Blood sugar problems have been linked to behavourial problems in young children, and delinquency and aggression in adolescents.

---

## Trigger Happy

If our diet contains too many refined foods, glucose levels may stay high or fluctuate between highs and lows. Either way, the body responds by over-producing insulin; a condition known as hyperinsulinaemia, which I've already mentioned briefly. The poor old pancreas becomes 'trigger happy', squirting out insulin in a vain attempt to get those glucose levels down. But if we keep on eating those unhealthy foods, we just keep putting more pressure on the pancreas. This means that there is nearly always an excess of insulin in the blood which has to be converted into those triglycerides we were talking about earlier and dumped into fatty tissue. Insulin has been called the hormone that makes us fat.

And there's another problem . . .

## Insulin Resistance

Over time, continual over-production of insulin can cause the body to become 'resistant' so that the insulin can no longer lower the glucose levels so efficiently. This is known medically as insulin resistance. When it works properly, insulin has access to a set of keys called insulin receptors which allow it to 'unlock' cells so that the glucose can be pushed inside. If someone is 'insulin resistant', the cells that usually take up and store glucose resist the efforts of the insulin by pushing against the door. The insulin receptors are powerless to help. More insulin is secreted to try to persuade the glucose to move into the cells but this isn't always successful. So glucose builds up in the blood because it has nowhere else to go.

## Long-term Damage

When excess glucose is allowed to float around in the blood on a more or less permanent basis, rogue molecules called free radicals are generated. If left unchecked, they can cause all kinds of havoc. They oxidise our cells, aggravate the ageing process and reduce our immunity to disease. The whole process of oxidative damage could be likened to rusting metal or perished rubber. It's this kind of degeneration that is also associated with some of the complications of diabetes such as furred arteries and damage to the nervous system, the eyes and the kidneys. And all the time, excess glucose keeps on being stored as fat. Eventually, the pancreas and the adrenal glands become exhausted. Either insulin production slows dramatically or the insulin that is already there is much less effective. One way or the other, the early stages of diabetes may be unavoidable.

**High risk**

If you are more than 14 pounds (6.5kg overweight) your risk of becoming diabetic is one in three – or one in two – depending on which research results you believe. Around 80 per cent of all diabetics are already significantly overweight. The risk of type II (adult-onset) diabetes increases as we age. There are already around one and a half million diabetics in the UK, with a further 100 people being diagnosed *every day*!

## Ultra Sensitive?

Doctors have known about insulin resistance for a long time but a new theory is suggesting that people who are insulin resistant might over-produce insulin *particularly dramatically* when they eat any kind of carbohydrates (simple sugary stuff or complex starches such as whole-wheat pasta or brown rice), predisposing them to obesity and diabetes.

One explanation as to why extra glucose is so readily converted into fat stores could be evolution. Remember I mentioned in the chapter on weight loss how, in times of plenty, the body would hang on to excess calories so that it had something to live off when food became scarce? Now there are no lean times, we don't need to store fat. But no one told the pancreas about this change. The trouble is that, because of the tendency that so many of us have to eat too many sugary foods, insulin is still being over-produced, increasing the likelihood of insulin resistance and obesity.

## A Healthy Lifestyle does Reduce Risk

One of the most important ways of fighting insulin resistance is to eat healthily, exercise sensibly every day or every other day, food combine, and get your bodyweight under control. The heavier you are, the less responsive you are likely to be to the glucose-lowering effects of insulin. Losing excess weight helps reduce sensitivity. By taking regular exercise, it seems we help to open up those blocked doorways into muscle cells, allowing insulin to transfer glucose to those cells more effectively. Muscles are big glucose-users because they need lots of energy.

## Confusing and Conflicting Advice

Because of the renewed interest in the link between insulin resistance and diabetes, there is now a new debate raging that the advice to diabetics to eat a diet rich in complex carbohydrates could be wrong. Once upon a time, diabetics were encouraged to eat high-protein diets. Protein certainly sustains the appetite well and reduces the risk of hypo attacks. But too much protein can damage the kidneys, already a potential weak spot in diabetics.

So the advice was turned on its head and complex carbohydrates were the thing. Now they, too, are also under the microscope. Why? Well, if they increase insulin resistance, are they the best thing for diabetes or for anyone with weight problems? Concern has been expressed by some diabetologist researchers that high carbohydrate, low-protein diets could be *more* likely to trigger diabetes than diets that have higher levels of poultry, fish or lean meat.

### Maintaining the status quo?

On the other hand . . .

The majority of health professionals still believe that complex carbohydrates should constitute the bulk of the diet. It's not that they don't see insulin resistance as a problem – estimates suggest it could affect as much as 25 per cent of the population – but they're not convinced that insulin resistance necessarily leads to diabetes in everyone or that the condition is made worse by eating carbohydrates. The jury is still out on this one but, in the meantime, the best advice, as always, is balance. Keeping your blood sugar in shape not only helps you to control your weight, energy levels and brain power, it may also reduce the risk of diabetes and cardiovascular disease.

**Author's note**

Diabetics suffer probably more than any other group as a result of constantly changing dietary advice. Over the years, diabetics have been advised to eat high-protein diets, to avoid high-protein diets, to eat high-carbohydrate diets and, more recently, to reconsider protein yet again. So what about the latest flip-flop that suggests increasing (yes, increasing) fat might be helpful because fat doesn't trigger over-production of insulin? I'd be cautious. Watch this space.

## QUESTIONNAIRE

**How you respond to the following questions should give you a fairly good idea whether or not you are sugar-sensitive:**

- ▶ Do you have a sweet tooth? ☐

- ▶ Do you crave foods like bread, jam, sweet breakfast cereals, cakes and biscuits? ☐

- ▶ Do you feel you could never live without bread? ☐

- ▶ Do you feel you couldn't live without sweet foods? ☐

- ▶ Do you often feel irritable or angry without real cause? ☐

- ▶ Do you feel sluggish and unable to get going first thing in the morning? ☐

- ▶ Do you need coffee, tea or cigarettes to start the day? ☐

- ▶ Are you more than 14 pounds (6.5kg) overweight? ☐

- ▶ Do you have difficulty losing weight? ☐

- ▶ Do you diet regularly for weight loss? ☐

▶ Do you suffer with an energy slump mid-morning or after lunch? ☐

▶ Do you *really need* your cup of coffee or tea mid-morning? ☐

**If you go for more than three hours without eating, do you:**

▶ Suffer from mood swings? ☐

▶ Feel irritable for no apparent reason? ☐

▶ Feel shivery? ☐

▶ Feel hollow in the stomach? ☐

▶ Find it difficult to concentrate? ☐

▶ Bump into things or drop things more often than usual? ☐

▶ Feel very thirsty? ☐

▶ Yawn? ☐

▶ Feel spaced-out? ☐

▶ Suffer dizziness? ☐

▶ Forget things? ☐

▶ Have difficulty focusing? ☐

▶ Get a headache? ☐

If you answered 'yes' to more than six of the above questions, there's a likelihood that your body is struggling to maintain a stable blood sugar. Following the advice in this chapter should help to eradicate these symptoms.

## Reasons for Susceptibility to Blood Sugar Imbalance

No one really knows why some people are more susceptible to blood sugar imbalances than others. However, there are a number of possible factors.

### Dieting

Dieters are definitely a high-risk group. If you are 'always on a diet', the chances are that you are either not eating enough or you're filling up on foods that provide fast-releasing sugars, such as white bread, white rice, low-fibre cereals, buns, cakes, chocolate – or both. Either way, it's likely that your blood sugar will be swinging violently between high and low, putting a strain on your adrenal glands, pancreas and the production of the blood sugar hormones that are trying to keep your system in balance.

### Missing meals

It's easy if you're extra busy to miss a meal and tell yourself it doesn't matter. Occasionally, it's fine – if you *don't* have a blood sugar problem, that is. If you have a tendency to hypo, it's especially important to eat proper meals on a regular basis.

### A fondness for sugar

If you have a sweet tooth, you don't need me to tell you how difficult it can be to say no to the dessert, the biscuits with the coffee or the cake at teatime. But sugar isn't just 'pure, white and deadly', it can be pure, brown and deadly too. It's the one food where being brown doesn't make it healthier, unless it is unrefined dark molasses or dark cold-pressed raw honey, both of which do contain some trace nutrients. Refined sugar provides the body with nothing more than empty calories. It has absolutely no nutritional value of its own and is well known for robbing the body of vitamins and minerals because it uses up such a lot of them during absorption. Stacks of sugary foods in your diet also put a real strain on all the blood sugar machinery, and could be programming your body for a diabetes diagnosis later in life.

It can be truly worthwhile – and a real long-term health investment – to cut right back on the sweet stuff. Keep a food diary for a week and then be honest about how much sugar you have eaten. It can sometimes be quite a shock to see it all there in one list. Then, over the next few months, be systematic about reducing your intake. Be aware that sweetened yoghurts, cola, 'fruit' drinks, canned foods, breakfast cereals and bottled sauces often contain lots of sneaky sugar.

## Artificial sweeteners

Don't be tempted to turn to artificial sweeteners because you think they are healthier than sugar. Studies suggest that they can disturb the appetite just as much as sugar.

## Stimulants

In reasonable, sensible amounts, coffee, tea, cola, alcohol and salt are unlikely to cause severe health problems – but in excess, they put just as much strain on the system as sugar does. Enjoy – but go for the healthiest alternatives whenever you can. Use my **Swap Sheet** (pages 80–1) as a guide to upgrade the quality of your food and drink.

## Vitamin and mineral deficiency

Low levels of some nutrients can increase the risk of blood sugar imbalances. The B group of vitamins are essential for the release of energy but are often destroyed by cooking and food processing. Wholefoods contain far richer supplies of B vits than their factory-refined relations. One way to increase intake of the B complex group is to cut right back on processed and packaged foods, ready meals and anything that is 'fortified' or 'enriched' (terms that usually indicate food that needed unnatural improvement!), and increase intake of wholegrains, nuts, seeds, vegetables, fish, eggs, yoghurt, peas and beans.

The minerals chromium, magnesium, manganese and zinc are vital for a long list of body processes including blood glucose balance. However, studies show they are often at below normal levels in the average diet. Chromium, in particular, is an essential part of the insulin pathway and, yet, is often found to be depleted.

### Mineral-rich foods to choose from:

All the foods listed here are rich in the minerals needed to support the body's glucose mechanism. Including more of them regularly in your diet could help to improve blood sugar control. If they are not part of your regular shop already, why not add at least some of the following to your weekly menu?

| | |
|---|---|
| Almonds | Ginger (fresh root) |
| Apples | Grapefruit |
| Asparagus | Honey (cold-pressed) |
| Avocado | Lamb (lean) |
| Beetroot (raw) | Lamb's liver |
| Blackberries | Lemon juice (fresh) |
| Blackstrap molasses | Olives |
| Brazil nuts | Peas and beans |
| Cashew nuts | Pineapple |
| Cheese (good-quality) | Pumpkin seeds |
| Chestnuts | Sea vegetables (including seaweed |
| Chicken (free-rangeand organic) | and spirulina) |
| Coconut | Shellfish |
| Eggs (free-range andorganic) | Vegetables (green leafy) |
| Fish | Wholegrains (especially oats, brown |
| Fruits (dried) | rice, whole rye and wholewheat pasta) |

Unfortunately, chromium is not well absorbed from food. It has, in fact, been suggested that only around 2 per cent of the chromium in our diet might actually be utilised. Up to 80 per cent of chromium can be lost as a result of food processing, making people who use a lot of processed food more at risk. Long-term illness, pregnancy, diabetes, prolonged stress, excessive exercise and repeated low-calorie dieting all call heavily upon chromium reserves. To make matters worse, we absorb less chromium as we age and store less reserves of it in our tissues. So, at the time of life when we are most at risk from conditions such as adult onset diabetes, one of the most important – potentially protective – minerals is in short supply. Because chromium is so hard to come by, it is often recommended that those with blood glucose problems take a chromium supplement. In studies where chromium supplements were given to patients with non-insulin dependent diabetes, they reported significantly improved diabetic control. I used to suffer quite seriously with hypoglycaemia in my teens and twenties, but have had no further problems since taking a six-month course of chromium polynicotinate.

**Vitamin C** is needed for hundreds of different body processes. One of them is converting food substances into energy. Most fresh vegetables and fruit contain vitamin C. In addition, it can be worth taking a vitamin C supplement. (I take at least one gram (1000mg) a day and double up if I'm travelling and exposed to traffic pollution – or have stressful deadlines to meet.)

**Vitamin E**, like vitamin C, is known as an antioxidant nutrient that helps protect cells against the degeneration caused by free radicals. In particular, vitamin E has been shown to dramatically reduce the risk of heart disease. If the levels of vitamin E in blood serum are low, the likelihood of heart problems is that much greater. Insulin resistance is known to be associated with cardiovascular disease, high blood pressure and elevated blood fats. Since recent studies continue to recommend the use of vitamin E in reducing cardiovascular disease, and since insulin is known to deplete vitamin E, nutrition experts are suggesting that those with blood sugar problems take extra vitamin E in supplement form. The amount usually recommended is 200iu–300iu daily.

---

**IMPORTANT NOTE**

Anyone taking anti-clotting medication should consult their doctor before taking supplements. Diabetic patients should supplement chromium and other nutrients *only under medical supervision.*

---

## Medication

Some types of prescribed medicines can disturb blood glucose balance in those who are ultra sensitive. If you are experiencing any of the hypoglycaemic symptoms listed on page 302 and are taking diuretics, tranquillisers, the contraceptive pill or hormone replacement therapy, ask your health centre, surgery or hospital clinic for advice.

## Stress

Unrelenting negative stress puts a huge strain on the adrenal glands which are, remember, responsible for producing the hormones that raise blood glucose. If you are suffering from exhaustion, overwork, low back pain, indigestion, palpitations, irritability, or any other stress-related symptoms such as difficulty sleeping or relaxing, it could be that your adrenals are trying to tell you something. The adrenal glands are the body's shock absorbers. When they are overworked or worn out, we lose our ability to cope not only with stressful situations but with everyday life events. However, squandered adrenals can be restored if the body is fed with less junk, especially less sugar and other stimulants, and is supported by good stress management, a nourishing diet and, if necessary, good-quality supplements. Try the advice in this book and also take the opportunity to talk to your doctor or health centre about stress management. More on coping with stress on pages 301–15.

## Family history

It is generally accepted that diabetes runs in families. It may also jump a generation. But no one really knows if the same can be said of insulin resistance or reactive hypoglycaemia. If you have a weight problem or have been suffering with any of the symptoms listed on page 302, do please talk to your doctor. *In particular, if you have a family history of diabetes and are also experiencing unquenchable thirst, unexplained weight loss or weight gain, tiredness, tingling or numbness in the limbs or itchy skin, you should see your doctor without further delay.*

# Help for the Hypo

The good news amongst all the gloom that I've just been giving you is that reactive hypoglycaemia is not difficult to treat. Some experts are convinced that it only survives and thrives because of our dependence upon high sugar diets. The information given below has helped many people overcome blood sugar problems. I hope it will help you too.

## MY TRIED AND TESTED TIPS FOR BALANCING BLOOD SUGAR

### Make an appointment with your doctor

Don't forget that the first thing you need to do if you suspect blood sugar problems of any kind is to see your doctor. A simple test of urine and blood, carried out at the surgery, is all that is needed to confirm or eliminate diabetes. If you have a family history of diabetes, you should be tested regularly. It's easy to detect high levels because when glucose stays high all or most of the time, it spills over into the urine. Detecting reactive hypoglycaemia is not always so simple. So, if symptoms persist, further more detailed tests may be required. Because of the erratic nature of low blood sugar, a single blood test is unlikely to be sufficient or accurate enough to tell you whether you are hypoglycaemic or not. A standard glucose tolerance test (GTT) may not be conclusive because it measures only glucose. Some practitioners suggest that the glucose insulin tolerance test (G/ITT) is more accurate and reliable.

### Food combine

Try it. I've seen it help many people to get their blood sugar under control.

### Never miss breakfast

It really is important. A decent amount of food at the start of the day can keep you going until lunchtime. If you honestly can't face food first thing, at least have a piece of fresh fruit and then eat a late breakfast or early lunch when you feel more like it.

### Don't miss out on lunch or your evening meal

It's easy to convince yourself that, if reducing calories is supposed to encourage weight loss, then missing a meal altogether could mean faster results. Not so. Regular meals encourage more efficient metabolism and better calorie burning. They are also one of the best ways to beat cravings, especially if you avoid the common allergens listed on page 211. Choosing foods that satisfy the appetite and sustain you for longer periods does not mean that you will put on weight. In fact, the opposite is more likely. And, if your appetite is satisfied, you are far less likely to hanker after snack foods. Research also shows that meals taken in smaller amounts, but more frequently, are better not just for balancing weight but for cholesterol levels, too.

### Eat good-quality protein

This does not mean eating large quantities of meat or fat. Free-range chicken and eggs, fish, pulses, yoghurt and good-quality cheeses are all excellent protein sources that don't put a strain on insulin production and so keep blood glucose on an even keel. Because proteins help to sustain the appetite for longer periods, they also reduce the risk of our reaching for not-so-healthy quick fix snacks.

### Use cold-pressed oils

Use extra-virgin olive oil for cooking and other cold-pressed oils such as safflower, sesame and walnut for dressings. Special nutrients known as essential fatty acids (see page 144) in vegetable and seed oils are believed to be beneficial to blood glucose balance.

### Eat proteins at breakfast and/or lunch

Those who suffer with hypoglycaemia often say that eating protein foods earlier in the day – for example, scrambled or boiled eggs for breakfast, fish or chicken for lunch – helps them to stay more energised and alert. Because starchy foods are more calming, potato, rice and pasta dishes may be better eaten later in the day. Include plenty of pulses and wholegrains in your diet. They release their fuel more slowly into the body, helping to keep glucose levels in check.

## Eat fresh vegetables and salad foods

Whatever your main ingredients, always add plenty of fresh vegetable and salad foods. Apart from containing many of the nutrients needed to balance blood glucose, they also have valuable dietary fibre which does the same.

## Eat more dietary fibre

Brown rice, oat bran, pulses, seeds (especially linseeds), psyllium husk, fresh vegetables, fresh fruit and dried fruit are more effective and more gentle than coarse wheat-bran fibre. They make you feel fuller for longer and, again, help to control your blood glucose levels.

## Don't be regulated by someone else's mealtimes

If you are genuinely hungry, eat something. If a meal is only minutes away and you are tempted to snack on junk while you're waiting, a glass of water can, temporarily, stave off hunger pangs. Diluted fruit juice can give a quick boost and is good to drink while you are waiting for a meal to be served. But don't drink fruit juice with other foods.

## Dilute your juices

Pure fruit juice is a healthier and delicious alternative to squashes or colas, but because it's no longer buffered by the fibre that is found in the whole fruit, it can still cause rapid changes in blood sugar. Make it less concentrated by topping up half a glass of juice with filtered or bottled water.

## Improve your digestion

If you're sure that you are eating a good-sized meal but are still feeling hollow or spaced-out soon afterwards, then it could be that you're not digesting or absorbing your food very well. The information on pages 168–70 will help you to decide if your digestive system is working properly or not.

### Avoid foods that are made with refined sugar and white flour

Nothing pushes up glucose levels faster than sugary baked goods, soft drinks and sweets. They release their energy too quickly into the system and can aggravate hypoglycaemic symptoms.

### Consider the possibility of food intolerances

Sensitivity to certain foods is believed to aggravate – or may even be the cause of – hypoglycaemia in some people. Common problem foods include bread, wheat-based or corn-based breakfast cereals, sugary breakfast cereals, anything made with wheat flour such as cakes, biscuits and buns, baker's and brewer's yeast, eggs, cow's milk, cow's milk cheese, packaged orange juice, coffee and chocolate. (See pages 202–18 for more information.)

### Snack before bedtime

If you eat supper early in the evening take a light snack, such as yoghurt or crispbread, about an hour before bed. This helps to keep blood glucose balanced during the night. Avoid heavy meals late at night.

### Go easy on the alcohol

And don't drink on an empty stomach. Drink wine with meals but steer clear of beer and spirits. Alcohol can interfere with the liver's ability to release sugar stores and keep blood glucose in balance.

### Keep healthy snacks nearby

If you can reach for fresh or dried fruit, Brazil nuts, almonds or pumpkin seeds, you'll be less interested in cream cakes and doughnuts. If a sweet tooth lets you down, choose natural liquorice, dried figs, sesame halva or wholegrain cereal bars (all available in health stores) instead of boiled sweets or chocolate.

## Try giving up coffee

Some sufferers say that it makes hypos – and cravings – worse. If you are a regular coffee drinker, ease off slowly; otherwise you could experience withdrawal from the caffeine. Don't go for decaf as an alternative. Coffee contains around 500 chemicals and some of these can be just as stimulating as caffeine. Decaffeinated coffee may be no better for you; the manufacturing process uses chemicals that are also used for degunking cars. It's best to dump the instant stuff altogether and find an alternative beverage. Enjoy real filtered coffee as an occasional treat.

## Watch that cola

Be aware that cola is not only high in sugar but also in caffeine. Low-cal fizzy drinks are sweetened artificially and are therefore best avoided.

## Don't forget to watch out for salty foods

Salt can upset blood glucose just as much as too much sugar. Remember to look out for the 'hidden' salt that is added to so many packaged foods.

## Take supplements

Add a one-a-day multi-supplement and 500–1000 milligrams of extra vitamin C to your diet. A good multi should include vitamin A, vitamin E, the B group, and minerals, especially chromium, magnesium, manganese and zinc. My own clinical experience is confirmed by a number of other practitioners and by nutritional research that, even when the diet is of very high quality, additional supplements can be extremely helpful in restoring blood glucose balance. Health stores have a good range of specialist supplements. Worthwhile products usually cost more because they are backed up by good research and development and contain high-quality ingredients. So buy the best that you can afford. The address list on page 400 can help you to find stockists.

## Understanding the GI Factor

A new yardstick for measuring the effect that foods have on your blood sugar is called the glycaemic index or GI factor. You may have read about this in a women's or health magazine recently. We are now being beseeched by a variety of different health gurus to remember the GI rating of every food. This is, of course, in addition to committing calories and fat grams to memory, along with a whole load of other nutrition cautions and exhortations that come our way almost daily. Here's what it's all about.

For several years now, health experts have advised that wholegrain products, pasta, oats and pulses, all known as complex carbohydrates, are better for us than simple carbohydrates (refined, processed and sugary foods). This is because complex carbohydrates release their natural sugars more slowly into the bloodstream and don't cause rapid or wild fluctuations in blood glucose.

More recently, scientists have found that even some of the complex carbohydrates that we thought were OK have glycaemic ratings high enough to disturb the levels of a particular type of cholesterol known as high-density lipo-protein or HDL cholesterol. HDL is the good guy in the cholesterol story. Unlike its sticky, we-could-do-with-less-of-it partner, low-density lipo-protein or LDL, we need HDL because it helps to keep LDL under control. We've all been told that fat, especially saturated fat, increases LDL and, as a result, multiplies the likelihood of heart disease. Some researchers now think that wayward glucose levels and excess insulin production upset HDL so much that they could be strong predictors of whether or not we keel over prematurely with a heart attack – even more so than fat! – which is why they are worried about the glycaemic rating of particular foods.

The discovery adds yet another complication to the ever-changing guidelines on what we should be eating to stay healthy.

It's an unfortunate fact of life that, because nutritional advice takes so many U-turns, it's difficult to know whether the glycaemic theory is worth following or not – or if someone else in another lab in another part of the world is going to go public tomorrow with a completely opposite view that is just as scientifically valid as all the ones that have gone before. And another possible downside to this latest research is the way in which different people have interpreted it.

## Let's Look at How it Works

In the world of glycaemic indices, foods are usually rated from 1 to 100. Anything below 50 is said to be good GI food because it releases its natural sugars slowly into the system and doesn't over-stretch those blood sugar hormones. Foods that score between 50 and 70 should not be eaten too frequently and only then with a low-scoring (below 50) food. All foods above 70 are really best avoided but may (or may not) be OK (depending upon which GI book or article you are following) if they are also mixed with a low-scoring food.

The ratings are worked out on the basis of what type of carbohydrate each food contains and how quickly the simple starches in that particular food are absorbed. High glycaemic carbohydrates are characterised by a rapid rise in glucose levels and a correspondingly rapid production of insulin. The serious aspect of all this is, as I explained earlier on, that if the food we eat produces lots of glucose and lots of insulin at more or less every meal, it's likely to result in increased insulin resistance which, in turn, increases the risk of a number of health problems.

It should come as no surprise to find that refined, processed or fibre-stripped foods, such as white bread, sugary breakfast cereals, white rice, cakes and biscuits attract a high score because they contain starches that are fast releasing. (This is not new knowledge. We've known for years that these foods are not healthy.) All proteins have low scores – less than 50 – because cheese, eggs, chicken, fish and soya don't trigger an insulin response.

Nothing wrong with any of that except . . .

## It's not a very reliable system

To begin with, the scoring is not consistent. I have come across several different GI lists that clearly don't agree with each other. For example, sugar shows up in one list as 75 (in other words, avoid it), and in another list as 59 (OK if you mix it with something). A third glycaemic directory uses figures above 100 for some foods and scores maltose (a type of sugar) at 152! White spaghetti rates at 50 in one index and 65 in another. Frosties get a 70, which you would expect because each packet contains nearly 50 per cent pure sugar. But Shredded Wheat, which we all know is advertised as completely sugar-free (and has been marketed on the basis that it supports heart health!), is only marginally better for us at 67. Then, most suprisingly, brown rice logs in at 66. But in many cultures and dietary systems, for example in macrobiotic philosophy, brown rice is considered to be one of the most balanced of foods.

## Fruit is a sticky one to deal with

The predominant sugar in most fruit is fructose. It has a similar chemical structure to glucose but doesn't need insulin to be absorbed, so it doesn't put anything like the same strain on the pancreas as sucrose or glucose. That's a fact of life whether you are a GI convert or not. As a result of their fructose level, grapefruit, apples and oranges are classed as low scorers. But, in addition to fructose, other fruit (pineapples, melon, bananas) also contain glucose and so, we are warned, they attract a higher rating. It would be easy to get the idea that, because of this scoring system, we should eat only fructose-rich, low-scoring fruit and ignore the rest. And yet common sense tells us that all fruit, whatever its type, is one of the most nourishing foods around.

### It gets even more confusing

How about grapes? Surely, they must be OK because, at a score of 46, they fall well below the threshold of 50. But you'd be wrong. In another list they are 62, accompanied by instructions reminding us that grapes contain glucose and shouldn't be eaten on their own. Sure, half-a-dozen grapes will whiz through the system pretty quickly, but a good-sized bunch of grapes can make a healthy light breakfast or sustaining snack. And other research has found that grapes contain a natural chemical called resveratrol that might be protective against cancer. Grapes are also brilliant foods for cleansing the system and figure in my detox programme (see page 231).

## Low numbers are better than high numbers

To be fair, the rules do tell us that high-rated foods are less of a problem if they are mixed with low-rated foods, i.e. new potatoes (70) are OK as long as they are accompanied by carrots (49) or peas (40). But how is it that a jacket potato attracts a whopping don't-touch-it-with-a-bargepole rating of 95, along with French baguettes and – you'll never guess what – Lucozade! This is despite recent research from Australia that showed potatoes, baked in their jackets or boiled in their skins, are three times more satisfying than white bread. And yet most GI listings have white bread scoring better than potatoes!

I thought that the humble spud, especially with its skin, was good solid nourishment. The various compilers of the glycaemic scoring system obviously can't agree one way or another. Although one list does advise that potatoes with skins attract a lower rating than those without, another doesn't differentiate at all between skins on and skins off.

We are supposed to guess, I guess.

Yet another tells us that baked potato (again we are left to wonder whether or not skins are included) scores 135, in between sugar at 138 and honey at 126.

Oh, for goodness sake!

What it probably comes down to is that boiled potatoes may be better than a baked potato because some of the starch that contributes to its high rating is lost in the cooking water. New potatoes, which are less starchy than old potatoes, are better still if cooked and eaten in their skins. Baked potatoes in their jackets should attract a lower score if you eat the skin because the extra fibre slows up the absorption rate.

OK, let's cut to the chase. We've been told for ages that brown foods are supposed to be better than white. Then the glycaemic index comes along. It confirms that refined foods are bad for us – so far so good. But could someone tell me, please, how a Mars bar at 68 can attract a rating nearly the same as a high-fibre muesli (66)? Any dietary advice that tells me chocolate and sugar have better scores than jacket potatoes and sweetcorn has me confused and bemused.

## Bad reputations

The upshot is that foods we once thought were good for us have had their reputation smeared by GI. In fact, the whole glycaemic concept has developed an inference that foods scoring above 50 are harmful in some way and that we should concentrate on those that score 49 or less. But I find it bothersome that, as there are so many potentially nourishing foods that score higher than 50, this could lead to a diet that lacks variety.

## What about nutritional value?

The most disturbing thing about this system is that it pays no heed to a food's nutritional value. Parsnips are a no-no at 97, but carrots are cool at 49. 'Ninety-seven' in GI-speak tells us that we shouldn't eat parsnips on their own and that they are better for our blood sugar if they're mixed with a low-scoring food. Such as roast chicken, perhaps? Or other vegetables? I don't see this as a problem, do you? How many people have you spotted since, say, last Christmas, chomping a parsnips-only meal or yum-yumming over a raw parsnip instead of a doughnut? It's nonsense that we should give up parsnips because they might give us heart disease and switch to carrots because they don't. Parsnips are not only rich in dietary fibre, they're loaded with nourishment. Apart from worthwhile amounts of calcium and magnesium, they're an especially valuable source of beta-carotene and of folic acid (a nutrient now known to be protective against neural tube defects *and* – guess what? – heart disease).

Sweetcorn is said to have a similar glycaemic profile to parsnips and to chocolate. Oh, dear. No more parsnip-flavoured, chocolate-covered corn-on-the-cob for me, then.

## Where Does GI Fit Into Food Combining?

You could say I'm biased because GI is difficult to follow if you're a food combiner. The glycaemic index suggests that the fast-releasing sugars in high-rated foods, such as cereals, will be slowed down if they're mixed with milk and that potatoes are less likely to disturb blood glucose if they are eaten with chicken or fish; in other words, mixing proteins with starches. If you are not a food combiner you're probably doing this already. Unless you eat your breakfast cereal dry, your parsnips all by themselves, and your baguette without any kind of filling, chances are that you will already be mixing high-scoring foods with low-scoring ones, which makes a bit of a nonsense of having an index in the first place.

Food combiners are no more at risk from eating too many high-scoring foods than anyone else. The whole essence of food combining is that it achieves balance. Food combining law wouldn't be recommending a diet of chocolate, refined breakfast cereals, sugar or jelly beans anyway. And if a recipe recommends a jacket potato, it's nearly always going to be accompanied by another food such as hummus (made from chickpeas), avocado or baked beans – all low-scoring foods. Rice, for example, would be slowed down by pulses or salad. *The Complete Book of Food Combining* leads you away from high-scoring starches and encourages you towards a more natural diet of lean proteins, vegetables, pulses and fruit. As anti-food-combining ammunition, the glycaemic index just doesn't hold up.

## Individual Needs are Important

There is plenty of evidence that a high-carbohydrate diet can encourage insulin resistance, hypoglycaemia and weight problems in some people. If you have a serious blood sugar imbalance, or if you're involved in an intensive training programme and need to keep a tight watch on blood glucose balance during exercise, I can see that this index may be useful. But I think it is misleading to suggest that everyone should live by it. The concept is good but the scoring system stinks. I have a rule about new fads and crazes. Leave them alone until they are proved, either by long-term usage or several consistent scientific studies, to be safe and successful.

And whether or not you believe that eating apples instead of potatoes is going to reduce your chances of an early demise, there is never going to be one diet or one piece of dietary advice that will suit every single person on the planet. Just because I have seen amazing successes brought about by food combining (effective weight loss, improved energy levels, better digestion, better elimination and less likelihood of food intolerance are just a few), it doesn't mean that I support it exclusively at the expense of other dietary ideals. But it has to be said that food combining has an excellent track record and, as a result of years of positive feedback, we know it works well for a great many people.

We are all different and all of us have individual nutritional needs. In the same way that I don't believe everyone needs to food combine, it is also the case that not all of us have an insulin problem and not everyone needs to follow a low-carbohydrate diet. I leave you to make your own judgements.

If you think the glycaemic index might work for you, by all means give it a try but do take care not to restrict your diet. Whatever dietary system you choose to follow, the keys to success are moderation, variety and flexibility.

# 15

# Easy Ways to Ease the Effects of Stress

**Stress** *noun*, strain; a constraining influence; physical, emotional or mental pressure

**stress'or** *noun*, an agent or factor that causes stress

**stressed-out** *adjective (colloquial)*, exhausted or incapacitated by psychological stress

Why is it that some people seem to suffer so much as a result of stress, while others in more or less the same situations appear to cope well with life's ups and downs? The answer could lie not so much in the type or the level of stress, but in how well the body handles it. Stress isn't actually caused by any particular event or experience but by how a person perceives the situation. To a certain extent, how we cope with stressful situations is, like so much else in our lives, determined by our genetic make-up and family history. However, it is also true that exhaustion, overwork, low self-esteem, poor health and poor eating habits can leave us less able to deal with life's ups and downs.

Introducing food combining into your life is one good way to improve the level of nourishment your body receives and so help guard against the damaging effects of stress.

# Investigating Stress

Stress, whether it's physical, mental or emotional, is said to be a leading cause of illness. Some experts have suggested that the effects of prolonged negative stress could cause more health problems than poor diet and lack of exercise put together. We all know of people who have eaten terrible food, high in fat and sugar, never done a stroke of exercise, smoked heavily and consumed vast quantities of alcohol, but lived long and apparently healthy lives because they appeared to be unaffected by stress. Then there are other perpetually anxious and frazzled types who seem to do all the right things, eat sensibly, exercise daily, never smoke, drink only moderately or not at all, and yet suffer with all manner of health disorders. Contrarily irritating, isn't it?

## Signs of stress

### Physical symptoms associated with stress:

Body odour

Chronic fatigue

Cramps

Diarrhoea

Food cravings

Headaches

High blood pressure

Indigestion or heartburn

Jaw pain

Joint and muscle pains

Lack of appetite

Loss of interest in sex

Muscle spasms

Nail biting

Neck tension

Palpitations

Poor co-ordination

Problems sleeping

Reduced resistance to infections

Restless limbs

Sour breath

Sweating

Tearfulness

### Mental and emotional symptoms associated with stress:

Being argumentative

Being irritable with others

Feeling neglected

Feeling spaced-out

Being irritable with yourself      Inability to concentrate

Depression      Loss of self-esteem

Fear of being alone      Mood swings

Fear of closed spaces      Not enjoying yourself

Fear of disease      Not wanting to join in

Fear of failure      Poor memory

Fear of open spaces

## So How Does Stress Wreak Such Havoc?

The body responds to stressful events by releasing a whole range of substances including hormones and neurotransmitters which interact with cells in the immune system. Moderate levels of certain types of stress – such as sensible levels of exercise, laughter or occasional crying – are believed to have a beneficial effect on immunity but prolonged and persistent stress will have the opposite effect, suppressing resistance and leaving us more prone to illness.

## Stress on the Increase?

We're all familiar with the classic list of stressors that includes death of a loved one, divorce, separation, moving house, serious accident or illness and unemployment. But what about those other everyday hassles that can wind us up into a serious frenzy? How about the stress of being late, not being able to find a parking space or getting a parking fine? Or computer stress. You're writing an important document on your computer and it crashes half-way through, or you start to download information you need urgently from the Web and then get a little screen message telling you it's only going to take another 38 minutes! There are other things that can get us down on a daily basis, too, such as arguments at work or at home, or noisy neighbours. More seriously, stress can be caused or compounded by bullying, harassment, discrimination, violence or abuse, excessive exercise programmes or extreme dieting. Any kind of stressful situation that is ongoing and has no let-up is likely to have a negative effect on our immunity. Chronic negative stress also shuts down the digestive system so that, if we eat when we are stressed, we don't properly digest or absorb the nutrients from our food.

## Stress Can Make Us Fat

If we are exposed to long and unrelenting periods of stress, we may not feel like eating and so could find ourselves losing weight. Short bursts of stress can have the opposite effect, causing appetite-stimulating hormones to flood the blood and brain, encouraging attacks of comfort eating or bingeing. The situation isn't helped by the fact that sweet and starchy foods – such as cakes, biscuits, ice cream and choco-late – have a calming effect on the body. That's why we so often find ourselves craving for those not-so-healthy foods when we are going through a bad patch. Stress can also promote the storage of fat. More stress hormones hang around in abdominal fat than in any other fatty areas of the body.

## All in the Family?

Our reactions to stress can also have a lot to do with heredity. We are likely to inherit either laid-back or coiled-spring traits from one or both of our parents. But, having said that, good nutrition and lifestyle habits adopted now can go a long way to protect our bodies from the dam-aging effects of stress, as well as improving our response to stressful life events. Eating right is vital at any time of life but is especially important if we are under pressure. Unfortunately, the irony of stress-ful situations is that the quality of our diets can plummet at the very time our nutritional needs are highest.

# Coping with Stress

For many of us, looking after ourselves properly, taking time off, or allowing ourselves some personal space without feeling guilty isn't always a simple matter. There are so many unavoidable and time-consuming commitments that come first in our lives. Like a runaway train, we can't stop even if we want to. And if we're particularly stressed, it can seem an impossible task to 'let up and let go'.

Suggest to someone that 'quiet time' is important and most people will laugh at the suggestion. Not because they don't think it's important, but because they see it as unachievable. It's true that the peace and tranquillity of being responsible only to ourselves is something that few of us seem to manage these days. There is always so much to do, and so many other people who demand our attention, that we often reach bedtime with no time left for ourselves.

It's a familiar scenario. And sometimes it can get out of hand. It's almost as if we are being held to ransom by other people's needs. You don't have enough time to pace *yourself* properly and do things for *you* but you're always available when someone else shouts. Your boss, a neighbour in need, your children, your partner, an elderly relative. 'Could you just . . .?' 'It'll only be for an hour or two.' 'Can you take me to . . .' Your inner voice responds with 'I can't let them down' or 'I'll feel guilty if I don't' or 'What will they think/do/say if I say "no"?' So you go right along getting more and more stressed, speeding up the vicious cycle. If this sounds like you, don't despair.

Here are a whole heap of ideas that are designed either directly to lighten your load, or to help support and protect your body against the effects of stress and overwork. See which ones fit best into your lifestyle and then introduce one positive change at a time.

## MY TIPS FOR FORTIFYING YOUR STRESS DEFENCES

### Food combine

If your digestion is good and your body well-nourished, you'll be much more able to cope with the effects of stress. So go on, de-stress those insides!

### Breathe properly

Right now, before you do anything else, check your breathing. Shallow or rapid breathing increases anxiety. Throughout the day, bring your thoughts back to your breathing. Take a *s-l-o-w* deep breath and let out a huge sigh. Be aware of how calming this can be. Read the information on pages 262–72 about the health benefits of proper breathing.

## Be unavailable once in a while

It's not a crime. Proper rest and relaxation are as important as regular exercise and a healthy diet. At a lecture I once attended on stress management, the main speaker opened his talk with this sentence. 'The inability to say "No" could be one of the greatest health hazards of our time.' He went on to explain that people who don't give themselves space often do so on the basis that they believe themselves to be far less important than those they are putting first. But by not giving themselves any kind of 'quiet time', they are leaving their own health at severe risk, increasing the chance that they won't stay well enough or live long enough to be there for other people anyway.

## Prioritise your day

Give all tasks a rating from one to five. Anything with a top priority rating is number one on your list of must-dos, but jobs with a three, four or five rating really don't need your immediate or urgent attention. *They really don't.* If you have difficulty deciding what's important and what is not, simply ask yourself if leaving the task undone is going to make a seriously important or life-threatening difference to you or your loved ones today, tomorrow, next year or in a hundred years' time.

## Don't overload your day

Leave an extra five or ten minutes between appointments to allow for hold-ups.

## Take a break

Don't spend hour after hour in front of your computer terminal or at the wheel of your car without taking proper and regular breaks.

## Programme your leisure time in advance

Don't look upon relaxation and recreation as luxuries; treat them as necessary parts of a healthy lifestyle. It isn't enough to assume that you might have a few minutes' unwinding time at the end of the day if you're not too busy. Make sure you plan your free time as carefully as you would a business appointment.

## Make self-care an important part of your routine

Book yourself a regular massage or reflexology session. Take yourself off to the hair or beauty salon. Make time for a pampering session at home. A deeply soothing and relaxing bath, a manicure or a facial can do wonders for your self-esteem and your coping skills.

## Recognise your stressors

What is it that stresses and worries you the most? By acknowledging the factors in our lives that cause us the most anxiety, we can deal with them more easily. Worrying wastes time and rarely achieves anything. When we're anxious and stressed, we're far less productive and so we manage our time less efficiently. If you're always tired, don't sleep well, sigh a lot or get bored easily, stress could be the cause.

## Get help online

If you don't know what is causing your stress or are really flummoxed as to how best to deal with your situation, have some stress-free fun online. There are plenty of interesting websites that offer advice on how to recognise stress and how to improve the way we cope with its effects. How about *www.stresstips.com/physical_stresstest.htm* – an interactive stress test that gives a summary of your condition. Or *www.optinutri.com/test.htm* – a question-and-answer session which will warn you if your nutritional status isn't up to scratch. You could take a look at www.drkoop.com – an advice and news site with emphasis on how stress can lead to depression. Or learn how to slow down by studying *www.theflow.org/meditate.htm* – a site offering an array of different meditation techniques.

### Don't let your imagination get the better of you

When we're stressed, our reasoning and perspective goes out of the window and we begin to create all kinds of unlikely scenarios in our minds. Assess the situation realistically and remind yourself that worst case scenarios hardly ever happen.

### Talk over your worries with a friend

Choose a person who knows you well – outside your family. Someone you can trust – but who is not going to be influenced or biased – can often put your anxieties into perspective and decide whether or not your fears are exaggerated.

### Think hard about what worrying does to you

It is a completely wasted emotion. Be concerned about important issues such as the health and welfare of your family and friends, but don't let anxiety eat away at your life and your emotions. Take it from one who knows. I was born a worrier and will always be one. It's probably in the genes. I worry mostly about things beyond my control such as war, famine, injustice, cruelty, destruction of the environment and what a needless waste it all is. But I'm far less anxious about things now than I was in my teens, twenties and thirties. I always keep in mind the advice of the world-famous healer Matthew Manning who asks you to ask yourself 'Did worrying all night make any difference?'. Ask yourself if it is going to matter in a hundred years' time? Or in a hundred hours or a hundred minutes? A better approach is to live life as you would wish the whole world to live theirs, with kindness, gentility, loyalty and fairness. One person's actions do make a difference to the bigger picture. *Small pebble thrown into small pond make big splash and big ripple.*

### Get walking

It's one of the best de-stressors. Before you start work in the morning, or sometime during the evening, go for a walk around the block.

Check the distance. A mile (1.6 kilometres), at a reasonable pace, should take 15–20 minutes. A slower stroll, just over half an hour. Make it your quiet time. Don't think about work or worry about anything while you're walking. Even wet weather doesn't need to beat you. Just don some waterproof boots and a raincoat, and go for it. Being outside has other benefits too. Natural light is known to improve mood. It also seems to strengthen our resistance to stress. If it's dark or impossibly inclement, I'll do indoor exercises on my rowing bike or rebounder. Daily exercise like this gets the circulation moving, makes the skin glow, and improves concentration and efficiency during the day. Once you start, you get hooked. It's really great fun and something to look forward to. And you can make time for it.

## Use an atomiser

If you're flagging over the task in hand, need a break and can't get one, feel hot or flustered or just need a lift, spray your face with an atomiser. Use one that contains either water with uplifting essential oils or a mineral water spray. Page 341 has some suggestions.

## Let water out and take water in

Go to the bathroom/washroom. Empty your bladder. Wash your hands. And then savour a long drink of water.

## Take definite meal breaks

Try to take breaks away from your working area. Is there a grassy area, park bench or garden where you could take your lunch on a fine day? Eating standing up or on the move can play havoc with your digestion and reduces the amount of nourishment you are likely to absorb from your food.

## Avoid racing and rushing

Slow down. You'll reach your destination just as quickly. The driver who over-took you in such a hurry is only two cars ahead. It gained nothing but an increased stress level. The same rule applies to everyday tasks at work and at home.

## Stop and stare

However hectic your day, it can be really good to do absolutely nothing every now and then. Even a few minutes of mind-wandering can calm us down and rest the mind. Stare into the distance. Look out of the window. Close your eyes and imagine yourself in a place you like to be. Anything is good as long as it takes you away from the task in hand for a couple of minutes or even a few seconds.

## Decide what's important

Sorting your needs from your necessities and counting your blessings are two good ways of restoring your perspective on life and deciding what's really important. Having enough to eat, being clothed, and having enough money to pay the bills are necessities. Any other advantages that come along are a bonus.

## Be better organised

Most people will say that finding time for themselves is impossible because they're too busy. The key to resolving this is to be just a bit better organised so that you can actually 'manufacture' a few minutes each day to use for your own needs.

## Think ahead to save yourself time

▶ Always leave a pad and pen by the telephone.

▶ Fill your petrol tank well before you reach the warning-light stage.

▶ Keep your first-aid box up to date.

▶ Buy a book of stamps when you are next out shopping. Most supermarkets sell them at the customer service desk. Then you'll have a stamp available for that urgent envelope so you don't have to make a special trip to the Post Office. Think of the time you'll save by not having to stand in line with all those other people who are queuing for a single stamp!

▶ Make a list of the ten most important telephone numbers in your life and put them next to the telephone or programme them into your mobile phone so that you don't have to look them up when you're in a rush.

▶ Have some spare light bulbs and batteries in the house.

▶ In case of a power failure, put candles, candle holders, a torch and matches or lighter somewhere safe, where you know you can find them in the dark!

These suggestions may seem simple now, perhaps not even worth bothering with – but will save you a great deal of anxiety if emergencies do arise.

## Plan your menus

Plan your week's menus *before* you do the shopping, and then make out a shopping list. It saves time at the store, saves money because you buy only what you really need, and there's no last minute panic about what to have for lunch/tea/dinner/supper.

## Buy yourself a piggy bank

Feed it occasionally with your smallest of small change and then, every now and then, empty it out and put whatever you've saved towards some quiet time just for you. Rent a video; buy a book or magazine; choose a plant from the local nursery; make an appointment at the hairdresser; have a manicure; or visit your favourite gallery or museum.

## Try not to rely on stimulants to keep you high

Too much tea, coffee, cola, chocolate or sugary foods will put even more stress on a body that is already hyper.

### Don't be afraid to cry

Some people cry easily. Others cry only occasionally. A few don't do it at all. Never hold back the tears on the basis that you'll embarrass yourself – or someone else. Men rarely show emotion and, unfortunately for many sons, the idea that boys shouldn't cry is passed down through the generations. Weeping is weak. Being macho is the thing. What many people don't realise is that tears are nature's way of getting rid of built-up tension, fear and anger. They also release chemicals that, if left inside the body, go on to cause more stress. People who bottle up their emotions and never let go are believed to be more at risk from serious illness. Crying can actually be calming and restoring. Notice how, even though a good cry can make you feel completely washed out at the time (and does terrible things to your make-up), it also re-jigs your perspective and helps you to see situations more clearly.

### Use relaxation tapes

Invest in some relaxation tapes or soothing music to play before you settle down to sleep. Use a player that switches off automatically.

### Laugh more. Smile more

It doesn't have to be at anything in particular. The very action of putting your face into a smile position can send positive messages to your cells. Try it now and see how you feel. Seeing the lighter side of life, say researchers, helps the body to cope more efficiently with the negative effects of stress and is less likely to lead to mood disturbance and depressive states.

### Nurture yourself

Remember that you are special and valuable and need to look after yourself.

ESSENTIAL READING

> ▶ Read Paul Wilson's *The Little Book of Calm* (Penguin). It's got lots of advice to inspire you and help you to regain calm and inner balance.

> ▶ Enjoy *Meditations for Women Who Do Too Much* (Harper San Francisco) by Anne Wilson Schaef

## Use essential oils

Essential oils can be a wonderful adjunct to other stress protectors such as good food, quality supplements and sensible exercise. Try the following oils individually to begin with, adding four drops only into a warm bath, to the water in a burner or diffuser, or to 25 millilitres of carrier oil such as grapeseed or apricot for massage purposes.

▶ **Lavender** (*Lavendula officinalis*) is probably the best known of all the fragrant oils, useful for relieving headaches, calming an over-active mind and encouraging soothing sleep.

▶ **Juniper** (*Juniperus communis*) is a good choice if anxiety and exhaustion have made you feel vulnerable and exposed. Good for lifting lethargy.

▶ **Clary sage** (*Salvia sclarea*) is mood lifting and helpful to anyone who is shattered but restless as a result of overwork. It's also good if you are nervous or depressed.

▶ **Ginger** (*Zingiber officinale*) is soothing for winter stress, that cold-ness that invades your whole being when you are chilled to the marrow. It's a strong oil so take care to use only small quantities.

▶ **Sandalwood** (*Santalum album*) is the oil for you if your stress is making you bottle up your feelings. It's helpful, too, if you are afraid or over-sensitive, or if you suffer from throat problems.

▶ **Frankincense** (*Boswellia thurifera*) is probably my favourite oil because I just adore its wonderful smell. That's a clue to which oils are right for you. If you don't like the aroma, then you may not absorb its therapeutic benefits. Frankincense is good for calming fears and insecurities, and for soothing emotional distress. It imparts a protective quality that can ease the trauma of particularly stressful situations. Good if you are a shivery type who feels the cold.

## ESSENTIAL READING

▶ If you are new to essential oils or want to learn more, there are a number of excellent introductory and self-help books available. Why not start with a simple and inexpensive booklet such as *Aromatherapy Stress Management – A Guide for Home Use* by Christine Westwood (Amberwood Publishing) and move up to Franzesca Watson's *Aromatherapy Blends and Remedies* (Thorsons).

## Try stress-busting supplements

There are several really useful vitamins, and minerals that can calm an over-active mind, help the body cope more effectively with stress, make it easier to relax, or encourage a good night's sleep.

▶ **Vitamin C** is vital for producing anti-stress hormones and for fortifying immune cells. One of the most concentrated areas of vitamin C is in the adrenal glands where it is readily available to help when a stressful situation occurs. It is used up in large amounts when we are frightened, severely traumatised, injured or suffering significant mental or emotional stress, leaving the body more prone to infection; one of the reasons why we tend to go down with colds when we're stressed. Most mammals are able to produce their own additional supplies of vitamin C when their bodies are in these circumstances. Unfortunately, humans have lost the ability to produce vitamin C internally, so it has to be provided daily from dietary sources. That would be fine if we all ate a diet rich in vitamin C. Nearly all fruit and vegetables are rich sources of vitamin C but, sadly, most of us don't even meet the minimum recommended requirements for this absolutely essential nutrient, let alone consume enough for optimum health. If you know you don't cope well with stress, suffer with persistent infections, are exposed to cigarette smoke (your own or others), drive in or walk near to heavy traffic or live or work near a busy road, or for any reason don't eat at least five servings of fresh fruit and vegetables every day, I would strongly recommend taking 500 milligrams of vitamin C twice or three times daily *in addition to your regular multivitamin.*

▶ **The B complex vitamins** are needed for a healthy nervous system and, like vitamin C, for adrenal support. If you are short of Bs, especially B1, B3, B5, B6, B12, choline and folic acid, you could be more easily affected by stress, anxiety and pressure. There is no need to take a whole load of different B vitamins separately, or take them in large amounts. A good multivitamin/ mineral (see page 400 for recommendations) should supply your everyday needs along with essential minerals such as magnesium (see below).

▶ **Magnesium** is known generally as a calming mineral. Unfortunately, it gets used up in large amounts every time the body produces stress hormones. Anxious worriers have higher levels of stress hormones in their bloodstream than more laid back types and so often have a higher requirement for magnesium. This mineral is found in a wide range of foods but especially in green vegetables and fruit.

## Get herbal help

Herbal remedies can also provide welcome support for all kinds of stressful situations. In my experience with patients, they can be just as effective as tranquillisers and sleeping pills but without the associated drowsiness or risks of dependence.

▶ **Passiflora/Passionflower** (*Passiflora incarnata*) is probably one of nature's best tranquillisers. Really good for relieving severe anxiety and for the kind of insomnia that keeps your mind as active as a hamster on a wheel. It's also a soothing remedy for any kind of extreme emotional upset, and can help to relieve headaches associated with nervous tension and muscle spasms. Passiflora hails from Mexico where the Aztecs prized its sedative properties. The Spanish Jesuits who gave it the name 'passionflower' brought seeds to Europe. Use this herb for 'accumulated' stress disorders; in other words, it you haven't been sleeping properly for months or are under persistent daily pressure. Passiflora is neither addictive nor habit-forming and has been used, in some cases, gradually to replace traditional drug treatments such as hypnotics and anti-depressants.

▶ **Valerian** (*Valerian officinalis*) does sound similar to the drug valium, and is used to treat similar symptoms, but the two are not related. Well known for its relaxing effect on the body, valerian is often used by herbalists to treat anxiety, depression, panic attacks, muscle cramps and nervous tension. It can be used with other calming herbs, such as passiflora, or on its own. Valerian can be taken during the daytime, as well as at night, without the risk of sleepiness.

▶ **Kava kava** (*Piper methysticum*) is less well known but is excellent for relieving muscle tension and for nervousness, anxiety and insomnia. Taken before bed, it can help to calm an over-active mind and promote sound sleep. The active ingredients are called kava-lactones which have anti-anxiety, muscle relaxing and pain-relieving effects. A native of the South Seas (and known there as sakan), it has been used by the Polynesian islanders as a popular beverage for thousands of years. Captain Cook was responsible for bringing kava kava to England.

---

**Before using herbal supplements**

Anyone already taking anti-depressant medication should consult their doctor before using herbal or other supplements.

---

In some countries, kava kava has been withdrawn from sale, following reports that this herb might have caused liver toxicity. Having read a considerable was of the available data, I'd like to express my own very personal view which is that the evidence against this helpful herb seems flimsy to say the least. In only three cases reported in the UK, at the time of this update, none has been proved to be definitely caused by kava kava. It appears two of those concerned were also taking prescribed drugs and the third had a higher than average alcohol intake. I took kava kava regularly and found it to be of huge benefit. Used wisely, it has proved to be an effective and side-effect free alternative to drug-based muscle relaxants, sleeping pills and painkillers for many people. However, until there is any definite prood one way or the other, kava kava remains unavailable here.

▶ **St John's wort** (*Hypericum perforatum*) is a well-researched plant medicine now recognised as an effective treatment for depression. But it can be a useful remedy if you are feeling 'raw' or 'wiped out' emotionally, or under exceptional stress. Studies suggest that the effectiveness of St John's wort may be down to its ability to increase levels of the calming brain chemical, serotonin. It's certainly a good muscle relaxer and has a generally soothing effect on the body. I have talked to several people who say it also helps to relieve chronic pain, especially if taken with kava kava. Don't use it if you are sunbathing, using a light box (to treat SAD) or are otherwise exposed to ultraviolet rays. There have been a few cases reported where St John's wort has caused photosensitivity.

▶ **Camomile** (*Matricaria recutita*) is best known for its calming qualities. Make a 'pot pourri' by tying dried camomile into a piece of muslin or other loosely woven material or even into a cotton sock or handkerchief and dropping it into the bath as you run the water. Drink camomile tea before bedtime. Camomile flowers are also available in capsule form. This herb can be especially helpful if your workload is making you anxious, jumpy or hyperactive, or is causing headaches, digestive disturbances including unsettled stomach, heartburn or irritable bowel.

▶ **California poppy** (*Eschscholtzia californica*) can be a valuable herb when stress is preventing someone from sleeping or where anxiety is leading to bad dreams or nightmares. This plant, which is a native of California, is a natural hypnotic which encourages peaceful and, restful sleep. It has no side-effects and is non-addictive.

Information on where to find the supplements mentioned here is on page 400. There is no need to use all these supplements. Start with a basic one-daily multivitamin/mineral that contains the major anti-oxidant vitamins A, C and E, all of the B group, and selenium, magnesium, chromium and zinc. Add California poppy for anxiety and St John's wort for depression and follow this programme for at least eight weeks before assessing any improvements. If you are not feeling better, use valerian and passiflora instead. If there is still no improvement, I would very strongly recommend that you see your doctor for a health check and possible referral for specialist advice.

**If you are taking prescribed drugs of any kind, don't use herbal medicines at the same time unless you have taken advice from your doctor or other qualified health care professional.**

---

### And, finally

When you are stressed, overworked or anxious, it could help to remember that pressure is what it takes to turn chunks of coal into diamonds!

# PART THREE

# Over 50 Fabulous Food Combining Recipes

# CHAPTER 16

# Tried and Tested Favourites

**W**elcome to the recipe section of *The Complete Book of Food Combining* where you'll find plenty of quick and easy meals to get you started. There's no complicated cordon bleu here, just simple and adaptable eatables that take no time at all to prepare from ingredients that are widely available. They're tasty and they work. Each of my recipes was created especially for this book and has been tried and tested many times before qualifying for inclusion. I have also included a handful of recipes from friends and colleagues who already enjoy food combining.

A major feature of all the meals is that they are high in nourishment and easy on preparation. They are all either suitable for vegetarians or offer vegetarian options. Every recipe will tell you its serving size. Most main courses and snacks serve two but if you are cooking for one, simply halve all the ingredients. You'll find that some quantities make enough to provide a leftover second serving which can be used for a next-day lunch, snack or supper, saving you time on particularly busy days. However, do make sure you refrigerate everything overnight and, if you're serving it hot, that you reheat it *thoroughly* before dishing up.

▶ **Breakfast Ideas** kick off on page 350.
▶ If you're looking for **Soups**, turn to page 354.
▶ For ideas on **Salads**, see page 365.
▶ You'll find **Scrumptious Snacks** and **Quick Lunches** on page 366.
▶ If it's **Simple Suppers** you need, go to page 401.
▶ For other **Mouthwatering Main Courses**, try page 386.

If you'd prefer ideas for a whole week, pages 418–19 gives you two simple seven-day plans that you can follow to the letter or amend to fit your own schedule.

Where possible, aim for one protein-based meal and two starch-based meals, per day – or the other way around – e.g. one starch and two protein meals, making sure you include plenty of fresh vegetables and salad foods. Try to avoid three of a kind; in other words, don't go for three protein meals a day or three starch per day. If you are trying to lose weight, it can help to include one alkaline-forming course of just salad, just vegetables or just fruit, with the remaining two meals as one protein and one starch. Each recipe is clearly marked so you know immediately whether it is protein (P), starch (S) or versatile (✓) and if it's suitable for vegetarians.

---

**Remember:**

Buy organic produce whenever possible.

Wash all fruit and vegetables really thoroughly before use – whether they are organic or not.

Avoid overcooking.

Don't deep fry.

Never reheat ready meals and takeaways.

---

**Author's note**

My grateful thanks to Magimix, Moulinex and Bosch for kindly loaning equipment to assist in the preparation of recipes for *The Complete Book of Food Combining*. We used the Magimix Le Duo Juicer, Magimix Cuisine 4100 Processor, Moulinex Avatio 3 Duo Processor/Blender and the Bosch Concept. Thanks also to the following who kindly supplied some of their favourite food combining recipes: Rose Rosney; Jean Cooper; Patricia Hubbard; Muriel Dubourdieu; Jan Robinson; Vera Garschagen; Mary King; Carol Newton; Margaret Stuart-Turner; and Alan R Johnson.

# Healthy Breakfasts

I cannot stress too strongly the importance of starting the day with nourishing food. Many people worry that a large breakfast will make them put on weight, not realising that missing out altogether presents a far greater risk. A whole day without proper food means that you are much more likely to load up with a large meal late in the evening, which actually increases the risk of weight gain! And the other fact is that eating soundly and sensibly first thing helps to maintain the balance of glucose in the blood, so that you don't feel hungry between meals. As a result, you're far less likely to reach for those diet-wrecking fatty, salty or sugary snacks.

But the first meal of the day can still be a problem. Let's face it, breakfast borders on the boring. Same old starchy cereal soaked in milk, an unsustaining wafer of toast that contains more fresh air than real goodness, a cup of coffee or tea and that's about it. Zero imagination!

Apart from the fact that breakfast can be a notorious mix of poor protein /starch combinations, it's also an assortment of common allergens – wheat, yeast, gluten and cow's milk – all being consumed at the same meal. Breakfast is also a very acid-forming meal that can leave some people feeling slouchy and grouchy with that *hung-over, can't-get-going feeling*. Couple all this to the fact that it's usually eaten in a rush, the after-effects of what is said to be the most vital meal of the day can be a kind of indigestible emptiness.

It's often the case that, by 10.30 or 11.00 o'clock in the morning, if we aren't gripped by heartburn, we're affected by severe stomach rumbling, hollow hunger and low blood sugar. Concentration as well as co-ordination are either diminished or completely out of the window. No wonder we resort, in desperation, to biscuits, chocolate or other not-so-healthy food or drink to fill us up while we long for lunch.

Why not broaden your breakfast horizons – and improve nourishment intake – by making a few changes? Here are some suggestions on how best to start your day:

## Fresh fruit

There's a lot more information on pages 23–33 about the benefits of eating fruit and enjoying fresh juices. Make sure you eat enough, though. One piece of fruit is unlikely to sustain you until lunchtime. Try a fruit platter or fruit salad, using the list on page 29 as a guide.

Remember that fresh fruit is best eaten on its own, away from proteins and starches.

## Dried-fruit compote

Dried fruit is packed with vitamins, minerals, natural sugars and dietary fibre. Some health stores and delicatessens sell packs of mixed dried fruits that you can soak overnight in either apple juice or water. Or you could buy individual fruits such as dried apricot, banana, date, fig, peach, pear, raisins and sultanas and make your own dried fruit salad. Serve it with a generous dollop of plain sheep's yoghurt or a good teaspoon of crème fraîche. Where possible, choose organic dried fruits. Buy them in small quantities and use them up within a week or two, then buy again.

## Hunza apricots

Hunzas are a delicious type of apricot with a distinctive sweetness. They are not very often stocked by supermarkets but are widely available in health stores. When dry, they resemble small scoops of concrete. Once soaked for a few hours, they change into the most delicious round fruits. A bowl of hunzas is high in nourishment and in dietary fibre.

## Cereals

Supermarkets and grocery stores sell a mind-blowing range of breakfast cereals in all kinds of guises, tempting us with words like 'fortified' or 'high in dietary fibre' or suggesting that a particular brand can make us enviably slim. But labels can be deceiving. The reality is that many packet cereals contain large quantities of well-disguised sugar and salt, and most are wheat-based. As I've explained earlier in *The Complete Book of Food Combining*, an overload of wheat in your diet can be a major handicap to successful weight loss. Wheat can also cause digestive and bowel discomfort in some people. And it's high in gluten, another common allergen. If you have a favourite cereal, it's worthwhile checking the ingredients to make sure you're not being duped. Go for whole oat cereals which are much lower in gluten than wheat, or rice or millet which are gluten free.

## Home-made muesli

This recipe is one that I have developed over the years and found to be an excellent alternative to the commonly available wheat-based packet cereals. It's easier to digest and far more nourishing. I use oatmeal or oat-bran as a base and then add sultanas, raisins, chopped dates, figs and apricots, pine nuts, chopped walnuts, pumpkin seeds, sunflower seeds and linseeds. The best thing to do is to buy the individual items and make up your muesli every morning. You can adjust the quantities to suit your own appetite. A dessertspoon of each ingredient is usually more than enough, and the mixture is even more delicious if you add a grated carrot and slice up a fresh banana. Moisten the whole lot with rice milk or almond milk or a teaspoon of single cream diluted in 100ml (a mean ¼ pint) of water. For those who prefer ready-prepared cereals, health stores usually stock good-quality muesli and gluten-free mixes.

## Rice cakes

Everyone knows that rice cakes resemble polystyrene packaging. But keep an open mind. First of all, rice is free of gluten. Rice cakes are easy to digest and also very versatile in that they blend with sweet or savoury spreads. For breakfast, try them with a little butter or non-hydrogenated spread and the best-quality honey you can find. Your health store should have a wide range of honey brands. Remember that you get what you pay for. Cheaper priced honey may have been heat treated and will probably be no better than sugar. Real cold-pressed untreated honey nearly always costs more. I love the wonderfully rich flavour of New Zealand Manuka honey which also makes an excellent alternative – and probably much healthier sweetener – to sugar.

## Yeast-free soda bread

This is a more appetising option than the squashy and tasteless sandwich loaf. Close-textured breads, such as soda bread, even though they are made from wheat, are sometimes easier to digest because they contain less gluten and less – or no – yeast. Spread three good slices with a scraping of butter and some good-quality honey or organic preserve and you have a filling breakfast. See page 59 for more information on bread.

## Porridge

Use oat-bran for a really smooth porridge and jumbo oat-flakes to make a thicker and chunkier consistency. Follow the pack instructions but use water instead of milk (otherwise you'll be mixing starch with protein). Porridge is extra delicious if you add a spoonful of Manuka honey and some chopped banana just before serving.

## Scrambled, boiled or poached eggs

Scares about salmonella poisoning and high cholesterol make many people nervous about eggs. In fact, if correctly stored and properly cooked, fresh free-range, organic eggs make a really sustaining and nourishing breakfast food. There is absolutely no convincing evidence that eggs raise cholesterol, so the only reason for avoiding them is if you don't like them or have an allergy to eggs. A couple of scrambled, poached or boiled eggs make a filling protein meal without the need for bread or toast. For a weekend breakfast treat, you could add an extra-special flavour to scrambled eggs with 25 grams (1oz) of grated Parmesan cheese, or a few strips of smoked salmon. Or add a small fillet of undyed smoked haddock to poached eggs. If you prefer your eggs fried but are worried about fat, don't be. Pan-fried in a little butter and olive oil and served with grilled tomatoes, they're absolutely delicious and very good for you. Check out the information on eggs in **Eating for Better Health** (page 66).

## Bacon, mushrooms and tomatoes

Mention cooked breakfasts and most people see them at best as unhealthy and at worst as sinful. In fact, a cooked breakfast of grilled lean bacon (especially if it's organic), served with mushrooms and tomatoes makes a truly satisfying meal that will see you right through until lunchtime. For those of us who choose not to eat meat, some supermarkets now stock a bacon look-a-like made from soya protein.

# Super Soups

## Basic vegetable stock or soup

 VERSATILE

This versatile mixture can be strained to make a nutritious clear vegetable stock for adding to soups and sauces, or blended into a thick vegetable soup in its own right. The recipe makes about 1.5 litres (2¾ pints) of stock and a little more if you blend it into a thick soup. It freezes well and will keep for 3–4 days in the refrigerator.

2 large onions
1 medium swede (rutabaga)
2 medium carrots
2 medium turnips
2 medium parsnips
2 medium leeks
3 cloves garlic, whole, not crushed
2 litres (3½ pints) filtered water

♦ Peel and chop all the vegetables and put them, with the whole garlic cloves, into a large stock pot or saucepan with the water and bring slowly to the boil.

♦ Reduce the heat, cover and simmer for 2 hours.

♦ Allow to cool before straining the liquid and storing in the refrigerator or freezer.

**TIP** Reduce the risk of spills and make fridge storage easier by keeping the stock in glass bottles or jars in the door space.

---

### If you don't have time to make your own stock

If you don't have any home-made vegetable stock to hand and don't have time to make it, simply use a low-salt vegetable stock cube with 570ml (1 pint) of filtered water. If a recipe calls for 2 pints or 1 litre of stock, you'll need to use 2 cubes. If you can't find low-salt stock cubes in your local supermarket, try a health store.

# Celery and Roquefort soup

**P** PROTEIN AND VEGETARIAN

**MAKES 2–3 SERVINGS**

The cheese content makes this a protein soup and so it doesn't combine well with starch. If you want to serve bread or crackers, make the soup without the cheese. Celery and onion are versatile foods and so will combine comfortably with proteins or starches.

1 tablespoon extra-virgin olive oil
1 small head of celery, washed and chopped into chunks (discard the outer
    stalks and use only the inner tender stalks)
1 large onion, roughly chopped
570ml (1 pint) vegetable stock (see page 354)
1 tablespoon dry sherry (optional)
50g (2oz) Roquefort cheese
1 tablespoon single cream

♦ Heat the olive oil in a large pan. When hot, add the celery and onion and stir over a medium heat for 2 minutes. Next add the vegetable stock (and dry sherry if liked) and cover and simmer for 20 minutes. Allow to cool for long enough to safely blend the soup in a liquidiser, then return to the pan to warm through.

♦ Just before serving, crumble the cheese and stir it into the soup with the cream.

**TIP** I use Roquefort for this recipe because it is made from sheep's milk which I find much more digestible than cow's milk cheeses. Roquefort is expensive but has a strong flavour so you need only a small amount.

# Mushroom, onion and lager soup

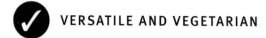 VERSATILE AND VEGETARIAN

**MAKES 2 GENEROUS SERVINGS**

Enjoy this soup on its own or as an interesting starter to either a protein or starch main course. If you want to make it a protein snack, it tastes terrific sprinkled with Feta cheese. Or serve croutons or crackers for a starch meal.

**1 tablespoon extra-virgin olive oil**
**2 medium onions, roughly chopped**
**1 medium leek, roughly chopped**
**1 clove garlic, crushed**
**200g (7oz) mushrooms, roughly chopped**
**300ml (½ pint) vegetable stock (see page 354)**
**1 teaspoon dark soy sauce**
**1 small can lager, stout or brown ale (approx 330ml)**

♦ Heat the olive oil in a large pan. When hot, add the onion, leek and garlic and fry over a medium heat for 5 minutes. Then add the mushrooms, vegetable stock, soy sauce and lager. Bring to the boil and then simmer gently for 20 minutes. Remove the pan from the heat and allow the soup to cool before blending in a liquidiser. Return the soup to the pan to reheat.

**TIP** This makes a delicious dinner party soup but make sure that guests know it contains alcohol.

# Spinach soup

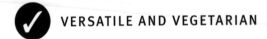 **VERSATILE AND VEGETARIAN**

**MAKES 2 SERVINGS**

To make this a starchy soup add a small can of butter beans, drained and well-rinsed.

**1 × 225g (½lb) bag baby spinach leaves**
**1 tablespoon extra-virgin olive oil**
**2 large onions, roughly chopped**
**570ml (1 pint) vegetable stock (page 354)**
**1 tablespoon single cream**
**freshly ground black pepper**

♦ Cook the spinach leaves in a large steamer (usually takes only 3–4 minutes), drain well and put to one side. Next, heat the oil in a large saucepan, add the onion and cook over a high heat for 2 minutes. Add the vegetable stock and the cooked spinach and simmer for 10 minutes. Pour into a food processor and blend for 2–3 seconds only. Stir in the cream just before serving and season with freshly ground black pepper.

# Eastern chicken soup

 PROTEIN

**MAKES 2 SERVINGS**

1 tablespoon extra-virgin olive oil
1 small onion, roughly chopped
200g (7oz) flat mushrooms, roughly chopped
½ teaspoon mild korma curry paste
2 teaspoons light soy or kelp sauce
½ teaspoon Thai 7 Spice Seasoning
4 spring onions, sliced into the thinnest possible strips
½ teaspoon crushed chillies
2.5cm (1in) piece of root ginger, peeled and freshly grated
½ teaspoon mango chutney
1 large or 2 small boneless free-range chicken breasts, skinned and cut into thin strips
1 × 400ml (14fl oz) can coconut milk
400ml (14fl oz) vegetable stock (page 354)
3 or 4 stalks lemon grass

♦ Heat the olive oil in a fry pan and, when hot, cook the onion for 2 minutes. Stir in the mushrooms, curry paste, soy or kelp sauce, Thai 7 Spice Seasoning, spring onions, crushed chillies, root ginger and mango chutney with the chicken strips and cook over a medium heat for 7–10 minutes.

♦ Meanwhile, in a separate pan, bring the coconut milk and stock to the boil. Bruise the lemon grass and add it to the milk (leave it whole, don't chop the stalks). Reduce the heat and simmer for 15 minutes. Then lift out and discard the lemon grass before adding the chicken and onion mixture. Continue simmering for a further 10 minutes. Remove the pan from heat and allow to cool for a few minutes. Then put the soup into a blender and process for, literally, 3 or 4 seconds. Reheat and serve.

**TIP** This filling, nourishing soup has a wonderfully warm spicy flavour and is a main meal in itself.

# Quick lentil and courgette soup

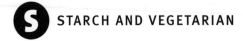 STARCH AND VEGETARIAN

**MAKES 2 SERVINGS**

1 × 400g (14oz) can lentils
1 tablespoon extra-virgin olive oil
1 medium onion, finely chopped
5cm (2in) piece of root ginger, peeled and freshly grated
2 medium courgettes, finely diced
570ml (1 pint) vegetable stock (page 354)
sea salt and freshly ground black pepper

♦ Drain and rinse the lentils. Heat the oil and cook the onion over a medium heat for 2 minutes. Then scoop up the grated ginger into a piece of cotton cloth or into the palm of your hand and squeeze the juice over the onion. You should get at least a teaspoon of ginger liquid from this. Discard the gratings. Add the courgettes, lentils and vegetable stock to the pan. Stir well. Bring to the boil and then simmer for 10 minutes. Mash gently for a chunky soup or put through a blender to make a smoother soup. Season to taste.

♦ Serve hot with matzo or rye crackers.

**TIP** For an even quicker soup, or for a change of flavour, leave out the courgette, use only half the quantity of vegetable stock and add a can of chopped tomatoes.

# Pea, mint and watercress soup

 **VERSATILE AND VEGETARIAN**

**MAKES 2 SERVINGS**

This soup makes an excellent starter to either a starch or a protein main course.

25g (1oz) butter
2 onions, finely chopped
1 clove garlic, crushed
100g (3½oz) bag or bunch watercress, washed really well and chopped
250g (9oz) frozen green peas
2 tablespoons freshly chopped mint
850ml (1½ pints) vegetable stock (page 354)
sea salt and freshly ground black pepper
1 tablespoon single cream

♦ Melt the butter in a large saucepan and fry the onion and garlic for 4–5 minutes over a medium heat. Add the watercress, peas, mint, vegetable stock and seasoning. Bring to the boil and then simmer for 15 minutes. Allow to cool for a few minutes before pouring the soup into a blender and processing until smooth. Return to the pan to reheat.

♦ Just before serving, stir in the cream.

**TIP** Fresh mint, watercress and peas are all excellent sources of carotene, folic acid and iron.

# Mild curried chickpea and vegetable soup

**S** STARCH AND VEGETARIAN

**MAKES 2 SERVINGS**

2 tablespoons extra-virgin olive oil
1 large onion, finely chopped
½ teaspoon mild curry powder
1 tablespoon tomato purée
1 head broccoli (250g/9oz approx) broken into small florets
2 sticks celery, chopped
2 carrots, peeled and chopped into small pieces
1 litre (2 pints) vegetable stock (page 354)
1 × 400g (14oz) can chickpeas

♦ Heat the oil in a large saucepan and sauté the onion with the curry powder for 3–4 minutes. Add the tomato purée, broccoli, celery and carrot and stir continuously over a high heat for 5 minutes. Next add the vegetable stock, bring to the boil and simmer for 15 minutes. Rinse and drain the chickpeas and add them to the soup. Cook for a further 5 minutes. Allow to cool sufficiently so that you can liquidise the soup safely.

♦ Heat through and serve with soda bread, rye crackers or matzos.

**TIP** Chickpeas are rich in dietary fibre and also contain worthwhile amounts of calcium and magnesium.

# Mediterranean soup

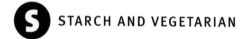 STARCH AND VEGETARIAN

**MAKES 4–6 SERVINGS**

This quantity makes 4 large or 6 small servings. It keeps well in the refrigerator for 3–4 days and is a good freezer standby, too.

2 tablespoons extra-virgin olive oil
1 large onion, finely chopped
1 clove garlic, crushed
2 sticks celery, cut into small pieces
2 carrots, peeled and chopped
1 red bell pepper, seeded and chopped
1 turnip, peeled and chopped
1 large can (approx 400g/14oz) chopped tomatoes
1 small can (approx 225g/8oz) red kidney beans, drained and rinsed
1 tablespoon finely chopped basil
1 tablespoon finely chopped parsley
1 teaspoon cold-pressed raw honey
1 litre (2 pints) vegetable stock (page 354)
freshly ground black pepper
125g (4½oz) small pasta shells such as fusilli or penne

♦ Heat the oil in large saucepan and cook the onion, garlic, celery, carrots, red pepper and turnip for 10 minutes over a medium heat next. Next, stir in the tomatoes, kidney beans, basil, parsley, honey, stock and black pepper. Bring to the boil, reduce heat, cover and simmer for 20 minutes. Add the pasta and simmer for a further 20 minutes until the pasta is tender.

**TIP** This soup is rich in vitamin C and carotenoids.

# Thick and creamy parsnip and butter bean soup

**S** STARCH AND VEGETARIAN

**MAKES 2 SERVINGS**

25g (1oz) butter
1 large onion, finely chopped
500g (1lb) parsnips, peeled and chopped
1 large potato, peeled and cut into small chunks
1 litre (2 pints) vegetable stock (page 354)
1 × 400g (14oz) can butter beans, drained, and rinsed
2 teaspoons single cream
½ teaspoon ground nutmeg
sea salt and freshly ground black pepper
freshly chopped chives to garnish

♦ Melt the butter in a large saucepan and cook the onion for 5 minutes over a medium heat. Add the parsnips and the potato, stirring continuously for a further 5 minutes. Then add the stock and the butter beans and simmer for 15 minutes. Leave the soup to cool slightly, then add the cream, nutmeg and seasoning. Blend in a processor until smooth.

♦ To serve, reheat and garnish with a few chopped chives.

**TIP** Not only are parsnips rich in dietary fibre, they're also a terrific source of potassium, folic acid and beta-carotene and have valuable amounts of calcium and magnesium, too.

# Special Salads

There's far more to a tasty salad dish than a bit of limp lettuce and half a tomato. Prepared with imagination, a salad can be a deliciously light meal on its own, or a nutritious addition to a main course. Make your salads using as many of the following ingredients as take your fancy. Bear in mind that most salads are more appealing if the contents are grated, chopped or sliced into small pieces. However, don't prepare salads in advance – once you've brought something out of the refrigerator into a warm room and cut or shredded it, the vitamin content begins to diminish. Go for organic alternatives whenever they are available. And remember to wash everything really thoroughly before use (see also page 36).

## Content ideas:

- Asparagus (lightly cooked and chilled)
- Avocado
- Beansprouts or seed sprouts
- Beetroot (raw and grated)
- Broccoli florets
- Carrots (grated)
- Cauliflower florets
- Celery
- Chicory
- Chinese leaves
- Cucumber (skinned)
- Dandelion leaves (young ones only)
- Lettuce (any kind but go for dark green leaves if possible)
- Peppers (red, green or yellow bell peppers or capsicums)

> **TIP** Add extra nourishment and flavour with fresh culinary herbs such as basil, coriander, fennel, mint or parsley, or by scattering seeds such as sunflower and pumpkin over your salads.

- Red cabbage
- Rocket
- Spanish onions
- Spinach (baby)
- Spring onions or scallions
- Tomatoes
- Watercress
- White cabbage

# Scrumptious Snacks, Starters and Quick Lunches

## Maggie's loaf (Margaret Stuart-Turner)

 **STARCH AND VEGETARIAN**

**MAKES 2 GENEROUS OR 4 SMALL SERVINGS**

This recipe makes a good snack or light lunch. It will keep for a day or two in the fridge and also freezes well.

1 French loaf
4 tablespoons extra-virgin olive oil
1 small red bell pepper, seeded
1 large onion
2 large flat mushrooms
12 stuffed green olives or pitted black olives
½ × 50g (1½oz) can anchovies
1 × 200g (7oz) can artichokes, drained and rinsed
2 sticks celery (use tender inner stalks for best results)
½ small cucumber, skinned and seeded

♦ Cut the loaf in half lengthways and remove the rounded ends. Scoop out the inside, leaving a thick shell. Crumble or process the bread-crumbs (not too finely) and put them to one side.

♦ Chop or slice all the other ingredients very finely. Next, heat 1 table-spoon of the olive oil in a pan and cook the red pepper, onion and mushroom over a medium heat until tender. This will take about 5 minutes. Remove from the heat. Then stir in the olives, anchovies, artichokes, celery and cucumber, together with the breadcrumbs and the rest of the olive oil. The mixture should be moist but not wet.

♦ Stuff the loaf from both ends until it is well packed with ingredients. Press the mixture firmly into the hollowed out halves, then put the loaf back together. Wrap it very tightly in greaseproof paper, tying it up with string or tape, making sure you secure both ends. Place the loaf in the refrigerator for several hours – or overnight – weight-ing it down with a heavy dish or plate.

♦ Slice and serve on its own or with crispy salad.

**TIP** You could ring the changes by adding an alternative filling such as hummus and tomatoes to the cooked ingredients instead of the anchovies, artichokes, celery and cucumber.

# Home-made hummus with crudités

**S** **STARCH AND VEGETARIAN**

**MAKES 2 PORTIONS**

Hummus is made from chickpeas which contain far more starch than protein, so class this as a starch meal. The hummus will keep well in a refrigerator for up to 3 days.

1 × 400g (14oz) can chickpeas, drained and rinsed
juice of a lemon (pre-packed lemon juice is not suitable)
4 tablespoons extra-virgin olive oil
2 tablespoons light tahini (pulped sesame seeds, available in most
  supermarkets)
1 clove garlic, crushed
2 tablespoons filtered water
freshly ground black pepper and sea salt to taste

♦ Mix all the ingredients with a hand blender or in a food processor until they resemble a paste. The mixture will keep well in a refrigerator for up to 3 days.

## For the crudités:

♦ Choose sticks of celery and carrot, slices of courgette and cucumber, plus spring onions (scallions), asparagus spears (lightly cooked and chilled), broccoli and cauliflower florets, and cherry tomatoes.

♦ Arrange the vegetables on a large plate or dish and serve the hummus in a small bowl.

**TIP** Ready-prepared hummus is widely available from supermarkets and delis or you could try this delicious easy-to-do recipe. Hummus makes a tasty snack with crackers or a jacket potato but is also a great party piece to serve with crudités and aperitifs.

# Bruschetta with char-grilled vegetables
(Rose Rosney)

 **STARCH AND VEGETARIAN**

**MAKES 4 SERVINGS**

1 large onion, cut into 8 wedges
2 cloves garlic, sliced
2 red bell peppers, seeded and cut into large chunks
2 yellow bell peppers, seeded and cut into large chunks
1 aubergine, cut into chunks
85ml (3fl oz) extra-virgin olive oil
sea salt and freshly ground black pepper
fresh basil to garnish

*For the base:*
2 small ciabatta, halved horizontally and halved again
50ml (2fl oz) extra-virgin olive oil
1–2 cloves garlic, crushed

♦ Preheat the oven to 200°C/400°F/Gas Mark 6. Put all the vegetables into a large roasting tin, drizzle with olive oil and mix thoroughly. Season with salt and pepper and roast in the oven for 25–30 minutes, stirring frequently.

♦ Arrange the ciabatta slices in a large roasting tin. Mix together the olive oil and garlic and spread half of this mixture over the bread. Bake for 5–8 minutes, then turn over and spread the rest of the mixture on the other side and put the ciabatta back in to the oven for a further 5–8 minutes.

♦ To serve, arrange the ciabatta on plates, top with the warm vegetables and garnish with fresh basil.

# Super salad soda bread

**S** STARCH AND VEGETARIAN

**MAKES 2 SERVINGS**

4 slices soda bread
½ ripe avocado, peeled and mashed
4 fresh dark-green lettuce leaves
1 large tomato, sliced
freshly chopped parsley
4 slices beetroot, cooked (see tip, page 384)
sea salt and freshly ground black pepper

♦ Cut 4 slices of soda bread. Spread 2 of the slices with ripe avocado, and then add the other ingredients in layers and season. Top off the sandwiches with the remaining slices of bread.

**TIP** Yeast-free soda bread can be a more easily digestible alternative to ordinary sandwich bread. Check labels before you buy. Not all soda bread is yeast-free.

# The best omelette

**P** PROTEIN. All fillings are suitable for vegetarians except the salmon.

**MAKES 1 SERVING**

Eggs are rich in protein, so don't serve any bread or toast with your omelette.

2 large free-range, organic eggs
filtered water
sea salt and freshly ground black pepper
small knob of butter
freshly chopped parsley to garnish

**To make the basic omelette:**

♦ Beat the eggs with a tablespoon of filtered water and season. You'll get a lighter mixture if you use an electric hand-blender instead of an ordinary whisk. Then melt a small knob of butter with a further teaspoon of water (no more) in an omelette pan until it just begins to sizzle. Add the egg and cook until the base is just set. Pile the filling (see below) on top and cook until the egg is just firm (usually takes about 3–4 minutes over a medium heat).

♦ Fold the omelette in half and then cut it in half. Garnish with fresh parsley to serve.

## Suggested fillings:

• Mushroom and onion filling – fried onions and mushrooms make a really tasty omelette filling.

• Lightly steamed spinach.

• Crumbled Feta cheese with chopped sun-dried tomatoes – quite salty so don't add any more seasoning to the egg.

• Fresh tomato slices.

• Smoked salmon – cut the salmon into strips and add to the omelette just before you tip it out of the pan.

• Mixed vegetables – for example, cauliflower, broccoli, carrot, red bell pepper, onion and peas. Chop all the first five ingredients very finely and cook them in a tablespoon of extra-virgin olive oil until tender. Cook the peas separately in a little boiling water. Drain them and stir them into the other vegetables. Make the omelette as above. Just before it sets, spread the vegetables over the omelette and fold it in half. Serve alone or with a crisp green salad.

# Spinach and curd-cheese soufflé

**(P)** **PROTEIN AND VEGETARIAN**

**MAKES 1 GENEROUS SERVING**

As well as making a tasty snack for 2 people, this can make a good protein main course for one.

1 × 225g (½lb) bag baby spinach
125g (4½oz) curd cheese
3 small egg whites
50g (2oz) grated Parmesan cheese
a little paprika

♦ Preheat the oven to 200°C/400°F/Gas Mark 6.

♦ Steam the spinach. When it is cooked, drain off the excess water. Lightly butter 2 ramekin dishes (150ml/5fl oz capacity) and mix together the spinach and curd cheese in a large bowl. Then whisk the egg whites in a separate bowl until they form stiff peaks. Fold the egg whites into the spinach and cheese mixture and spoon the mixture into the ramekins. Sprinkle with the grated Parmesan and a little paprika for extra colour. Place the ramekins on a baking sheet and bake for 20–25 minutes, or until well risen and golden brown. (Take care not to open the oven door suddenly during cooking, otherwise the soufflés may sink.)

♦ Serve with a mixed or green salad.

# Savoury potato slices

 **STARCH AND VEGETARIAN**

**MAKES 2 SERVINGS**

This is a starch snack, great on its own and a good companion to a starch or vegetable main course.

2 medium potatoes (organic if possible)
1 medium onion, finely chopped
2 tablespoons extra-virgin olive oil
½ teaspoon mild curry powder
sea salt

♦ Wash the potatoes and remove any eyes or blemishes but leave the skins on. Slice and rinse the potatoes again, then dry the slices on kitchen paper or a clean cotton cloth. Next peel the onion and chop it very finely. Heat the olive oil in a large flat-base fry pan or skillet, add the onion and the curry powder and cook for 1 minute. Then add the potato slices to the pan, and cook for about 4–5 minutes on each side, or until golden brown. Sprinkle with a little sea salt.

♦ To serve, cram the slices into ciabatta or a baguette, or eat with a crisp green salad.

**TIP** Makes a tasty, low-fat alternative to chips or French fries.

# Jacket potatoes

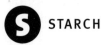 **STARCH AND VEGETARIAN**

Jacket potatoes can be one of the most satisfying and nourishing snacks. Great for lunch or supper, too. Don't dismiss them because you think toppings will be difficult. Cheese won't work for a food combined jacket potato because that would be mixing protein with starch. But there are plenty of other alternatives.

# Jacket potato with leek and mushroom filling
(Muriel Dubourdieu)

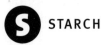 **STARCH**

**MAKES 1 SERVING**

1 large baking potato
1 tablespoon extra-virgin olive oil
1 small leek, cooked and finely sliced
2 large field mushrooms, washed and sliced
1 teaspoon potato flour
2 teaspoons single cream
1 teaspoon balsamic vinegar
a little vegetable stock

♦ Preheat the oven to 220°C/425°F/Gas Mark 7. Scrub the potato and pierce in several places with a thin skewer or a fork. Bake directly on the oven shelf for about 1¼ hours or until the potato yields to a gentle squeeze (remember to use an oven glove).

♦ Heat the olive oil in a frying pan and add the leek and mushrooms. Fry until the mushroom is just cooked and then add the potato flour. Stir until well mixed before adding the cream and balsamic vinegar to form a paste. Add a little vegetable stock to make a thick sauce and pour over the potato. Serve immediately.

## Other suggested fillings:

- Baked beans – organic baked beans are now available from some supermarkets

- A fresh green salad

- Avocado pesto (page 407)

- Creamy pea sauce (page 408)

- Quick pasta sauce (page 409)

- Chopped mushrooms – fry them in a little olive oil first.

- Crunchy mixed coleslaw (page 413)

- Hot couscous salad (page 414)

- Home-made hummus (page 368)

- Or just add freshly ground black pepper and a knob of butter

**TIP** If you're using organic potatoes, it's fine to eat the skins, providing they've been well scrubbed. If you're not using organic potatoes, leave the skin.

# Brown rice potato cakes

**S** STARCH AND VEGETARIAN

**MAKES 2 PORTIONS**

This makes a good stand-alone snack. Make it more substantial by serving with organic baked beans, or the bean salad (page 380), or a side salad. As a main course, serve with a generous helping of salad or vegetables. The quantities given below will make 4 large or 8 small cakes.

50g (2oz) brown rice
450g (1lb) large potatoes
4 tablespoons extra-virgin olive oil
1 large onion, chopped or sliced
freshly chopped chives or parsley as liked
1 tablespoon brown rice flour
sea salt and freshly ground black pepper

♦ Cook the rice according to the packet instructions, drain and put to one side in a bowl. Peel and boil the potatoes and then mash and add to the rice. Heat 1 tablespoon of the oil in a large fry pan and cook the onion gently for about 5 minutes into until soft. Then add the onion to the bowl containing the rice and potatoes and add the herbs. Mix thoroughly. Next, spread the rice flour on to a board, form the mixture into small-sized cake shapes and pat both sides of each cake in the rice flour. Heat the remaining oil in the same pan you used for the onion and cook each cake for 10 minutes each side or until golden brown.

♦ Serve with salad or vegetables (see suggestions above).

# Walnut avocado

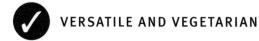 **VERSATILE AND VEGETARIAN**

**MAKES 1 MAIN COURSE SERVING OR 2 STARTER SERVINGS**

This versatile meal is good on its own or as a fresh tasting starter to a protein or starch main course.

1 ripe avocado, washed, halved and stoned
1 teaspoon fresh lemon juice
2 walnut halves to garnish

*For the filling*
¼ cucumber skinned and finely chopped
1 level tablespoon finely chopped walnuts
1 level tablespoon finely chopped mint
sea salt and freshly ground black pepper
1 tablespoon plain sheep's yoghurt
1 teaspoon balsamic vinegar

♦ Brush the cut avocado with lemon juice to prevent it browning. Put it to one side. Then place the cucumber, chopped walnuts, mint, sea salt and black pepper into a large bowl. Separately, whisk together the yoghurt and balsamic vinegar and add to the bowl with the cucumber, walnuts and mint. Finally, spoon the filling into the avocado centres and top each with half a walnut.

**TIP** Avocado is rich in monounsaturated oil which, researchers say, can help to keep cholesterol and blood glucose balanced. Walnuts contain special nutrients known as essential fatty acids, similar in structure to those found in fish oils.

# Melon, kiwi and grapefruit boats

## ALKALINE-FORMING AND VEGETARIAN

### MAKES 2 SERVINGS

This dish is best eaten away from proteins and starches.

½ **cantaloupe or galia melon**
1 **ripe kiwi**
1 **fresh grapefruit (or, if unavailable, use unsweetened canned segments)**
2 **tablespoons cold-pressed raw honey**
2 **teaspoons Cointreau (optional)**

♦ Cut the melon into 2 segments and remove the seeds. Peel and cut the kiwi into thin slices. Then lay the grapefruit segments and the kiwi slices across the top of each melon portion.

♦ If you are serving this as a starter at a special supper or dinner party, pour the Cointreau over the fruit before serving.

**TIP** Did you know that kiwi fruits are super-rich in vitamin C? Weight for weight, a kiwi fruit can contain twice the vitamin C of an orange.

# Simple and quick Greek salad

 PROTEIN AND VEGETARIAN

**MAKES 2 SERVINGS**

2 large, ripe tomatoes, each one sliced into 8
100g (4oz) Feta cheese, cut into chunks
¼ cucumber skinned and chopped or sliced
8 black olives

*For the dressing:*
2 tablespoons extra-virgin olive oil
1 tablespoon cider vinegar (or, for more sweetness, use balsamic vinegar)
1 teaspoon, finely chopped fresh oregano or ½ teaspoon dried oregano,
(chopped parsley or mint are good alternatives if oregano is unavailable)

- Arrange the tomatoes, Feta cheese, cucumber and olives in small salad bowls or plates.

- Put all the dressing ingredients into a screw-top jar and shake until well mixed. Then pour over the salad.


**TIP** It can be cheaper to buy Feta cheese off the block from the cheese counter rather than in small pre-packaged chunks

# Easy Caesar salad (Jan Robinson)

 **PROTEIN**

**MAKES 2 SERVINGS**

8 crisp lettuce hearts
a handful fresh chives, chopped
1 tablespoon roasted pine nuts
grated Parmesan cheese, to taste

*For the dressing:*
1 very fresh egg (free-range, organic)
1 clove garlic, crushed
2 heaped teaspoons capers
4 anchovy fillets
1 heaped teaspoon Dijon mustard
1 tablespoon extra-virgin olive oil

> **IMPORTANT NOTE**
> Use the dressing the day it is made and keep refrigerated. Don't use raw eggs if you are pregnant or unwell.

♦ Break the lettuce hearts into a large dish and sprinkle over the chives, pine nuts and grated Parmesan.

♦ Place all the dressing ingredients into a jam jar and shake well. Slowly pour in some good quality cold-pressed extra-virgin olive oil until the mixture thickens like mayonnaise. Add a little more Parmesan, shake and drizzle over the salad before serving.

# Mixed bean salad

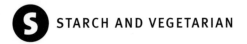 **STARCH AND VEGETARIAN**

**MAKES 2 SERVINGS**

This bean salad is quick to make from these basic ingredients – if you're pushed for time, buy a ready-prepared tub from the supermarket or delicatessen. Alternatively, buy a can of mixed pulses, drain and rinse them well, and toss them into the dressing with the onion and pepper. You can use any kind of beans for this recipe. Serve as a starchy starter or as a main salad ingredient. Great with cooked and chilled brown rice or couscous.

200g (7oz) cooked broad beans
1 × 400g (14oz) can mixed pulses, drained and rinsed
25g (1oz) butter
1 medium onion, finely chopped
1 red pepper, seeded and cut into very small pieces
1 tablespoon seeded raisins or sultanas
1 tablespoon freshly chopped chives
a few chopped fresh mint leaves (if available)
a generous twist of sea salt

*For the dressing:*
1 tablespoon extra-virgin olive oil
1 teaspoon horseradish sauce
¼ tablespoon balsamic vinegar
½ teaspoon cold-pressed raw honey
1 clove garlic, crushed

♦ Cook the broad beans in the usual way, allow to cool, and then mix with the pulses. Heat the butter in a fry pan over a medium heat, and cook the onion and red pepper until tender. This should take about 5 minutes. Put to one side and allow to cool. Meanwhile, make the dressing by putting the olive oil, horseradish sauce, balsamic vinegar, honey and crushed garlic into a jam jar and shaking well. Then stir all the ingredients together, not forgetting the raisins, herbs and salt, and serve.

**TIP** A mixed bean salad is nutrition rich. Apart from top scores for dietary fibre, this meal also provides valuable amounts of potassium, calcium, magnesium, iron and zinc, plus carotene and a number of B vitamins including folic acid.

# Egg salad with fresh herb dressing

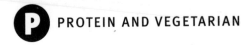 **PROTEIN AND VEGETARIAN**

**MAKES 2 SERVINGS**

4 hard-boiled eggs (choose free-range, organic eggs if possible)
8 good-sized lettuce leaves
4 small tomatoes
8 slices of skinned cucumber
1 carrot, finely grated
1 ripe avocado, peeled and sliced into quarters
a pinch of paprika

*For the dressing:*
100g (3½oz) plain sheep's yoghurt
2–3 tablespoons any chopped fresh herbs (I usually use an equal mixture of fresh parsley, mint and chives but basil, coriander and dill are also a good combination)
1 teaspoon balsamic vinegar
sea salt and freshly ground black pepper to taste

♦ Cut the eggs into halves and divide them between 2 plates with the lettuce leaves, tomatoes, cucumber, carrot and avocado. Put all the dressing ingredients into a jam jar and shake well. (For a smoother dressing, use a food processor and blend until smooth.) Spoon the dressing over the eggs and sprinkle with a little paprika.

# Easy tuna and caper salad (Jean Cooper)

 **PROTEIN**

**MAKES 2 SERVINGS**

2 × 185g (6½oz) cans tuna in oil, drained
1 tablespoon capers

- Mix the tuna and capers together.

- Serve on a bed of mixed green salad with either grated raw carrot, thinly sliced cucumber and several pieces of cooked baby corn for a colourful and nutritious meal, or with a thinly sliced avocado, several chopped black olives and sprinkled with lemon juice and freshly ground black pepper for a Mediterranean touch.

# Warm goats' cheese and walnut salad
(Jean Cooper)

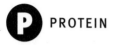 **PROTEIN**

**MAKES 2 SERVINGS**

This protein meal is ideal for a summer's day.

1 tablespoon extra-virgin olive oil
2 medium-sized field or open-cap mushrooms, washed
1 large yellow bell pepper, seeded and thinly sliced
12 walnut halves
12 black olives, halved
2 goats' cheeses, cut into rounds
mixed leaf salad

- Heat the olive oil in a wok or non-stick fry pan. Add the mushrooms, pepper and walnut halves and fry gently, turning regularly until the peppers have softened and are slightly brown. Then add the olives.

- Meanwhile, place a sheet of foil on a baking tray and lightly grease with more olive oil. Arrange the goats' cheese on the tray and place under a medium grill until lightly browned, but not melted.

- Arrange the salad leaves on a plate with the goats' cheese on top. Sprinkle the walnut and pepper mixture around the cheese and drizzle with the juices from the pan.

# Red, orange and green salad

### VEGETARIAN

### MAKES 2 SERVINGS

Eat this, salad either on its own, or as a starter to a protein or starch main course.

1 small eating apple, peeled and finely sliced
2 small beetroot, sliced (see tip below)
1 medium carrot, grated
a handful of lettuce leaves
8–10 sprigs of watercress
a handful of rocket leaves, if available
1 teaspoon mayonnaise

♦ Arrange all the ingredients on to serving plates and dress with a teaspoon of your favourite mayonnaise.

**TIP** Use either raw beetroot, home-cooked beetroot, or organic from the supermarket or grocery store. Don't use pre-cooked, pre-packed beetroot unless it's organic as most brands contain preservative.

# Avocado and green leaf salad (Vera Garschagen)

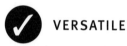 VERSATILE

**MAKES 1 SERVING**

This is a light, versatile salad ideal for lunch or a simple snack

a selection of salad leaves (spinach, watercress, rocket or any dark
  lettuce leaf)
1 ripe avocado, sliced
2 spring onions, finely chopped
6 shelled walnut halves
2 chestnut mushrooms (preferably organic)
fresh parsley

*For the dressing:*
juice of ½ lemon
1 tablespoon cold-pressed hazelnut oil or extra-virgin olive oil
1 clove garlic, crushed
sea salt and freshly ground black pepper to taste

◆ Lay the salad leaves on a serving plate and decorate with the
  avocado, spring onions, walnuts, mushrooms and parsley.

◆ Place all the dressing ingredients in a jam jar and shake until well
  blended. Pour over the salad and serve.

# Mouthwatering Main Courses

## Fast fish curry

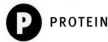 **PROTEIN**

**MAKES 2 SERVINGS**

This protein meal is mildly spicy and very quick to make.

1 small knob of butter (about a level teaspoon)
1 tablespoon extra-virgin olive oil
2 small onions, cut into quarters
2 teaspoons mild curry paste
½ teaspoon dried coriander powder
1 teaspoon mango chutney
1 teaspoon freshly grated root ginger
4 tablespoons white wine or Chinese cooking wine (optional)
150ml (¼ pint) coconut milk
2 small fillets or boned steaks of fish, skinned, washed and cut into chunks (I usually use cod, haddock or bass for this dish, but any firm white fish fillets or steaks will do)

♦ Melt the butter and olive oil in a fry pan. Next, add the onion, curry paste, coriander, chutney and ginger, and cook over a medium heat for 4–5 minutes. Slowly stir in the wine and coconut milk and simmer for a further 2 minutes. Finally, add the fish pieces and simmer for another 5 minutes.

♦ Serve with steamed spinach and mangetout.

# Tomato trout

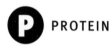 PROTEIN

**MAKES 2 SERVINGS**

2 fresh whole trout, gutted and cleaned
1 teaspoon softened butter
1 teaspoon freshly chopped parsley
1 large ripe tomato, skinned and sliced very thinly

♦ Preheat the over to 200°C/400°F/Gas Mark 6.

♦ Rinse the fish, blot them dry with kitchen paper and lay each one in the centre of a large square of foil or greaseproof paper (make sure it's big enough to wrap around the whole fish). Blend the butter with the parsley and spread the inside of each fish with half the mixture. Next, cram the thin slices of tomato along the inside of each fish and wrap the foil around the fish, forming long parcels. Lay the parcels on a baking dish and cook for 35–40 minutes. To check the fish are cooked, test them with a sharp knife. This should penetrate the flesh without resistance.

♦ Serve with a green salad (page 384) or green vegetables such as steamed broccoli and garden peas.

**TIP** For a dinner party or special occasion, garnish each fish with two or three pitted black olives, a sprinkling of halved or crushed blanched almonds and sprigs of fresh fennel just before serving.

# Baked stuffed peppers

**S** STARCH AND VEGETARIAN

**MAKES 2 SERVINGS**

2 large yellow or orange bell peppers
1 tablespoon extra-virgin olive oil
1 medium onion, finely chopped
100g (3½oz) flat mushrooms, chopped
2 tablespoons cooked brown rice (or couscous if you have no brown rice prepared)
1 medium tomato, skinned, seeded and cut into small chunks
1 carrot, grated
1 tablespoon of chopped fresh herbs (I use mint, chives and parsely from my window box)
1 teaspoon dark soy sauce
freshly ground black pepper

♦ Preheat the oven to 200°C/400°F/Gas Mark 6.

♦ Wash the peppers, slice off the tops (to make lids) and scoop out the pith and seeds. Heat the olive oil in a pan and fry the onion and mushrooms over a medium heat for 5 minutes. Remove from the heat. Next stir in the cooked brown rice, tomato, carrot, fresh herbs, soy sauce and a sprinkle of black pepper. When all the ingredients are well mixed, pack them into the hollow peppers and replace the tops. Put the peppers into a casserole dish with the remaining vegetable mixture spread around. Cover with a lid and bake for 1–1¼ hours until the peppers are tender.

♦ For serving suggestions, see tip below.

**TIP** Make this nourishing light meal or snack more substantial by serving with savoury potato slices (page 373) or crunchy mixed coleslaw (page 413). If you are making this just for yourself, it is worth knowing that the second pepper is delicious served cold the next day.

# Tomato rice (Rose Rosney)

 **STARCH AND VEGETARIAN**

**MAKES 4 SERVINGS**

This dish is a great starch variation on the classic risotto dish.

2 tablespoons extra-virgin olive oil
½ teaspoon onion seeds
1 onion, finely chopped
2 tomatoes, skinned and sliced
1 orange or yellow bell pepper, seeded and chopped
1 teaspoon freshly grated root ginger
1 clove garlic, crushed
1 teaspoon chilli powder
2 tablespoons freshly chopped coriander
1 potato, diced
50g (2oz) frozen green peas
½ teaspoon sea salt
400g (14oz) Basmati rice, washed
700ml (1¼ pints) filtered water

♦ Heat the oil in a large fry pan over a medium-high heat. Add the
onion seeds and fry for 30 seconds. Add the onion and fry for 5
minutes. Add the tomatoes, pepper, ginger, garlic, chilli, coriander,
potato and peas and season with sea salt. Stir-fry for a further 5
minutes. Add the rice and stir-fry for 1 minute. Pour in the water
and bring to the boil. Lower the heat to medium, cover and cook for
a further 12–15 minutes. Remove the pan from the hob and leave
to stand for 5 minutes before serving.

# Special vegetable brown rice (Mary King)

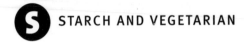 STARCH AND VEGETARIAN

**MAKES 2 SERVINGS**

This nutritious dish is filling and quick to make

350ml (¾ pint) filtered water
200g (7oz) brown rice
1 tablespoon extra-virgin olive oil
1 onion, peeled and finely sliced
4 tomatoes, washed and cut into quarters
1 red or green bell pepper, seeded and chopped
1 strip of Arame, soaked and well drained
a handful unsalted cashew nuts
2 teaspoons sunflower seeds

♦ Bring the water to boil in a large saucepan and add the rice. Cook for 20–25 minutes until tender.

♦ Meanwhile heat the olive oil in a wok or large frying pan over a medium heat. Add all the remaining ingredients apart from the sunflower seeds and toss for 5-6 minutes. Heap the rice on a serving dish, top with the vegetable mix and sprinkle with sunflower seeds. Alternatively, stir the rice and sunflower seeds into the wok and mix everything together before serving.

# Spiced bean goulash (Rose Rosney)

 **STARCH**

**MAKES 4 SERVINGS**

This variation of the traditional Hungarian dish is a wonderfully warming starch meal.

2 tablespoons extra-virgin olive oil
1 large onion, finely chopped
2 cloves garlic, crushed
1 large red bell pepper, seeded and chopped
1 large green bell pepper, seeded and chopped
3 sticks celery, sliced
1 tablespoon paprika (plus a little extra for a garnish)
1 teaspoon caraway seeds
1 × 400g (14oz) can chopped tomatoes
8 sun-dried tomatoes, halved
1 × 420g (15oz) can red kidney beans, drained and rinsed
1 × 420g (15oz) can chickpeas, drained and rinsed
1 low-salt vegetable stock cube

♦ Heat the olive oil in a large casserole dish. Fry the onion and garlic over a medium heat for 15 minutes until soft and golden. Stir in all the remaining ingredients, cover and simmer for 30 minutes, stirring occasionally to ensure the mixture isn't sticking. Add a little water if necessary.

♦ When the peppers are tender, serve the goulash in bowls, topped with a spoonful of crème fraîche and a pinch of extra paprika.

# Mary's quick meal pasta (Mary King)

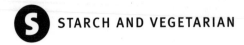 **STARCH AND VEGETARIAN**

**MAKES 2 SERVINGS**

A quick supper or lunch dish.

75g (2½oz) pasta
1 teaspoon extra-virgin olive oil
1 × 400g (14oz) can chopped tomatoes
1 × 400g (14oz) can organic lentils
¼ teaspoon mixed dried herbs

♦ Bring a large saucepan of water to the boil. Add the pasta and olive oil and cook for about 10 minutes or as per packet instructions.

♦ Meanwhile place the tomatoes, lentils and herbs in a saucepan over a medium heat. Cook until thoroughly heated through (about 5 to 10 minutes).

♦ Serve the pasta in bowls topped with the sauce and a generous side serving of green salad.

# Chicken waldorf salad

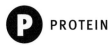 PROTEIN

**MAKES 1 GENEROUS SERVING OR 2 SNACKS**

2 boneless free-range chicken breasts, skinned, cooked and sliced
4 sticks celery, thinly sliced
16 mangetout, thinly sliced
12 walnut halves, broken into small pieces
1 ripe avocado, peeled and sliced
a couple of generous handfuls of mixed salad greens, torn into fine strips
fresh chives, parsley or mint to garnish

*For dressing: see page 413.*

♦ Simply arrange the ingredients in a large bowl, add the dressing and toss. Garnish with fresh herbs.

**TIP** Add extra vitamins and minerals to your menus by making more use of fresh culinary herbs. Even if you don't have a garden, growing your own is easy, indoors or out. All you need is a window box, tub or a few small pots. Failing that, nearly all supermarkets and grocery stores now sell fresh herbs.

# Mushroom and fresh herb-stuffed chicken

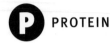 **PROTEIN**

**MAKES 2 SERVINGS**

1½ tablespoons extra-virgin olive oil
1 medium onion, finely chopped
1 clove garlic, crushed
1 small courgette, finely chopped
6 small flat mushrooms, finely chopped
1 teaspoon freshly chopped parsley
½ teaspoon freshly chopped mint
sea salt and freshly ground black pepper
2 boneless, free-range chicken breasts, skinned

♦ Preheat the oven to 200°C/400°F/Gas Mark 6.

♦ Heat a tablespoon of olive oil in a pan. Add the onion, garlic, courgette and mushrooms and cook over a medium heat for about 10 minutes, stirring or shaking occasionally. Stir in the parsley, mint and black pepper to taste. Remove the pan from the heat.

♦ Slice each chicken breast lengthways to make 2 thin slices from each piece. Place one slice in the base of a casserole dish and spread it with one third of the vegetable mixture. Sprinkle with a little sea salt and black pepper. Lay a second slice of chicken on top and then another layer of mixture, and season. Repeat with the third slice of chicken, spreading the remainder of the vegetables and topping with the last chicken slice. Secure the stack by inserting a cocktail stick at each end. Spread any remaining mixture around the base of the dish. Brush the chicken generously with the remaining oil and place the lid on the casserole dish. Bake for 30 minutes. Then, carefully remove the casserole lid and leave the chicken cooking for a further 15 minutes.

♦ Serve hot with green vegetables or cold with salad.

**TIP** Any leftover stuffed chicken makes a good lunchbox alternative to sandwiches.

# Pan-fried chicken breast (or Quorn substitute) with red onion and mushroom purée

 **PROTEIN** (chicken) although, suitable for vegetarians if you swap chicken for Quorn

**MAKES 2 SERVINGS**

2 tablespoons extra-virgin olive oil
2 small red onions, finely chopped
100g (3½oz) open mushrooms, finely chopped
2 medium free-range chicken breasts or Quorn fillets
1 clove garlic, chopped
2 tablespoons plain sheep's yoghurt

♦ Heat 1 tablespoon of olive oil in a pan and cook the onions over a medium heat for 5 minutes. Tip them into a bowl and put to one side. Heat the remaining oil in a fry pan and sauté the mushrooms over a medium heat for 5 minutes. Add the onions to the mushrooms and return the fry pan to the heat. Add the chicken breasts and cook for 6–7 minutes on each side. Remove from the pan and keep warm. Now put the cooked onions and mushrooms with the raw garlic into a blender and whizz until smooth. Add the yoghurt and any juices from the chicken pan to the blended mixture and reheat for 1 minute only. Finally, pour the purée over the chicken breasts.

♦ Serve with green beans and grilled tomatoes.

**TIP** This colourful, tasty recipe is quick to prepare. The purée is thick enough without the need for flour.

# Shepherds' moussaka

**S** STARCH AND VEGETARIAN

**MAKES 2 GENEROUS OR 4 AVERAGE SERVINGS**

A very nourishing, sustaining and really tasty one-course meal, low in fat and rich in dietary fibre. It takes a bit longer to prepare than the other recipes in this book but the effort really is worth it.

900ml (1½ pints) vegetable stock (page 354)
2 large aubergines, finely sliced
1 heaped tablespoon red lentils
2 large potatoes, suitable for mashing
25g (1oz) butter
1 level tablespoon crème fraîche
1 tablespoon extra-virgin olive oil
1 medium leek, finely sliced
1 medium onion, finely chopped
1 clove garlic, crushed
8 small flat mushrooms, chopped
½ yellow or red (but not green) bell pepper
1 medium carrot, grated
1 × 220g (7½oz) can chopped tomatoes
1 tablespoon tomato purée
1 × 440g (15½oz) can mixed pulses, drained and rinsed
1 teaspoon soy sauce
2 tablespoons dry white wine (optional)
1 large fresh tomato, thinly sliced
freshly ground black pepper

♦ Preheat the oven to 200°C/400°F/Gas Mark 6.

♦ Bring the stock to the boil and cook the aubergine slices in it for 2 minutes. Drain and save the stock. Pat the aubergine slices dry with kitchen paper and put them to one side. Return the stock to the pan and add the lentils. Cover and simmer for 30 minutes or until tender. All the water should be absorbed. Rinse them, drain and set aside.

◆ In a separate pan, cook the potatoes. Remove from the heat, drain and mash with the butter and crème fraîche. Put to one side and cover to keep warm.

◆ Heat the olive oil in a large fry pan. Add the leek, onion, garlic, mushrooms, pepper and carrot. Cook for 10 minutes, turning every few minutes. Then add the lentils, canned tomatoes, tomato purée, mixed pulses, soy sauce and wine. Simmer and stir for a further 10 minutes. Next, spoon half the mixture into a deep casserole dish and spread half the aubergine slices over the top. Make a second layer of the vegetable mixture and another with the remaining aubergine. Spread the mashed potato evenly over the whole dish, garnish with the tomato slices and sprinkle with black pepper. Bake for 1¼–1½ hours.

◆ Serve with extra vegetables if you like or on its own if you are pushed for time.

**TIP** If it's going to be a hectic week, I usually make up this casserole on a Sunday night and refrigerate it, so all I have to do when I get in on Monday evening is lift it out and pop it into the oven. Any leftovers will keep until next day as long as they are covered and kept in the fridge. It also freezes well.

# Patricia's 'mince' (Patricia Hubbard)

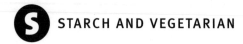 **STARCH AND VEGETARIAN**

**MAKES 4 SERVINGS**

This starch meal is a great alternative to beef mince.

**1 tablespoon extra-virgin olive oil**
**1 medium to large onion, finely chopped**
**350g (12oz) mushrooms, chopped**
**3 bell peppers (red, yellow or green), seeded and chopped**
**4–5 medium fresh tomatoes, skinned, seeded and diced or**
  **1 × 400g (14oz) can chopped tomatoes**
**sea salt and freshly ground pepper**

♦ Heat the olive oil in a wok or large fry pan. Add the chopped onion and cook for 1–2 minutes, then add the mushrooms. Stir in the peppers and cook for a few minutes more. Finally add the tomatoes and cook for another couple of minutes. If you are using canned tomatoes, adding ½ teaspoon cold-pressed raw honey helps to balance their acidity.

♦ Season to taste and serve with rice or pasta.

# Ten-vegetable stir-fry (Alan Johnson)

 VERSATILE

**MAKES 2 SERVINGS**

You can either serve this dish with meat or chicken to make a protein meal, or with rice, pasta or jacket potatoes to make a tasty starch dish.

1 dessertspoon extra-virgin olive oil
1 small onion, finely chopped
1 clove garlic, crushed
1 small chilli, seeded and finely chopped
a handful of white cabbage
a palmful each of carrot, mangetout, baby corn and dwarf beans, chopped
1 bell pepper, any colour, seeded and chopped
2 asparagus tips
225ml (8fl oz) filtered water
a pinch of cumin, turmeric, cinnamon and coriander to taste, or a dash of
  oyster sauce

♦ Heat the olive oil in a wok or large fry pan. Add the onion, garlic and chilli and cook over a medium-to-high heat until they begin to turn brown. (If you want to add meat to the recipe, you should add it at this stage. Lightly brown the meat or cook the chicken until white and soft.) Add all the other vegetables and stir-fry for a couple of minutes. Then pour in the water and spices or sauce. Stir gently and bring to the boil. Boil for about 3 minutes, continuing to stir gently all the time. Reduce the heat and simmer until the vegetables have softened and all the water has been absorbed, stirring occasionally.

**TIP** You don't have to stick to the vegetables suggested above. Experiment or use whatever is available.

# Favourite stir-fry vegetables (Jean Cooper)

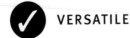 VERSATILE

**MAKES 1 SERVING**

This is a really versatile dish which can be eaten on its own or with protein such as chicken.

1–2 tablespoons extra-virgin olive oil
a pinch of dried or crushed chillies
25cm (1 in) piece of root ginger, finely chopped, or ½ teaspoon ginger
 powder
2 shallots *or* 1 small red onion, finely chopped
1 clove garlic, crushed
4 baby courgettes or 1 large courgette, sliced
6 baby corn-on-the-cob, cut into chunks
½ red bell pepper, seeded and chopped
½ yellow bell pepper, seeded and chopped
1 small carrot *or* ½ a large carrot, finely grated
sea salt
sesame and sunflower seeds

♦ Add the olive oil to a fry pan over a high heat. Put the dried or crushed chillies and ginger in the pan and then add the onion and garlic and fry for 1 minute. Add the rest of the vegetables except the grated carrot and stir-fry until the vegetables are almost cooked. Add the carrot and season with salt to taste.

♦ When the vegetables are lightly browned, serve sprinkled liberally with sesame and sunflower seeds.

# Simple Suppers

## Honey-roasted vegetables

 **VERSATILE AND VEGETARIAN**

**MAKES 2 SERVINGS**

To make this a starch meal, serve with brown rice or couscous. For a protein meal, add meat, poultry or fish – or enjoy the vegetables as a light but filling item on their own.

2 small carrots, cut into chunks
1 parsnip, cut into chunks
1 tablespoon cold-pressed raw honey
2 whole cloves garlic
1 courgette, cut into chunks
8 button mushrooms, cut in half
1 red onion, peeled and sliced into 8 wedges
1 small aubergine, cut into 8 segments
1 red or orange bell pepper, seeded and cut into 8 segments
1 large tomato, cut into quarters
3 tablespoons extra-virgin olive oil
sea salt and freshly ground black pepper

♦ Preheat the oven to 200°C/400°F/Gas Mark 6. You will need a large, flat baking dish for this recipe.

♦ Parboil the carrots and the parsnips together for 4–5 minutes. Drain, then tip them into a bowl and stir in the honey until the carrot and parsnip chunks are evenly coated. Then spread them randomly with the garlic cloves and remaining vegetables over the base of the baking dish. Drizzle the olive oil over the tops of all the vegetables and sprinkle the whole lot with a little sea salt and black pepper. Bake for 30 minutes. Then remove the dish from the oven to turn the vegetables. Return the dish to the oven for a further 30 minutes.

# Broccoli bake

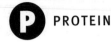 PROTEIN

**MAKES 2 GENEROUS SERVINGS**

The cheese content makes this a protein meal.

1 small cauliflower
1 head of broccoli
2 medium carrots
25g (1oz) butter
1 medium red onion, chopped
herb or celery salt and freshly ground black pepper
2 large free-range, organic eggs
100g (3½oz) any strong cheese, grated or crumbled
a little natural yoghurt or rice milk
2 large tomatoes, sliced

♦ Break the washed cauliflower and broccoli into florets and cut the carrots into chunks. Steam them until just tender (approximately 10 minutes). Drain. (*Note: Even when it is steamed, cauliflower can hold on to a lot of moisture – so make sure the vegetables are really well drained once cooked.*)

♦ Heat the butter in a small pan and fry the onion gently for 3–4 minutes. Tip the steamed vegetables and the onion into an open baking dish, mashing them gently down so that they are just broken up and evenly spread. Sprinkle with a little herb salt and black pepper. In a separate bowl, beat the eggs and mix with the cheese to make a thick 'cream'. If it seems too thick and won't pour, add a little natural yoghurt or rice milk. Pour over the vegetables, and arrange the sliced tomatoes over the top. Place under a hot grill until the tomatoes are cooked and the top is beginning to turn brown.

**TIP** Broccoli and cauliflower stems are an excellent source of calcium so don't discard the stalks unless they are very tough.

# Tasty stir-fry vegetables with brown rice

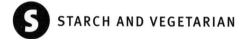 **STARCH AND VEGETARIAN**

**MAKES 2 GENEROUS SERVINGS**

If you wanted to make this a protein meal, skip the rice and add fried tofu, turkey, or chicken instead.

25g (1oz) butter
2 large flat mushrooms, each cut into quarters
1 tablespoon extra-virgin olive oil
1 small red onion, cut into 8 wedges
1 teaspoon freshly grated root ginger
1 clove garlic, crushed
1 quarter red or yellow bell pepper, finely sliced
½ teaspoon Chinese 5 Spice
2 tablespoons Chinese cooking wine
2 teaspoons Japanese shoyu
50g (2oz) mangetout
100g (3½oz) beansprouts
1 medium carrot, grated

♦ For this recipe you will need a large fry pan or wok and a second smaller pan to cook the mushrooms in.

♦ Melt the butter in the smaller pan and fry the mushrooms for 2 minutes. Put to one side, discarding any excess water. Then heat the olive oil in a large fry pan or wok. It needs to be hot but not smoking. Add the onion, ginger, garlic and bell pepper, Chinese 5 Spice and cook for 1 minute. Pour in the wine and the shoyu sauce and cook for a further 2 minutes. Then throw in the mangetout, beansprouts, grated carrot and the mushrooms and cook for a further 4–5 minutes, stirring all the time.

♦ Serve with brown rice

**TIP** To give the rice more flavour, add half a low-salt vegetable stock cube or a teaspoon of low-salt stock powder to the water during cooking.

# Mixed bean and cashew risotto

**S** STARCH AND VEGETARIAN

**MAKES 2 GENEROUS SERVINGS**

1 cup of brown rice
1 litre (1¾ pints) vegetable stock (see page 354)
1 tablespoon extra-virgin olive oil
¼ teaspoon dried mixed herbs
1 small red onion, finely chopped
½ bell pepper, any colour
200g (7oz) mixed mushrooms
1 × 200g (7oz) can mixed pulses
1 × 200g (7oz) can sweetcorn kernels
1 carrot, grated
50g (2oz) unsalted cashews
1 level tablespoon sunflower seeds
1 tablespoon sultanas
freshly ground black pepper

♦ Cook the rice in the vegetable stock. When cooked, drain the stock away and put the rice to one side. Heat the oil in a large fry pan and add the herbs, onion, bell pepper and mushrooms and cook over a medium heat for about 5 minutes. Add the mixed pulses, sweetcorn and grated carrot and stir for another 5 minutes until the mushroom has that delicious fried aroma and any excess water has evaporated. Mix in the rice, cashews, sunflower seeds, sultanas and black pepper and cook for a further 1 minute.

♦ Serve straightaway with a crisp green salad.

# Omelette pizza (Jean Cooper)

 PROTEIN

**MAKES 1 SERVING**

2 free-range, organic eggs
sea salt and freshly ground black pepper
extra-virgin olive oil
2 tablespoons grated goats' cheese
1 beef tomato, thinly sliced
black olives, halved
fresh or dried oregano

♦ Beat together the eggs, salt and pepper. Lightly brush a non-stick fry pan with olive oil and place over a medium heat. Pour in the egg mixture. Just as the omelette is setting, sprinkle over the goats' cheese. Turn down the heat and arrange the tomato slices and olives over the top. Sprinkle with oregano and a little more black pepper to taste.

♦ When the eggs are fully cooked and the cheese has melted, turn the omelette pizza out on to a plate and serve with a mixed salad or steamed broccoli.

# Colourful pasta

**S** STARCH AND VEGETARIAN

**MAKES 2 SERVINGS**

75g (2½oz) three colour fusilli (pasta twists)
1 teaspoon extra-virgin olive oil plus a further 1 tablespoon
1 small mild onion
1 clove garlic, crushed
½ teaspoon mild curry powder
½ red bell pepper, seeded and finely chopped
1 small carrot, grated
1 tablespoon Chinese cooking wine
8 black olives, pitted and chopped

♦ Bring a large saucepan to the boil. Add the pasta and 1 teaspoon of the olive oil. Cook for about 10 minutes or as per pack instructions. Then drain and set the pasta aside.

♦ To make the sauce, heat 1 tablespoon of olive oil in a large fry pan. Sauté the onion and garlic with the curry powder for 5 minutes. Add the red pepper, grated carrot and wine and stir to combine. Cook for a further 3–4 minutes. Finally, add the cooked pasta and black olives and continue to heat for another 2 minutes.

♦ Serve immediately.

**For alternative pasta sauces,** *see pages* 407–9.

**TIP** Cook some extra pasta for a great next-day salad. Simply add a tablespoon of mayonnaise or dressing to the chilled pasta and serve with a big green salad. Delicious!

# A selection of pasta sauces

The problem with pasta is that many pasta sauces contain meat or cheese. That's fine, but not if you're food combining because pasta is a starchy food and cheese and meat are proteins. The following three sauces make delicious alternatives and can also be used to top jacket potatoes.

## Avocado pesto

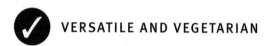 VERSATILE AND VEGETARIAN

MAKES 2 SERVINGS

1 clove garlic, crushed
1 tablespoon pine nuts
1 tablespoon freshly chopped basil (optional)
1 tablespoon freshly chopped parsley
2 tablespoons extra-virgin olive oil
1 tablespoon good-quality mayonnaise
1 ripe avocado, peeled and stoned
sea salt and freshly ground black pepper to taste

♦ Put all the ingredients into a blender and process until smooth. If you don't have a blender you can still make a 'chunkier' version of this sauce. Crush the nuts with a rolling pin, mash the avocado and then mix them together with all the other ingredients.

♦ Stir the sauce into hot pasta immediately before serving.

**TIP** Nearly all supermarkets now stock delicious organic, additive-free mayonnaise.

# Creamy pea sauce

✓ **VERSATILE AND VEGETARIAN**

**MAKES 2 SERVINGS**

25g (1oz) butter
1 medium onion, finely chopped
100g (3½oz) green peas, frozen or fresh
1 teaspoon finely chopped parsley
1 tablespoon finely chopped mint
sea salt and freshly ground black pepper
2 tablespoons single cream or crème fraîche

♦ Melt the butter in a pan and fry the chopped onion for 3–4 minutes. Add the peas, parsley, mint and seasoning and just enough water to cover the peas. Bring to the boil and then simmer for 5–6 minutes. Then, pop into a blender with the cream or crème fraîche and process for 10–15 seconds.

♦ Pour on to hot pasta immediately before serving.

# Quick pasta sauce

 **VERSATILE AND VEGETARIAN**

**MAKES 2 SERVINGS**

1 tablespoon extra-virgin olive oil
1 clove garlic, crushed
2.5cm (1in) piece of root ginger, peeled and freshly grated
1 medium onion, finely chopped
100g (3½oz) mushrooms, finely chopped
2 medium fresh tomatoes, or a small can of chopped tomatoes

♦ Heat the olive oil in a fry pan. Add the garlic, ginger and onion, and cook for 3–4 minutes. Then add the mushrooms and cook for a further 5 minutes. Finally, add the tomatoes and stir for an additional 2 minutes.

♦ Tip the mixture on to any freshly cooked pasta immediately before serving.

# Food combiner's chicken salad

**P** **PROTEIN** (chicken), although suitable for vegetarians if you swap the chicken for tofu or Quorn

**MAKES 2 SERVINGS**

This is a protein meal. Make it a vegetarian one by replacing the chicken with tofu (beancurd).

**1 pack or small bunch of cooked baby asparagus tips**
**1 cooked free-range chicken breast or 100g (3½oz) marinated tofu**
**½ teaspoon paprika**
**1 level tablespoon balsamic vinegar**
**1 small heart of crisp lettuce**
**100g (3½oz) mangetout**
**¼ red bell pepper**
**8 cherry tomatoes**
**fresh parsley to garnish**

♦ Cook the asparagus and the chicken in advance and allow to cool. Then slice the chicken into fine strips (or cut the tofu into small cubes) and place in a large bowl. Add the paprika and the balsamic vinegar. Stir until the chicken (or tofu) is coated and then place the bowl to one side.

♦ Wash the lettuce, mangetout, red pepper and tomatoes. Shred the lettuce very finely and slice the mangetout and red pepper into thin strips. Add all the remaining ingredients, except the asparagus, to the bowl containing the chicken or the tofu. Stir gently once or twice to combine the ingredients and then divide it into two salad bowls or individual serving dishes. Overlay each dish with the asparagus.

♦ Garnish with parsley to serve.

# Chilli Quorn

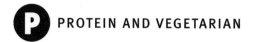 PROTEIN AND VEGETARIAN

**MAKES 2 GENEROUS SERVINGS**

Quorn is useful protein substitute for those who don't eat meat, but it can seem bland and usually benefits from additional flavourings. However, if you don't like spicy food, do try this recipe without the Thai 7 Spice Seasoning and chillies. Instead, soak the Quorn in vegetable stock for a couple of hours before use.

**2 tablespoons extra-virgin olive oil**
**200g (7oz) button mushrooms, chopped**
**1 medium onion (red onion gives colour and has good flavour)**
**¼ red bell pepper**
**2.5cm (1in) piece of fresh root ginger, peeled, grated and squeezed.**
**1 level teaspoon Thai 7 Spice Seasoning**
**¼ teaspoon crushed chillies.**
**200g (7oz) Quorn pieces (from the vegetarian chill-cabnet)**

(*Note: Instead of peeling and grating the ginger in the usual way, try grating it with the peel still on, then collect the gratings either into the palm of your hand or into a cloth and squeeze the juice into your ingredients. This still gives a good gingery taste without the 'bite'.*)

♦ Heat 1 tablespoon of olive oil in a medium-sized saucepan and sauté the mushrooms for 3–4 minutes. Put to one side. Peel the onion and cut into 8 wedges, and slice the pepper into strips. Heat the remaining olive oil in a large fry pan and sauté the onion, ginger and red pepper with the Thai 7 Spice Seasoning and crushed chillies over a medium-to-hot ring for 5 minutes. Then add the Quorn pieces and the mushrooms. Stir gently over a medium heat for another 6–8 minutes.

♦ Serve with a big green salad or at least 2 fresh non-starchy vegetables.

**TIP** Thai 7 Spice Seasoning and crushed chillies are available from most supermarkets and delicatessens.

# Tomato and garlic mushrooms

**(P)** **PROTEIN AND VEGETARIAN**

**MAKES 2 SERVINGS**

4 large open mushrooms (largest you can find)
4 spring onions (scallions), trimmed and finely chopped
1 sun-dried tomato, finely chopped
5cm (2in) chunk of cucumber, skinned and cubed
1 clove garlic, crushed
1 teaspoon freshly chopped parsley
2 teaspoons dark soy or kelp sauce
freshly ground black pepper
extra-virgin olive oil
1 large tomato cut into 4 slices
4 thin slices Parmesan or mozzarella cheese

♦ Preheat the oven to 200°C/400°F/Gas Mark 6.

♦ Carefully wash and dry the mushrooms. (If you aren't using organic mushrooms, you should peel them as well). Remove and cut the stalks into small pieces. Pop the stalks into a large bowl with the onions, sun-dried tomato, cucumber, crushed garlic, parsley, soy sauce and black pepper. Then spoon the filling into the open mushrooms. Brush the edges of the mushrooms with olive oil, place a tomato slice over each mushroom and then do the same with a slice of cheese. Arrange the mushrooms in the base of a casserole dish (you need to put a lid on to stop the mushrooms drying out) for 15–20 minutes, until the mushrooms are just tender and the cheese is melted.

♦ Serve at once on a bed of green leaves (anything you have to hand such as Chinese leaves, rocket, lettuce, watercress or baby spinach).

**TIP** You could add extra protein with marinated tofu pieces or lean bacon, grilled and chopped. Or remove the cheese and turn it into a starch meal by mixing in cooked brown rice or couscous.

# Crunchy mixed coleslaw

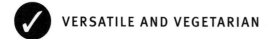 **VERSATILE AND VEGETARIAN**

**MAKES 2 SERVINGS**

This fine salad mix makes a deliciously light and nourishing snack on its own or, because all the ingredients are so versatile, can be combined with any starch or protein main course.

**1 mild onion**
**¼ small white cabbage**
**¼ small red cabbage**
**2 medium carrots, peeled**
**1 tablespoon sultanas**
**1 tablespoon crushed walnuts**
**1 teaspoon freshly chopped parsley**

*For the dressing:*
**3 tablespoons extra-virgin olive oil**
**1 tablespoon apple cider vinegar**

♦ With a sharp knife, cut the onion, cabbages and carrot into the thinnest of slices. (Instead of a knife, I use a Mandoline slicer. It has 3 easy-to-change blades for professional shredding and slicing. See page 438 for stockists) Add the sultanas, walnuts and parsley and stir lightly.

♦ Just before serving mix the dressing ingredients together and toss the coleslaw in it.

**TIP** Once you cut into a fruit, a vegetable or a fresh leaf of any kind, vitamin loss speeds up. So get the best nourishment from this salad by eating it as soon as it's ready. Don't prepare it more than a few minutes in advance.

# Hot couscous salad

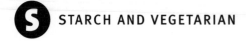 **STARCH AND VEGETARIAN**

**MAKES 2 SERVINGS**

225ml (8fl oz) vegetable stock (page 354)
100g (3½oz) couscous
1 teaspoon butter
½ red bell pepper, thinly sliced
1 small carrot, grated
2 small tomatoes, cut into 8 segments
1 ripe avocado, peeled, stoned and sliced
¼ cucumber, skinned and cubed
1 tablespoon pine nuts
1 tablespoon flaked almonds
1 tablespoon sultanas or raisins
1 tablespoon balsamic vinegar
1 tablespoon Chinese cooking wine

♦ Bring the vegetable stock to the boil and add the couscous. Remove from the heat and leave to stand for 10 minutes. (If you use the exact measures for vegetable stock and couscous given above, all the liquid should be absorbed and the couscous should be soft but 'dry'.) Next, heat the butter in a large sauté pan and cook the red bell pepper for 3–4 minutes. Then add the couscous, carrot, tomatoes, avocado, cucumber, pine nuts, flaked almonds and dried fruit, with the balsamic vinegar and the wine, to the pan and stir gently over the heat for 5 minutes.

♦ Serve with fresh crisp dark lettuce leaves.

*Note: vary this recipe by adding fried onion and mushrooms, chopped sun-dried tomatoes, mixed pulses and/or chopped walnuts.*

**TIP** Couscous is a creamy coloured grain made from semolina, which is a member of the Triticum (wheat) family. It makes a nice change from rice with the big plus that it is so quick to make up. A good source of vitamin B1 and iron, too.

# Garlicky mushroom salad

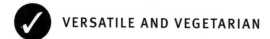 VERSATILE AND VEGETARIAN

**MAKES 2 SERVINGS**

Serve as a light snack, with tomatoes, crispy lettuce and slices of avocado or as an add on to a protein or starch meal.

**2 tablespoons extra-virgin olive oil**
**2 cloves garlic, crushed**
**2 red onions, finely chopped**
**200g (7oz) field mushrooms, cut into 4 or 5 slices**
**2 spring onions, finely chopped**
**juice of half a lemon**
**1 tablespoon freshly chopped parsley**
**1 tablespoon freshly chopped chives**
**freshly ground black pepper and sea salt to taste**

♦ Heat the olive oil in a fry pan. Add the onions, garlic and mushrooms and cook over a medium heat until the mushrooms have that delicious 'fried' aroma.

♦ Stir in the spring onions, lemon juice, chopped parsley and chives with a generous twist of pepper and salt. Serve at once with the salad.

# Hot potato salsa

**S** STARCH AND VEGETARIAN

**MAKES 2 SERVINGS**

1 large sweet potato
½kg (approx. 1lb) new potatoes
4 tablespoons extra-virgin olive oil
1 small red onion, finely chopped
1 clove garlic, crushed
¼ teaspoon cumin powder
½ teaspoon crushed chillies
2 tablespoons freshly chopped coriander leaves
2 tablespoons cold pressed sesame oil
½ teaspoon Tabasco sauce
30g (approx. 1oz) butter
zest and juice of 1 lime
sea salt and freshly ground black pepper

*For the salad:*
2 large ripe tomatoes
½ small cucumber, skinned and sliced
1 tablespoon your favourite oil and vinegar dressing

♦ Peel and chop the sweet potato and cook in salted water for 20–30 minutes until soft. Drain (saving the water) and mash, then put to one side. Using the same water put the new potatoes on to boil.

♦ Meanwhile, heat the olive oil in a frying pan and add the onion, garlic, cumin powder and crushed chillies, and cook until the onion is just beginning to brown. Tip this mixture into the sweet potato and mash them together with the coriander, sesame oil and Tabasco sauce.

♦ When the new potatoes are cooked, drain them and melt the butter over them. Fold the sweet potato salsa into the new potatoes and, just before serving, drizzle the whole lot with the lime juice and zest and season to taste.

♦ To make the salad: skin the tomatoes by plunging them into boiling water for 30 seconds (no longer) and then lifting them out on to a cold plate. The skins should lift easily away. Pop the tomatoes into the fridge for five minutes. Slice the tomatoes thinly and arrange with the cucumber on a serving plate and drizzle with your favourite dressing.

♦ Serve the hot potato salsa with the salad.

## Mustard mushrooms (Carol Newton)

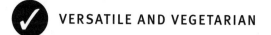 **VERSATILE AND VEGETARIAN**

**MAKES 2 SERVINGS**

A terrifically tasty and versatile snack

**4 large field or open-cap mushrooms, washed**
**extra-virgin olive oil**
**wholegrain mustard**

♦ Wash the mushrooms and remove the stalks. Brush all over with a little olive oil. Spread the inside with a coating of your favourite wholegrain mustard. Place on a tray under a hot grill until the mushrooms are cooked and mustard is bubbling (approximately 10 minutes). Serve with a mixed salad.

**TIP** Make this a protein meal be serving with chunks of Feta cheese

# Weekly Menu Plans

The following menu plans aren't set in stone, they are just to give you some ideas to get you started. If you don't like the sound of a recipe, simply swap it for another. Or make up your own menu plans.

| Menu 1 | Breakfasts | Lunches | Suppers |
|---|---|---|---|
| **Monday** | Home-made muesli (page 352) **S𝒱** | Red, orange & green salad (page 384) **A✓𝒱▼** | Shepherds' moussaka (page 396) **S𝒱** |
| **Tuesday** | Scrambled eggs with grilled tomatoes **P𝒱** | Jacket potato with fresh green salad **SA𝒱** | Tasty stir-fry vegetables with brown rice (page 399) **S✓𝒱** |
| **Wednesday** | Porridge with chopped banana **S𝒱** | Walnut avocado (page 377) **𝒱✓** | Fast fish curry (page 386) **P** or Chilli Quorn (page 411) **P𝒱** |
| **Thursday** | Rice cakes with butter & honey (page 352) **S𝒱** | Thick & creamy parsnip and butter bean soup (page 364) **S𝒱** | Honey-roasted vegetables (page 401) **A✓𝒱** |
| **Friday** | Fresh fruit salad with sheep's yoghurt **A𝒱▼** | Super salad soda bread (page 370) **S𝒱** | Mixed bean & cashew risotto (page 404) **S𝒱** |
| **Saturday** | Melon, kiwi & grapefruit boats (page 378) **A𝒱▼** | Celery & Roquefort soup (page 356) **P𝒱** | Tomato trout (page 387) **P** or Simple & quick Greek salad (page 379) **P𝒱** |
| **Sunday** | Hunza apricots or Dried-fruit compote served with crème fraîche (page 351) **A𝒱▼** | Pan-fried chicken with red onion and mushroom purée (page 395) **P** | Hot couscous salad (page 414) **S𝒱** |

| Menu 2 | Breakfasts | Lunches | Suppers |
|--------|-----------|---------|---------|
| **Monday** | Hunza apricots served with sheep's yoghurt (page 351) **P𝒗** | Hummus with crudités (page 368) **S𝒗** | Eastern chicken soup (page 359) **P𝒗** |
| **Tuesday** | 2 large boiled eggs **P𝒗** | Great big, fresh salad (choose from ingredients list on page 365) **A✓𝒗** | Colourful pasta (page 406) with avocado pesto (page 407) **S✓𝒗** |
| **Wednesday** | Half a fresh melon with slices of kiwi fruit (save rest of melon for tomorrow) **A✓𝒗** | Simple & quick Greek salad (page 379) **A✓** | Jacket potato (page 374) Choose your topping from pages 374–5 **S𝒗** |
| **Thursday** | Half a melon as yesterday **A✓𝒗** | Tomato trout (page 387) **P𝒗** | Hot couscous salad (page 414) **S✓𝒗** |
| **Friday** | Rice cakes with butter & honey **S𝒗** | Pea & watercress soup (page 361) **✓𝒗** serve with matzo crackers to make this a starch meal | Broccoli bake (page 402) **P𝒗** |
| **Saturday** | Slices of soda bread stacked with large grilled mushrooms **S𝒗** | Crunchy mixed coleslaw (page 413) **A✓𝒗** | Chilli Quorn (page 411) **P𝒗** |
| **Sunday** | Large bowl of millet or rice cereal served with oat milk or rice milk (page 321) **S𝒗** | Warm goat's cheese & walnut salad (page 383) **P𝒗** | Mediterranean soup (page 363) Serve with pitta bread or olive bread **S𝒗** |

---

**KEY**

**P** = protein

**S** = starch

**A** = alkaline-forming

**✓** = versatile, combines with proteins or starches

**𝒗** = suitable for vegetarians

**▼** = best eaten away from major proteins or starches

# Food Combining Chemistry

The area of acid-forming and alkaline-forming foods is a fascinating one that many practitioners believe may hold a vital key to improving and maintaining general health and well-being. Achieving the right balance of acid-forming to alkaline-forming foods is not an area exclusive to food combining and once explained, doesn't need any more of our attention. In fact, as it's perfectly possible to food combine successfully without knowing *anything* about acid-forming or alkaline-forming foods, you don't even have to read this appendix if you don't want to.

The only thing we need to acknowledge is that the right acid/alkali balance is essential to good health whether we food combine or not.

## Acid-forming, Alkali-forming

When food is metabolised, it leaves chemical and mineral residues that are either acid-forming or alkaline-forming. The reason that the phrase 'acid/alkali balance' has become synonymous with food combining is because early researchers, including Dr Hay, recognised that the more acidic the blood, the more likely it was that people would feel and look ill. Diets heavy with sugar, bread, cereals and meat but low in fresh vegetables and fruits, they suggested, created something called 'progressive acid saturation', whereas increasing the intake of fresh vegetable produce and fruit upped the alkalinity of the blood and brought about improved health and vigour. As a result, the phrase 'eat more alkaline-forming foods' is often listed in food combining books as one of the 'rules'.

So what does this mean in practical terms?

First of all, it helps to remember that:

**Foods fall into two main categories. They are either:**

**ACID-FORMING**

or

**ALKALINE-FORMING**

**Acid-forming foods include:**

| | | |
|---|---|---|
| Alcohol | Eggs | Poultry |
| Biscuits | Fish | Processed foods |
| Bread | Hydrogenated fats | Soft drinks |
| Cakes | Meat | Sugar |
| Canned goods (any) | Microwaved food | |
| Cheese | Pastry | |

**Alkaline-forming foods include:**

Dried fruits (nearly all)

Fresh fruits (nearly all)

Fresh fruit juices

Salad greens

Vegetables

Potatoes

**Other things that are acid-forming**

It's not just meat and bread that are acid-forming. Rich sauces, gravies, sugary, fatty foods and desserts are too. So are over-work, late nights, lack of sleep, stress, pollution, inactivity, poor circulation, anger, anxiety, envy, fear, irritability, panic and worry.

# Too Much Acid, Not Enough Alkaline

Acid saturation can be easy to reach, especially if you have a fondness for sweet biscuits, pastries, bread, buns and burgers or if you love meat, chicken and fish but never eat the vegetables. Nearly everyone eats too many acid-forming proteins and starches and not enough alkaline-forming vegetables and fruits. This puts strain on other internal systems that have to work overtime to mop up and deal with the acid. Loading up on the acid-forming stuff slows down the elimination of waste, causing a build-up of some rather smelly gases, such as sulphur, phosphorus and chlorine, which link up with other chemicals to form acids. I suppose you could look upon these acids as aggressive, since a build-up over a long period of time can lead to a variety of health problems. Some experts believe that over-acidity is responsible for a whole range of conditions common in the so-called civilised world, including rheumatism, arthritis, nerve pain, headaches, kidney stones, gallstones and even cellulite. It is even suggested that over-acidity could affect heart health. The theory is that when cells are too acid, they lose their flexibility and elasticity, impeding blood flow and increasing the risk of blockages by allowing cholesterol to build up in the arteries. Whether or not this turns out to be the case, research does already show us that a diet that is high in acid-forming foods is one of the potential risk factors for heart disease.

---

**Signs of an over-acid system include**

| | | |
|---|---|---|
| Body odour | Headaches | Sour taste in the mouth, |
| Constipation | Indigestion | especially first thing in the |
| Grey pallor | Oily or dull hair | morning |
| Halitosis | | |

---

**Health warning**

Some experts believe that too much acidity could aggravate conditions such as arthritis, diabetes, gout, gallstones, kidney problems, heart disease, muscle and bone disorders and poor lung function.

## Natural Balance

To prevent over-acidity from happening in the first place, the body calls up reserves of alkaline-forming trace elements (also called trace minerals) which help to clear up any excess acids. But that is only going to work if there are enough of those elements around to do the job. One of the best ways to make sure we have plenty is to increase our intake of vegetables, salads, herbs and fruits which are rich in the right kind of alkaline-forming minerals – potassium, magnesium, sodium and calcium.

This doesn't mean that foods such as fish, eggs, cheese or cereals are bad for us, just because they are acid-forming. Nor does it mean that we should eat nothing else but alkaline-forming vegetables and fruits. It's simply that, for good health, we need the right amounts of both! One of the great benefits of food combining is that, when we do it correctly, the acid/alkali thing balances itself automatically!

---

**Author's note**

It's easy to get the words *acid* and *acid-forming* mixed up. Foods such as grapes or apples may have an acid taste, but once they have been digested, absorbed and metabolised they leave behind a kind of mineral 'ash' that is said to be *alkaline-forming*. So, a food that is obviously acid before it's swallowed doesn't necessarily remain acid once it has been through the digestive system. On the other hand, when we eat obviously non-acidic or bland foods such as meat, fish, eggs, bread and cereals, they end up as *acid-forming* 'leftovers'. Put another way, acid-forming and alkaline-forming foods are classified not by how acidic or alkaline they are before being eaten, but by the residues they leave in the body after the digestive process has been completed.

---

## The Benefits of Alkaline-Forming Foods

When we combine foods correctly, we – almost unconsciously – increase our intake of alkaline-forming vegetables and fruits and reduce a little on those not-so-healthy, acid-forming processed and sugary foods. This should provide some really worthwhile health benefits:

▶ Alkalising vegetables and fruits can be especially helpful to anyone who is trying to quit smoking, cut back on alcohol or overcome cravings for sugar and chocolate. Balancing the blood pH ( see page 392 for more information) also reduces the acidity of urine. It seems that when urine is too acidic, cravings are more difficult to beat. It's an interesting point that the urine of a carnivore (such as a cat or a dog) is acid, whereas the urine of a herbivore (like the rabbit or a cow) is alkaline. Human urine can range from an acid 4.8 to a just alkaline 7.5. If our diet consists of some flesh foods and some vegetarian, our urine is usually edging on the acid side. A high meat intake could make it more acidic. The urine of a person who is vegetarian (or vegan) is likely to be nearer to neutral or alkaline than that of a dedicated meat eater, but not if the vegetarian diet relies too heavily on grains and pulses without the balance of additional vegetables and fruits.

▶ Eating more alkaline-forming foods has also shown an excellent response in patients with asthma, hayfever and other allergies. This may be because foods that mop up excess acid are helping to detoxify the blood and encouraging the liver to function more efficiently. Sensitivity to certain foods is more likely if the liver is sluggish. Page 186 has more on how food combining can help to relieve allergies.

▶ Some experts believe that serious health problems such as heart disease, stroke and high blood pressure may be aggravated by over-acidity. Another good reason for eating more vegetables, salads and fruit.

## Hunter-Gatherers had it Right

With absolutely no scientific or nutritional knowledge but plenty of gut instinct, it seems likely that our hunter-gatherer ancestors achieved near to perfect acid/alkali balance. Anthropological and archaeological evidence suggests that they ate very little in the way of meat (around 20–25 per cent of their diet was game) and that the other 75–80 per cent of their food was made up from fruits, roots, nuts, seeds and leaves. This lean protein, low-fat, lots of fresh produce approach supported surprisingly good health profiles, enhanced, more than likely, by the lack of pollution, stress and the trappings of modern-day living we like to call 'progress'.

Even though our bodies – and more particularly, our digestive systems – have evolved hardly at all since the days of the loin-cloth and the club, our present-day diets are vastly different to the hunter-gatherer diet. Today, most of us eat completely the opposite ratio; 25 per cent *or less* fruits and vegetables, and 75 per cent *or more* proteins, starches and sugars, much of it processed and chemically adulterated. Perhaps we would do well to take a leaf or two out of the Stone Age diet book and adjust the ratio a little in the other direction. I don't think anyone could disagree that the health profile of modern man, woman and child could do with a little improvement.

## Early Research

One of the earliest scientific studies into acid/alkali elements in food was begun in 1907, when researchers Sherman and Sinclair referred to the 'injurious effects' of having too much protein and not enough vegetable matter in the diet. Modern researchers have confirmed those early findings that the correct acid-alkali balance of the body is absolutely vital for our survival.

### A ratio of 4:1

Dr Hay recommended that for optimum well-being and to strengthen our resistance to disease, we should eat four-parts alkaline-forming foods to one-part acid-forming foods, i.e. 80 per cent vegetables and fruits to 20 per cent proteins and starches. Several health writers have followed this lead and included similar recommendations in more recent books. It is also sometimes suggested that one-fifth of our diet should be cooked food and the other four-fifths is better eaten raw. But is this realistic? If someone suggests to you that, for example, to be healthy, you have to eat only 20 per cent acid-forming foods (meat, cheese, eggs, grains etc) and 80 per cent alkaline-forming fruits and vegetables, it can seem a daunting prospect.

## Seems like a good idea?

There is little doubt that nearly everyone would benefit from eating more fresh fruits and vegetables and less of the rest. However, it isn't actually all that practical for most of us to follow a diet that is 80 per cent plant material. So impractical, that I wouldn't mind betting that even those who promote the idea don't always achieve it themselves. In fact, it might not always be appropriate. Why not? A diet containing a *very* high proportion of vegetables and fruits might, perhaps, be recommended to someone who is very physically active, since vigorous exercise creates a lot of acid in the system and lots of alkaline-forming stuff helps to counteract the acidity. People who are less active produce less acid, and so don't need so much alkalineforming food to mop it up. Someone in, say, a sedentary job, who takes a reasonable but not excessive amount of exercise, might be more comfortable with a diet consisting of 40 per cent proteins and starches, and 60 per cent vegetables and fruit. All this happens in that ideal world, of course. For most people, achieving a balance of 50:50 is worthy of a gold star.

## The pH Scale

This next section is interesting but, honestly, is not something you need to commit to memory so either stay with me or ignore the box and skip to page 428 if you want to.

> **! TECHNICAL STUFF**
>
> Acidity and alkalinity could be likened to the yin and yang of chemistry. They are opposites but are complementary to each other, like hot and cold, and night and day.
>
> Acids contain a large number of hydrogen ions (indicated by the letter H+). The more hydrogen ions a substance (in this case, a food) contains, the more acidic it is.

To determine the acidity or alkalinity of a substance, we calculate the number of hydrogen ions using a logarithm known as pH (which stands for Hydrogen ion concentration in solution to the Power of 10x a number).

To get a clearer picture of this, look at the pH scale below. You'll notice that it is marked from 1 to 14. The figure 7, right in the middle, indicates neutral – in other words, neither acid nor alkali. Water has a pH of 7. Anything from 6 down to 1 indicates increasing acidity and more hydrogen ions. For example, stomach acid is very acid indeed at 1.0–1.1. Anything from 8 up to 14 indicates increasing alkalinity, and less hydrogen ions. Sea water is only just alkaline at 8.1 but caustic soda is very alkaline at 14.

## The pH scale

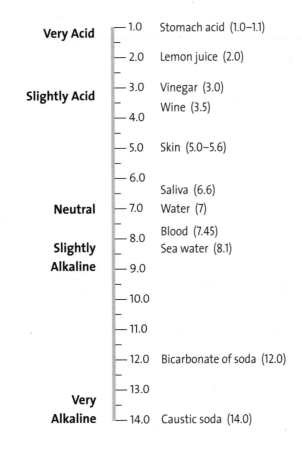

| | | |
|---|---|---|
| **Very Acid** | — 1.0 | Stomach acid (1.0–1.1) |
| | — 2.0 | Lemon juice (2.0) |
| **Slightly Acid** | — 3.0 | Vinegar (3.0) |
| | | Wine (3.5) |
| | — 4.0 | |
| | — 5.0 | Skin (5.0–5.6) |
| | — 6.0 | |
| | | Saliva (6.6) |
| **Neutral** | — 7.0 | Water (7) |
| | — 8.0 | Blood (7.45) |
| **Slightly Alkaline** | | Sea water (8.1) |
| | — 9.0 | |
| | — 10.0 | |
| | — 11.0 | |
| | — 12.0 | Bicarbonate of soda (12.0) |
| | — 13.0 | |
| **Very Alkaline** | — 14.0 | Caustic soda (14.0) |

## pH and the Skin

I expect almost everyone will be familiar with the letters pH, even if they can't remember where they last saw them. The most likely place is on the labels of pH-balanced skin-care products, shower gels or shampoos. Secretions from the sweat and sebaceous glands, together with the protein-coating of the skin, form what is known as the acid mantle. The pH value of this protective coating is between 5.0 and 5.6. If the mantle is disturbed or damaged by anything more acid or more alkaline than this, skin becomes more prone to dryness or oiliness, infection and ageing and takes on an uneven texture. If it comes into contact with anything extremely acid or extremely alkaline, the skin may be permanently damaged.

The idea behind pH-balanced products is that if the pH of, say, your moisturiser, matches your skin pH, the natural skin surface is less likely to be irritated or inflamed. The reason that ordinary soap can cause itching and dryness is because it is usually very alkaline and disturbs the skin's slightly acid defences.

Damage to skin pH can show up quite quickly. External and internal factors such as too much sunlight, excessive perspiration, unbalanced cosmetics, poor skin hygiene, a digestive upset or other health problems can alter pH within as little as 24 hours. Sallow, oily or flaky skin is often an early sign of some internal imbalance or illness.

One of the most ignored areas of likely skin damage is a VDU screen. If you don't already know that computers can affect skin health, you might find the following information useful.

The air around us is full of electrically charged atoms. Outside air is composed, mostly, of beneficial atoms called negative ions. Inside buildings, especially those that have a lot of static and electrical and electronic equipment, the air is usually charged with positive ions that can disturb the natural pH balance of the skin. Bacteria are then more likely to be attracted to the skin's surface, increasing the likelihood of spots, blemishes, eczema-like dryness and redness. The health of the eyes can also be detrimentally affected by the emissions from desktop computers. The problem is compounded by sitting in front of the screen for hours at a time without a break.

Here's how to reduce the risks:

▶ Invest in a best-quality filter for your VDU. Good ones will not only reduce the likelihood of skin sensitivity but also reduce eye-strain, headaches, stress and tiredness. Bear in mind that inexpensive filters are not always designed for extended use. If you spend a lot of time in front of a screen, go for a top-of-the-range anti-radiation, anti-static, anti-glare filter that cuts out 99.9 per cent of VLF and ELF (very low frequency and extremely low frequency) electro-magnetic field (EMF) radiation. Specialist office equipment supplies and catalogues have a range of filters for different sized screens. Or you might consider upgrading to a laptop. The LCD (liquid crystal display) screen on a laptop (or notebook) – or flat-screen monitor – produces negligible EMFs compared to the cathode-ray tube of a desktop computer. They're more expensive to buy than ordinary monitors but could be a worthwhile health investment.

▶ Don't wear plastic or rubber-soled footwear whilst working at your VDU.

▶ Plug an ioniser unit into a socket near your desk. It helps to increase the negative ions in the atmosphere. Available from good electrical stores, drug stores, some pharmacies and from selected mail order outlets (see page 438).

▶ Rinse or spray your face regularly throughout the day with fresh water. An atomiser is useful for this. Or use one of the prepared skin fresheners that contain essential oils (page 438 has details). Re-apply moist- uriser. A pure aloe-vera gel or natural sunscreen product can also add a protective layer.

▶ Work with windows open if you can.

▶ Take a ten-minute break every couple of hours from whatever you are doing. Move around, change the scene and get out into the fresh air, if possible.

▶ Stretch and yawn.

▶ Breathe more deeply.

▶ Drink plenty of mineral water throughout the day.

▶ Take plenty of exercise every day.

## Healthy Blood, Healthy Body

The reason for explaining the pH scale in some detail, especially in relation to acid-and alkaline-forming foods, is that I need to tell you how important it is for healthy blood.

There's a bit more scientific stuff here. I hope you'll find it useful but if you'd rather skip it, turn to page 431.

## Balanced Diet, Balanced Blood

The body relies upon a nourishing food supply to keep pH levels in the blood precisely tuned. It is especially interested in the type of mineral residue that different foods leave behind after they have been digested, absorbed and metabolised. As I explained earlier, meat, fish, cheese, sugars, bread, cereals, pulses and pasta are called acid-forming because they form acid ash deposits of chlorine, iodine, phosphorus and sulphur. Most fruits, vegetables, herbs, and most nuts and seeds, leave behind an alkalising (alkaline-forming) ash of minerals such as calcium, iron, magnesium, potassium and sodium. If your diet is

**! TECHNICAL STUFF**

While healthy skin needs to be very slightly acid, healthy blood needs to be very slightly alkaline; between 7.35 and 7.45. Even a small change upwards or downwards can affect us. For example, a pH of 6.9 could lead to coma and 7.7 to convulsions. But these dangers are only likely to occur in extreme circumstances. The body has some very precise control mechanisms, including special buffering systems, which call up reserves of particular minerals to keep blood pH finely balanced.

When the levels of acids in the bloodstream rise, they are:

**a.** neutralised and excreted via the kidneys, lungs and skin;

**b.** sent to the stomach to form hydrochloric acid; while the remainder is . . .

**c.** balanced and buffered by alkalising minerals – such as potassium, calcium and magnesium – obtained from our food supply.

unbalanced and any minerals are in short supply, in the wrong quantity or missing altogether, the stabilising system is disturbed.

## Could I Become Too Alkaline?

A long-term regime of a raw-food diet could lead to the 'floaty', spaced-out feelings and lack of grounding associated with an over-alkaline state. However, although it is possible for blood to become too alkaline as a result of a diet, this rarely happens because most of us eat far too many acid-forming foods. In any event, the body is well capable of recovering short-term excesses. If you have ever done a raw-food or fruit-only diet and wondered why, at the end of it, you could kill for a bar of chocolate or a biscuit, it may be your body is telling you that you have been eating alkaline-forming foods in too large a quantity, or for too long, and that it needs some acid-forming foods to restore the balance!

## The Importance of Good Breathing

The one situation that is much more likely to cause over-alkalinity is a condition known as BPD or breathing pattern disorder (chronic hyperventilation or fast, shallow breathing). BPD has been linked to many different diseases and may be a causative or aggravating factor in high blood pressure, ischaemic heart disease, coronary insufficiency, cardiac arrhythmia, asthma, ulcers, rheumatoid arthritis, colitis, over-active thyroid, and many more. In theory, if all those acid-forming cakes and fry-ups that we love so much are acid-forming, you might think you could counter their effects and increase alkalinity by hyperventilating! Not a good idea! The best way to maintain a healthy equilibrium is to eat a balanced intake of acid-forming and alkaline-forming foods and by breathing steadily and deeply. You'll find more information on how the right kind of breathing techniques can improve health by turning to page 262.

## Acid-forming Foods Aren't all Bad News

It's much easier to become over-acidic than over-alkaline. For most people, being too acid is nearer the norm. But don't get the idea that all acid-forming foods are bad just because pretty much everything that is alkaline-forming is good for you. To maintain an ideal balance, we need both kinds of foods. That's because acid and alkaline mineral deposits perform different, and equally vital functions. Some acid-formers, like sugar, soda drinks, sticky cakes and ready meals, are clearly not going to do us a lot of good if eaten to excess. However, lean organic meat, real cheeses, oily fish, free-range chicken and turkey, free-range eggs, and all kinds of pulses – even though they are also acid-forming – contain valuable nourishment and should form part of a healthy balanced diet.

There are a number of other lifestyle factors, apart from choosing the right food, that can help keep our blood healthily alkaline. Fresh air, fun, good companions, laughter, love, regular exercise, rest, relaxation, slow steady breathing, peace of mind, positive thoughts and emotional stability are all said to be alkaline-forming.

## Exceptions to the Rule

Now I know I've told you that *nearly* all fruits, vegetables and salad foods are alkaline-forming and *nearly* all proteins and starches are acid-forming. So that means there are going to be exceptions. Well, why wouldn't life be complicated? I'm going to tell you what they are but then, because they are small in number and not likely to affect your own acid/alkali balance, I suggest that you forget about which category they belong to and, to make the whole thing really easy, stick to the basic rule that:

ALL proteins, starches and sugars are acid-forming
and
ALL vegetables, salads and fruits are alkaline-forming

If you're still unsure, use the chart on pages 435–6 as an easy reference.

### Fermented foods are alkaline-forming

Fermented foods are valuable acid-buffers. Salted black bean, tempeh, miso, shoyu (soy sauce), nam pla fish sauce, cultured buttermilk and yoghurt are all believed to be buffering or alkaline-forming. Fermentation changes the nature of a food completely. Flavours become stronger, richer and sometimes sharper. Nutritional status is also markedly improved because the natural fermentation organisms added to the food benefit digestion and absorption. One of the most important things these bacteria can do is to encourage friendly intestinal flora which, in turn, helps to synthesise more enzymes and vitamins and improves the digestibility of proteins and starches. The organisms are especially helpful for making vitamin B12 (a nutrient sometimes lacking in vegan and vegetarian diets) more available to the body. It is this change in the microbiological and nutritional status of these foods that alters them from acid- to alkaline-forming.

### Potatoes are alkaline-forming

For food combining purposes, potato is classified as a starch but when it comes to the chemistry category, it is very definitely alkaline-forming.

### Other alkalisers

Amongst the normally acid-forming grains, millet is contrarily alkaline-forming. Grain-based coffee substitutes and cold-pressed raw honey are also alkalising.

### Acid-formers

Asparagus, artichokes, olives, butter beans, lentils, and mustard and cress are usually classified as acid-forming. They are also, as it is easy to see, exceptionally nutritious. As I mentioned earlier, acid-forming foods are just as important in the diet as their alkaline forming counterparts – as long as the balance is right.

So ...

I suggest that, if it is vegetable in origin, you treat it as a healthy, great-to-eat-it food.

## What about fats and oils?

Oh dear! Here's yet another frustration. I've spent a considerable time collecting as much data as possible on this aspect of food combining and, guess what, found, yet again, that most references disagree to one extent or another on where fats should be included. The first book I picked up stated 'all fats except butter are extremely acid-forming'. The second listed butter under 'Acid Dairy' but made no mention of any other fats in any category at all. In a third, butter and vegetables oils are 'neutral' and all other fats are 'acid-forming'. Yet another has margarine as 'neutral'. Several books avoided the issue entirely by simply not mentioning fats at all. Not very helpful.

By the end of a week of flip-flopping in, out and around the accumulated data, I found myself getting extremely irritable, a sign, apparently, that I needed to eat more alkaline-forming foods. I opted instead for a deep breath, a glass of red wine and what I hope is some common sense.

So what did I decide?

### It's the quality of the fat that matters

In actuality, some fats are acid-forming but the likely level of acidity will depend upon how *stripped* or *processed* the fats are. For example, mass-produced, chemically refined cooking oils should be considered acid-forming but cold-pressed flax oil or cold-pressed extra-virgin olive oil or the oil in a fresh avocado are alkaline-forming. Butter is believed by some leading food combining experts to be neutral.

### Advice on how to deal with fats and oils

▶ Use them wisely and in sensible, not excessive, quantities.

▶ Don't eat any kind of fat or oil to excess.

▶ But don't avoid them altogether. Some are essential to our health.

▶ Include the good ones (cold-pressed oils, a little butter or non-hydrogenated margarine spread).

▶ Say no to the bad ones (hydrogenated margarine, processed cooking oils).

▶ Avoid any obviously fatty foods such as cream cakes or anything deep-fried.

▶ Remember that, for the purposes of food combining, fats and oils appear in the **Versatile** column and so will mix with either proteins or starches, and with salads and vegetables.

# Here's What to Do About Acid- and Alkali-Forming Foods

The main thing to remember is to keep it simple. The following chart will help. Use it for quick reference.

## HERE'S A RECAP

### Acid-forming foods include:

| | | |
|---|---|---|
| Alcohol | Fish | Poultry |
| Biscuits | Heat-treated honey | Processed foods |
| Bread | Hydrogenated fats | Pulses |
| Cakes | Meat | Rice |
| Canned goods (any) | Microwaved food | Shellfish |
| Cereals | Oats | Soft drinks |
| Cheese | Pasta | Soya beans |
| Dried peas | Pastry | Soya milk |
| Eggs | Pasteurised milk | Sugar |

### Alkaline-forming foods include:

| | | |
|---|---|---|
| Buttermilk | Millet | Seeds |
| Cold-pressed raw honey | Miso | Shoyu (soy sauce) |
| Fruit (fresh and dried) | Nam pla fish sauce | Spices |
| Garden or green peas | Nuts | Tempeh |
| Green beans | Potatoes | Tofu (beancurd) |
| Grain-based coffee substitutes | Salad foods | Vegetables |
| Herbs (fresh and dried) | Salted black bean | Yoghurt |
| Kudzu | Seaweed | |

**What about fats?**

Keep fats to a minimum and don't worry about their category. Think of good-quality fats and oils, such as butter and extra-virgin olive oil, as neutral – neither acid nor alkaline. Fats and oils are versatile enough to combine with proteins or starches.

## MY TIPS FOR ACHIEVING A HEALTHY BALANCE OF ACID- AND ALKALI-FORMING FOODS

▶ Ease up on your intake of meat and bread.

▶ Avoid any fatty or deep-fried food.

▶ Use extra-virgin olive oil for cooking and salad dressings, and small amounts of butter or non-hydrogenated margarine for spreading.

▶ Avoid added sugar, sugary foods and artificial sweeteners.

▶ Use cold-pressed raw honey as an alternative sweetener. ('Cold-pressed' means that the honey hasn't been subjected to heat or processing.)

▶ Follow the fruit rule on page 12 and aim to eat at least two, preferably three portions of fresh fruit each day, taken between or just before meals.

▶ Replace some cups of tea or coffee with diluted fresh fruit juice, herbal teas or green teas.

▶ Plan more fresh vegetables into your daily menu. Try to include at least two fresh vegetables with your main meal of the day.

▶ Add a side salad to every lunch and dinner, whether you are including cooked vegetables or not.

▶ Prepare more vegetable stir-fries and vegetable soups.

And finally, it's equally important to:

- Get plenty of fresh air, regular exercise, rest and sleep.

- Enjoy good company.

- Listen to joyful music.

- Breathe more deeply.

- Laugh more.

- Smile at nothing.

- Think positive thoughts.

- Count your blessings.

---

### For hassle-free food combining, Kathryn Marsden says:

Treat ALL fruits, vegetables, salads, herbs, spices and fermented foods as alkaline-forming. Treat ALL starches, sugars, pulses (legumes), and proteins as acid-forming.

# Resources: Useful Addresses

Healthy eating can be a powerful tool to getting well again and food combining has proved itself many times to have been a catalyst, encouraging the body to heal itself. There are times, however, when you may need additional support such as a particular nutrient supplement or herbal remedy. If your health problem is a longstanding one, qualified help from a nutrition-oriented practitioner should be considered essential. The following resource directory is compiled from personal experience.

**Important note:** *Don't take vitamins, minerals or herbal preparations at the same time as prescribed medication without first taking advice from your health care professional. In particular, St. John's Wort should not be combined with certain drugs.*

Independent health food stores should stock most of the items recommended in *The Complete Book of Food Combining*. To find your nearest stockist or to order by mail, use the contact list below. To find a practitioner, see page 000.

### All Ages Vitamins
4 Kings Walk, Nottingham NG1 2AE
Website: www.all-ages-vitamins.co.uk
Stockists of a wide range of vitamin and herbal products from reputable manufacturers including Bioforce, Higher Nature, Pharma Nord and Solgar. Also for Ainsworths homoeopathic medicines.

### Arkopharma
7 Redlands Centre, Coulsdon, Surrey CR5 2HT
Tel: 020 8763 1414
Website: www.arkopharma.com/english
Email: e-mail sales@arkopharma.co.uk
Stockists of a Wide range of herbal supplements and cold-pressed flax oil liquid and capsules. Write or email with your name and address for price list and order form.

### Bach Flower Remedies
Consumer order line: 020 7495 2404
Website: www.bachremedies.com
or www.bachcentre.com

### Biocare
Lakeside, 180 Lifford Lane, Kings Norton, Birmingham B30 3NU
Tel: 0121 433 3727
Fax: 0121 433 3879
Website: www.biocare.co.uk
Wide range of vitamin, mineral and herbal products. Specialists in digestive enzymes, probiotics.

*Bioforce*
2 Brewster Place, Irvine,
Ayrshire KA11 5DD
Tel: 0845 6085858 (Helpline)
Website: www.bioforce.co.uk
Herbal medicines
Echinacea drops
Silicea liquid
Organic food seasonings
Papayaforce
Organic herbal tinctures and tablets
Alfred Vogel's Swiss Muesli
Jan de Vries Bowel Essence

*Bio-Health*
Medway City Estate, Rochester,
Kent ME2 4HU
Tel: 01634 290115
Quality herbal medicines

*Blackmores*
Consumer order line: 08707 700979
Website: www.blackmores.com.au

*Bodywise Uk Ltd*
See *Natural Woman Ltd*

*Complementary Medicine Services*
9 Corporation Street, Taunton,
Somerset TA1 4AJ
Tel: 01823 325022 (advice desk)
or 01823 321027 (orders)
Specialist suppliers of foods for people
suffering allergies. Allergy Care
brochure available.

*Ecozone*
Unit 1, Tannery Close, Beckenham,
Kent BR3 4BY
Tel: 0208 662 7200
Fax: 0208 662 7222
Website: www.ecozone.co.uk
Email: info@ecozone.co.uk
Specialist in eco-friendly products
Enzymes

Probiotics
Stockist for *Green People* and
*Biocare*

*G&G Vitamin Shop*
Vitality House, 2-3 Imberhorne Way,
East Grinstead, West Sussex RH19 1RL
Tel: 01342 312811
Website: www.gandgvitamins.com
Digestive Complex
Green Walnut tincture
Clove capsules
Wormwood capsules

*Green & Blacks Organic Chocolate*
Website: www.greenandblacks.com
From health stores and some
supermarkets

*Green People Company*
Brighton Road, Handcross,
West Sussex RH17 6BZ
Tel: 01444 401444
Website: www.greenpeople.co.uk
Organic Omega 3&6
flax/pumpkin/borage oil mix
Organic Omega 3&6 flax seed sprinkle
Organic skin care products
See also *Ecozone*

*Healthy House*
The Old Co-op, Ruscombe, Stroud,
Gloucestershire GL6 6BU
Tel: 01453 752216
Website: www.healthy-house.co.uk
Email: info@healthy-house.co.uk
E-mail, write or phone for product
brochure
Specialist products for people with
allergies
Organic paints
Anti geo stress products
Water filters
Non-toxic toiletries
Natural bedding

### Higher Nature

The Nutrition Centre, Burwash
Common, East Sussex TN19 7LX
Tel: 01435 882880
Website: www.higher-nature.co.uk
Details also available on food allergy
testing. Excellent product brochure
available.
Flax seed and oil products
Hemp seeds oil
Psyllium
Probiotics
Aloe Vera drinks and topical gel
Cleansing products including Paraclens

### Homoeopathic Medicines

Ainsworths Homoeopathic Pharmacy,
38 New Cavendish Street,
London W1M 9FG
Tel: 0171 935 5330
Available from some chemists, most
health food stores and by mail from
the address above.

### Foods Matter at The Inside Story

Berrydale House, 5 Lawn Road, London
NW3 2XS
Tel: 020 7722 2866
Website: www.foodsmatter.com
Email: info@foodsmatter.com

I highly recommend this excellent
newsletter, an essential reference for
anyone suffering food sensitivity or
allergies. It's packed with useful
articles, recipes, latest findings and an
extensive list of self-help and support
groups. Contact them at the address
above enclosing a large s.a.e. for
subscription details.

### Jurlique

Website: www.apotheke20-20.co.uk
Jurlique specialist herbal teas
Organic skin care products
Essential oils

### Kiki Health

Chequers House, 9 Stratton Road,
Hainford, Norwich NR10 3AZ
Tel: 08450 60 10 60
Website: www.kiki-health.com
E3Live blue green algae
Nature's Biotics probiotic supplements
(also available from *Natural Woman
Ltd.*).

### Kiwiherb

Kiwiherb products are available
through all independent health food
stores and by mail order through
*Xynergy Health* (see below).
Meadowsweet & Aniseed
Ginger & Kawakawa syrup
Valerian Root Extract
Echinacea

### Lakeland Ltd

Alexandra Buildings, Windermere,
Cumbria LA23 1BQ
Tel: 015394 88100
Website: www.lakelandlimited.com
Blenders
Food mixers
Juicers
Mandolin slicer
Stay fresh food bags

### Lichtwer Pharma herbal products

Tel: 01202 780 558
Website: www.lichtwer.co.uk
Available from in the UK from Boots,
Superdrug, The Nutri Centre and from
health food stores.

### Linusit Gold Linseeds

Vacuum packed nutritional quality
linseeds.
Available from some supermarkets and
most health food stores.

### Manuka Honey Products

Look for Comvita Manuka, available

from good health food stores and by mail from *Xynergy Health*. In case of difficulty, contact *Xynergy* or *New Zealand Natural Food Company.*

## Natural by Nature Essential Oils
Website www.all-ages-vitamins.com or www.auravita.com

## Natural Woman Ltd.
86 Shirehampton Road, Stoke Bishop, Bristol BS9 2DR
Tel: 0117 968 7744
Website: www.natural-woman.com
Udo's Choice products
PelvicToner stockist
Bodywise bleach-free products
Biocare stockist
Nature's Biotics from Kiki Health

## New Zealand Natural Food Company
Unit 7, 55-57 Park Royal Road, London NW10 7JP
Tel: 0181 961 4410
Website: www.comvita.com
or www.kiwiherb.com
Products also available from *Xynergy Health*.

## Neal's Yard
29 John Dalton Street, Manchester M2 6DS
Tel: 0161 831 7875 or 020 7627 1949 (Customer Services)
Website: www.nealsyardremedies.com
Wide range of herbal tinctures such as Echinacea and dried herbs including Slippery Elm
Natural skin care products
Essential oils

## Nutshell Natural Paints
P.O. Box 72, South Brent TQ10 9YR
Tel: 01364 73801
Website: www.nutshellpaints.com

## Pharma Nord
Spital Hall, Mitford, Morpeth, Northumberland NE61 3PN
Tel: 01670 519989
or Freephone: 0800 591756
Extensive range of vitamin, mineral, and other supplements.
Probiotics
Q10 Skin care products

## Potters Herbal Medicines
Leyland Mill Lane, Wigan, Lancashire WN1 2SB
Tel: 01942 405100
Website: www.herbal-direct.com
or www.all-ages-vitamins.com

## Savant Health
Quarry House, Clayton Wood Close, Leeds LS16 6QE
Tel: 0113 230 1993
Fax: 0113 230 1915
Website: www.savant-health.com
Udo's Choice Beyond Greens
Udo's Choice Super 5 and Super 8
Probiotics
Udo's Choice Digestive Enzyme Blend
Udo's Choice Ultimate Oil Blend

## The Soil Association
Bristol House, 40-56 Victoria Street, Bristol BS1 6BY
Tel: 0117 314 5000
Website: www.soilassociation.org
Regional Guides available giving organic producers/stockists, opening times, types of produce sold, delivery and mail order services county by county. Send large s.a.e.

## The Soil Association Scotland
18 Liberton Brae, Tower Mains, Edinburgh EH16 6NE
Tel: 0131 666 2474
Website: www.sascotland.org

### Solgar Vitamins
Albury, Tring, Hertfordshire HP23 5PT
Tel: 01442 890355
Website: www.solgar.com
All international addresses for Solgar
can be found under the International
menu on the website.
Gold label range
Vitamins, minerals, enzymes, psyllium,
probiotics and other specialist
supplements

### The Stamp Collection
Buxton Foods, 12 Harley Street,
London W1G 9PG
Tel: 020 7637 5505
Website: www.stamp-collection.co.uk
Fabulous range of no-wheat, no-cow's
milk foods. Available from Sainsbury's,
Tesco, Waitrose. ASDA and health
food stores. Website has product
information, recipes and useful links to
other sites.

### Virani Food Products Ltd
10-14 Stewarts Road, Finedon Road
Industrial Estate, Wellingborough,
Northamptonshire NN8 4RJ
Tel: 01933 276483
Specialist foods including a wide range
of flours suitable for wheat-free and
gluten-free diets.

### Viridian Nutrition
31 Alvis Way, Royal Oak, Daventry,
Northamptonshire NN11 5PG
Tel: 01327 878050
Website: www.viridian-nutrition.com
Digestive Aid
Psyllium
Acidophilus Complex
Cold-pressed oils
Vitamins, minerals, herbals.

### Xynergy Health Products
Lower Elsted, Midhurst, West Sussex
GU29 0JT
Tel: 01730 813642
Green foods
Aloe Vera products
Stockist for Kiwiherb and Manuka
products
Stockist for Pukka ayurvedic herbals &
essential oils

# Resources: Product Information

## Vitamin, mineral and herbal supplements
Biocare
Bioforce
Viridian
Pharma Nord
Solgar
All Ages Vitamins
Higher Nature
Natural Woman

## Probiotics
Biocare
Higher Nature
Savant Health
Natural Woman

## Atomisers
Jurlique Aromamist or Jurlique Rosewater Facial Spray
Xynergy Health Rose Water Spray
Evian Mist (from chemists and some beauty counters)

## Skin care and hair care products:
The Green People Company
Ecozone
Xynergy Health
Pharma Nord
Spiezia Organic Care

## Honey
Comvita Manuka Honey
From health stores

Also
Xynergy Health
New Zealand Natural Foods

## Linseeds
Linusit Gold is now available from most health food stores, some chemists and supermarkets
Linoforce linseeds are available from health stores. Contact Bioforce for information.
Cold Milled Flax seeds – Higher Nature

## Organic chocolate – health stores. See Green & Black.

## Organic herbal and regular teas –
health stores, some supermarkets.
Also
Jurlique
Eco-zone

## Spirulina/green juice
Try Apotheke 20:20
Xynergy Health
Higher Nature
& Health food stores

## Help for allergies
*Anti-allergy bedding, organic cottons, filters, air purifiers, anti-pollen and anti-vapour masks, ionisers, emf protection, water purifiers, light boxes, detergent-free clothes washing products*

The Healthy House
Ecozone
Savant Health (ceramic laundry discs)

### Specialist foods for people with wheat, gluten & dairy allergies
Stamp Collection & Virani Food Products (see main address list for details)

The following brands are also available from most health food stores and some supermarkets. A number of them supply foods by direct mail. An Internet search will provide web addresses and e-mail contacts for:
Orgran, The Village Bakery, Everfresh, Trufree, Doves Farm, Goodness Direct, Kallo, Lyme Regis Foods, St. Helen's Dairy, Delamere Dairy, Raven's Oak Dairy & Woodlands Park Dairy.
See also
Foods Matter, a superb resource for food allergy sufferers.

### Bleach-free sanitary protection
See Bodywise and Natural Woman

### Juicing Equipment
Lakeland Limited
Savant Health
& from most electrical retailers

### Mandolin slicer
Lakeland Limited
& Hardware stores

### Natural toothcare
Green People Company
Weleda
Biocare
Ecozone
& Health food stores

### Stay-fresh vegetable bags
Lakeland Limited

# Resources: How to Find A Practitioner

If you live in London, the following multi-therapy centres have a staff of qualified practitioners and offer a wide range of services and valuable information:

### The Wren Clinic,

All Hallows House, Centre for Natural Health, Idol Lane, London EC3R 5DD
Tel: 020 7283 8908 Monday to Thursday.
Website: www.wrenclinic.co.uk
Nutrition therapy, McTimoney chiropractic, acupuncture, homoeopathy etc.

If you are outside London, All Hallows will try to help you find a practitioner nearer to your home.

### Apotheke 20-20

296 & 300-302 Chiswick High Road, London W2H 1PA
Tel: 020 8995 2293 (appointments)
Website: www.apotheke20-20.co.uk
Qualified practitioner support os also available by telephone to those who cannot travel to London. Personal consultations in London. Visit website and click Naturopathic Clinic.

Jane McWhirter's Book *The Practical Guide To Candida (page 218)*
This contains a UK directory of practitioners who treat candidiasis with natural medicine. It costs £11 and is available from 93 Ram Gorse, Harlow, Essex CM20 1PZ.

### The Hale Clinic

7 Park Crescent, London W1B 1PF
Tel: 0870 167 6667
Website: www.haleclinic.com

### Health Interlink

Unit B, Asfordby Business Park, Welby, Melton Mowbray, Leicestershire LE14 3JL
Tel: 01664 810011
Website: www.health-interlink.com

Health Interlink offers diagnostic/testing services to practitioners for conditions such as candidiasis, digestive malfunction, intestinal permeability, parasites, bacterial overgrowth, food sensitivity and more. This company isn't able to give telephone advice or discuss individual cases but it is happy to tell you if it knows of a practitioner in your area.

### Stress

Tel: 020 7233 5566
Email: ken@chihealthcentres.com
The Safeline (listed above) is primarily for confidential guidance and information on stress. If you're under

pressure and want to talk to a qualified therapist or counsellor, or if you're trying to find a practitioner in your local area, then try this number or use the email address given above.

The following UK-based organisations hold lists of registered practitioners:

Check with your GP or local Family Health Service Authority (in the 'phone book) to find out which, if any, alternative and complementary therapies are available through your NHS practice.

### Governing Bodies/Institutes/ Associations of Alternative Medicine

Website: www.britishservices.co.uk

### British Naturopathic Association

2 Goswell Road,
Street, Somerset BA16 0JG
Tel: 08707 456985
Website: www.naturopaths.org.uk

### National Federation of Spiritual Healers

Old Manor Farm Studio, Church Street, Sunbury-on-Thames,
Middlesex TW16 6RG
Tel: 0845 123 2777
Website: www.nfsh.org.uk

### McTimoney Chiropractic

The McTimoney Chiropractic Association, 21 High Street, Eynsham, Oxford OX8 1HE
Tel: 01865 880974
Website:
www.mctimoney-chiropractic.org

### The British Chiropractic Association

17 Blagrave Street, Reading,
Berkshire RG1 1QB

Tel: 0118 950 5950
Website: www.chiropractic-uk.co.uk

### General Chiropractic Council

344-354 Gray's Inn Road, London
WC1X 8BP
Tel: 020 7713 5155
Website: www.gcc-uk.org

### British Medical Acupuncture Society

12 Marbury House, Higher Whitley, Warrington, Cheshire WA4 4QW
Tel: 01925 730727
Website: www.medical-acupuncture.co.uk

### The UK Homoeopathic Medical Association

6 Livingstone Road, Gravesend, Kent
DA12 5DZ
Tel: 01474 560336
Website: www.homoeopathy.org

### British Homeopathic Association

15 Clerkenwell Close,
London EC1R 0AA
Tel: 020 7566 7800
Website: www.trusthomeopathy.org
(when looking for websites, be aware of the two different spellings of the word homeopathy/homoeopathy)

### British Complementary Medicine Association

P.O.Box 5122, Bournemouth,
Dorset BH8 0WG
Tel: 0845 345 5977
Website: www.bcma.co.uk

## Other Useful Addresses

### Digestive Diseases Foundation

3 St. Andrew's Place, Regents Park,
London NW1 4LB
Tel: 020 7486 0341
Website: www.digestivediseases.org.uk

**Hyperactive Children's Support Group (HACSG)**
71 Whyke Lane, Chichester, West Sussex PO19 2LD
Website: www.hacsg.org.uk
Really valuable information for allergy sufferers and for those with allergic and/or hyperactive youngsters. A very dedicated, non-profit-making organization. Please send large stamped addressed envelope and £1 donation towards expenses.

**National Association for Diverticular Disease**
7 Cambridge Road, Orrell, Wigan, Lancashire WN5 8PL
Tel: 01942 213572
Website: www.ukselfhelp.info

**What Doctors Don't Tell You**
Website: www.wddty.co.uk
Groundbreaking journal that lives up to its name.

**Women's Environmental Network**
P.O.Box 30626, London E1 1TZ
Tel: 020 7481 9004
Website: www.wen.org.uk

For those interested in keeping up to date with environmental issues. Send large stamped addressed envelope for details. Membership available.

**Self-Help Website**
Website: www.ukselfhelp.info
Go to the website above and click on the alphabet letter you need.

If you are concerned about animal welfare and factory farming and are interested in supporting and receiving information from non-violent pressure groups, contact:

**Compassion in World Farming (CIWF)**
5A Charles Street, Petersfield, Hampshire GU32 3EH or
CIWF, P.O.Box 206, Cork, Ireland
Contact either address for their Action Pack and membership details. CIWF also have a youth group called FarmWatch.

**Farm Animal Welfare Network**
P.O. Box 40, Holmforth, Huddersfield, West Yorkshire HD7 1QY

## APPENDIX FIVE

# Sources of Reference

## Introduction

Deckelbaum, R J *et al*, 'Unified dietary guidelines – summary of a consensus conference on preventive nutrition: paediatrics to geriatrics', copy of American Heart Association conference proceedings, 18 June 1999.
'Eight guidelines for a healthy diet', Food Sense document published by HMSO, 1990.
'National food survey on household food consumption, expenditure and nutrient intake', second quarter 1998, Government Statistical Service, published by the Ministry of Agriculture, Fisheries and Food, 7 September 1998.

## Food Combining – Then and Now

Cohen, Mark Nathan, *Health and the Rise of Civilisation*, Yale University Press, 1989.
Grant, Doris and Joice, Jean, *Food Combining for Health*, Thorsons, 1984.
Hay, Dr William Howard, *A New Health Era*, 1934.
Hay, Dr William Howard, *Health via Food*, Harrap, 1934.
Marsden, Kathryn, *Food Combining in 30 days*, Thorsons, 1994.
Marsden, Kathryn, *The Food Combining Diet*, Thorsons, 1993.
Schepper, Luc de, *How to Dine like the Devil and Feel like a Saint*, Full of Life Publishing, 1993.
Schonfield, Hugh, *The Essene Odyssey*, Element Books, 1984.
Shelton, Dr Herbert M, *The Myth of Medicine*, Lodi Books, 1995. Originally published as *Rubies in the Sand*, 1961.
Shelton, Dr Herbert M, Willard, Jo and Oswald, Jean A, *The Original Natural Hygiene Weight Loss Diet Book*, Keats Publishing, 1986.
Shelton, Dr Herbert M, *Orthobionomics – Volume 1 of the Hygienic System*, published by Dr Shelton's Health School, 1934.
'Why we need a healthy plate of slushy greens', article from the *Daily Mail*, 3 June 1999.
Wolfe, David, *The Sun Food Diet Success System*, Maul, 1999.

## Going into Detail: Fruit

Diamond, H and Diamond M, *Fit for Life*, Bantam Books, 1985, pp 61–77.
Diamond, M, *A New Way of Eating*, Bantam Books, 1987, pp 5 and 10–11.

Marsden, Kathryn, *The Food Combining Diet,* Thorsons, 1993, pp 77–81.

McCance & *Widdowson's The Composition of Foods* (fifth edition), Fruit and Nuts Supplement, Royal Society of Chemistry, 1992.

McCance & *Widdowson's The Composition of Foods,* Milk Products and Eggs Fourth Supplement, Royal Society of Chemistry, 1997.

Notes provided to the author by Dr David Chappell MB.BS FRCS (Glasgow) MF Hom., DO., MGO (Lond.).

Shelton, H, *Food Combining Made Easy,* Willow Publishing, 1979.

Wolfe, D, *The Sun Food Diet Success System,* Maul, 1999, pp 212–14 and 296.

## Food Combining for Good Digestion

Burdon M L *et al,* 'A comparison of the glycaemic and insulinaemic effects of an Asian and European meal', *Practical Diabetes,* 1994; 11 : pp 208–11.

Colbin, A, *Food and Healing,* Ballantine Books, 1986, p 78.

Eastwood, M A *et al,* 'Physical properties of dietary fiber that influence physiological function: a model for polymers along the gastrointestinal tract', *American Journal of Clinical Nutrition,* 1992;55 : pp 436–42.

Eastwood, N A, Brydon, W G and Anderson, D M W, 'The effect of the polysaccharide composition and structure of dietary fibers on meal fermentation and fecal composition', *American Journal of Clinical Nutrition,* 1986; 44 : pp 51–5.

Englyst, H N and Cummings, J H, 'Improved method for measurement of dietary fiber in non-starch polyscchardies in plant foods', *Journal of the Association of Official Analytical Chemists,* 1988; 71 : pp 808–14.

Francis, C Y, 'Bran and IBS: time for reappraisal', *Lancet,* 1994;344 : pp 39–40.

Gibson, G R *et al,* 'Selective stimulation of bifidobacteria in the human colon by oligofructose and inulin', *Gastroenterology,* 1995; 108 : pp 975–82.

Grant, Doris, 'Food combining – it works', *International Journal of Alternative and Complementary Medicine,* January 1994, pp 17–19.

Guyton A C, *Textbook of Medical Physiology* (eighth edition), WB Saunders, 1991, pp 727–35.

Letter to the author from Doris Grant, dated 14 March 1996.

Spiller, R C, 'Cholesterol fibre and bile acids', *Lancet,* 1996; 341 : pp 415–16.

Stephens, A M and Cummings, J H, 'Mechanism of action of dietary fibre in the human colon', *Nature,* 1980; 284 : pp 283–4.

Thompson, W C T, 'Doubts about brain,' *Lancet,* 1994; 344 : pp 3.

Trowell, H, 'Ischemic heart disease and dietary fiber', *American Journal of Clinical Nutrition,* 1972; 25 : pp 926–32.

Vander, Arthur J, *Human Physiology – The Mechanics of Function,* McGraw Hill, 1986, pp 459–503.

Wason, H S *et al,* 'Fibre supplemented food may damage your health', *Lancet,* 1996; 348 : pp 319–20.

Wunsch, H, 'Link between fibre and colorectal cancer debunked in largest-ever study', *Lancet,* 1999; 353 : pp 385.

Guyton, Arthur C, *Textbook of Medical Physiology,* W B Saunders, 1991, pp 709–42.

# Food Combining and Blood Glucose

Anderson, R A *et al*, 'Supplemental chromium effects on glucose, insulin, glucagon and urinary chromium losses in subjects consuming low chromium diets', *American Journal of Clinical Nutrition*, 1991; 54: pp 909–16.

Anderson, R W and Lev-Ran, A, 'Hypoglycaemia: The standard and the fiction', *Psychosomatics*, 1985; 26: pp 38–47.

Baker, B, 'Chromium supplements tied to glucose control', *Family Practice News*, 15 July 1996, p 15.

'Bioavailability of chromium', update, *UK journal of Alternative and Complementary Medicine*, August 1994, p 32.

'Chromium-niacin food supplement lowers serum cholesterol in university study', *The American Chiropractor*, June 1991, pp 22–4.

'Chromium picolinate', special report, *Tufts' University Diet & Nutrition Letter*, October 1996, pp 4–6.

Cunningham, J J, 'The glucose/insulin system and vitamin C: implications in insulin-dependent diabetes mellitus', *Journal of the American College of Nutrition*, 1998; 17: pp105–8.

Data presented at the 57th Annual Scientific Session of the American Diabetes Association, Boston, Massachusetts, 23 June 1997.

'Dietary allowances for chromium announced', report, *Townsend Letter for Doctors*, January 1990.

Editorial: 'Chromium deficiency – 90 per cent of your patients may be at risk', report in *The American Chiropractor*, Sept/Oct 1992, pp 22–4.

'Enhanced insulin action and chromium picolinate', report presented by the Diabetes Comprehensive Care and Research Program at the Bowman Gray School of Medicine, Wake Forest University, to the 57th Annual Scientific Session of the American Diabetes Association, Boston, 23 June 1997.

Flowers, S W, 'Absorption of simple sugars', *Townsend Letter for Doctors*, July 1992; p 594.

Freund, H *et al*, 'Chromium deficiency during total parenteral nutrition', *Journal of the American Medical Association*, 1979; 1241 [51]: pp 496–8.

Frost, G *et al*, 'The effect of low glycaemic carbohydrate on insulin and glucose, response in vitro and in vivo in patients with coronary heart disease', *Metabolism*, 1996; 45: pp 669–72.

Frost, G *et al*, 'Insulin sensitivity in women at risk of coronary heart disease and the effect of a low glycaemic index diet', *Metabolism* 1998; 47: pp 1245–51.

Frost, G *et al*, 'Glycaemic index as a determinant of serum HDL-cholesterol concentration', *Lancet*, 1999; 353: pp 1045–8.

Gaby, A R and Wright J V, 'Nutritional regulation of blood glucose', *Journal of Advancement in Medicine*, 1991; 4(1): pp 57–67.

Hackman, R M, 'Chromium and cholesterol', parts 1 and 2, *Townsend Letter for Doctors*, Aug/Sept 1991 and Oct/Nov 1991.

Hadii-Georgopoulos, A, Schmidt, M L I, Margolis, S and Kowarski, A A, 'Elevated hypoglycaemic index and late hyperinsulinism in symptomatic postprandial hypoglycaemia', *Journal of Clinical Endocrinology and Metabolism*, 1980; 50 : pp 371–6.

Harris, S, 'Hyperinsulinism and dysinsulinism', *Journal of the American Medical Association*, 1924; 83 : p 729.

Harris, S, 'The diagnosis and treatment of hyperinsulinism', *Annals of International Medicine*, 1936; 1010 : p 54.

Heaton, K W, Marcus, S N, Emmett, P H and Bolton, D H, 'Particle size of wheat, maize, oat test meals: effects on plasma glucose and insulin responses and rate of starch digestion in vitro', *American Journal of Clinical Nutrition*, 1988; 471: pp 675–82.

Hofeldt, F D, 'Reactive hypoglycaemia', *Metabolism*, 1975; 24 : pp1193–1208.

Hudspeth, W J, Peterson, L W, Soli, D E and Trimble, B A, 'Neurobiology of the hypoglycaemia syndrome', *Journal of Holistic Medicine*, 1981; 3[10]: p 60.

'Intense sweeteners do not decrease appetite,' *Obesity 91 Update*, May/June 1991; fig 4.

Liu, V J and Abernathy, R P, 'Chromium and insulin in young subjects with normal glucose tolerance', *American Journal of Clinical Nutrition*, 1982; 25[4]: pp 661–7.

Mason, P, 'Handbook of Dietary Supplements (Blackwell Science, 1995), USA gives chromium an official RDA', update, *UK Journal of Alternative and Complementary Medicine*, May 1990, p 24.

Matsen, Dr John, *Eating Alive*, Crompton Books, 1987.

O'Hare, J A, 'The enigma of insulin resistance and hypertension', *American Journal of Medicine*, 1988; 84 : pp 505–10.

Reaves, G M, 'The role of insulin resistance in human disease', *Diabetes*, 1985; 37 : pp 1595– 1606.

Shah, S *et al*, 'The significance of the flat glucose tolerance test', *Journal of the Kansas Medical Association*, November 1975; pp 263–7.

Stebbing, J B, Turner M O, and Franz K B, 'Reactive hypoglycaemia and magnesium', *Magnesium Bulletin*, 1982; 2 : p 131.

Taylor, L and Rachman S, 'The effects of blood sugar level changes on cognitive function, affective state and somatic symptoms', *Journal of Behavioural Medicine*, 1988; 11[3]: pp279–91.

'The slimming scandal', *The Food Magazine*, Feb/Apr 1992; pp 8–9.

Velussi, M *et al*, 'Long-term treatment with an antioxidant drug silymarin is effective on hyperinsulinemia, exogenous insulin, need and malonidaldehyde levels in cirrhotic diabetic patients', *Journal of Hepatology*, 1997; 26 : pp 871–9.

'Vitamins and minerals: A scientific evaluation of the range of safe intakes', draft prepared by Dr Derek Shrimpton, 1996.

'Weight – get yourself a healthy body', video produced by Iron Bridge Film and Television Ltd., 45 Muswell Road, London N10 2BS, telephone 020 8444 9574.

'Wright, J V, 'The glucose-insulin tolerance test and its relevance to "essential hypertension" and HDL/LDL cholesterol abnormalities', *International Clinical Nutrition Review*, 1990; 10[3]: pp 381–2.

## Food Combining Chemistry

Acid/alkaline food lists provided to the author by Dr David Chappell MB.BS FRCS (Glasgow) MF Hom., DO., MGO (Lond.).

Best, S, 'VDUs: The eyes get it', *What Doctors Don't Tell You*, Wallace Press, 1999;10[7]: p 12.

Blackmore, M C H, *Mineral Deficiencies in Human Cells*, Blackmores Communications Service, 1983.

Cohen, K S, *The Way of Qigong*, Ballantine Books, 2000, pp 131–5.

Colbin, A, 'Food and Healing', Ballantine Books, 1986, pp 73–81.

Fisher, Dr Leslie, *The Clinical Science of Mineral Therapy*, Maurice Blackmore Research Foundation, 1991.

Sherman, H C and Sinclair, J E, 'The balance of acid-forming and base-forming elements in foods: a preliminary paper', *Journal of Biology and Chemistry*, 1907; 3 : pp 307–9.

Thompson, Peter and Thompson, Donna, *Complete Food Combining*, Bloomsbury, 1996, pp 29–30.

Ultmann, John E (Ed), *The Blood Handbook*, Hartley & Marks, 1991.

## Food Combining and Eating Disorders

Author telephone conversation with the Mental Health Foundation.

Author telephone conversation with the Eating Disorders Association, 9 and 10 June 1999.

Bryce-Smith, D and Simpson, R, 'Case of anorexia nervosa responding to zinc sulphate', letter to the Editor, *Lancet*, 1984; 2 : 350.

Bryce-Smith, D and Simpson, R, 'Anorexia, depression and zinc deficiency', *Lancet* 1984; 2 : p 1162.

Dinsmore W W *et al*, 'Zinc absorption in anorexia nervosa', letter to the Editor, *Lancet* 1985; 1 : pp 1041–2.

*Eating Disorders: A guide for primary care*, Eating Disorders Association, 1995.

Hoek, H W, 'The incidence and prevalence of anorexia nervosa in primary care', *Psychological Medicine* 1991; 21 : pp 455–60 (quoted from *Mental Health Research Review 4*, April 1997).

Hoek, H W, 'Review of epidemiological studies of eating disorders', *International Review of Psychiatry*, 1993; 5 : pp 61–74 (quoted in Eating Disorders: *A guide to purchasing and providing services*, Eating Disorders Association, 1995.

Howlett, M, McClelland, L and Crisp, A H 'The cost of the illness that defies', *Postgraduate Medical Journal*, 1995; 71 : pp 36–9 (quoted from *Mental Health Research Review 4*, April 1997).

Palmer, R L, *Understanding Eating Disorders*, Family Doctor Publications, 1996.

Thomas, P, 'Eating Disorders – starved of the right foods', *What Doctors Don't Tell You*, Wallace Press, 1998; 8[10]: pp 1–4.

'Eating Disorders', council report CR14, Royal College of Psychiatrists, 1992.

Turnbull, S, Ward, A, Treasure, J, Jick, H and Derb, L, 'The demand' for eating disorder care: An epidemiological study using the general practice research database', *British Journal of Psychiatry*, 1996; 169: pp 705–12.

## Food Combining Detox

Chaitow, L, *Amino Acids in Therapy*, Thorsons, 1985, pp 88–90.

Cohen, Mark Nathan, *Health and the Rise of Civilisation*, Yale University Press, 1989.

Cox, Peter and Brusseau, Peggy, *Secret Ingredients*, Bantam Books, 1997.

Erdmann, R and Jones, M, *The Amino Revolution*, Century, 1987.

Guyton, Arthur, C, *Textbook of Medical Physiology*, W B Saunders, 1991.

Kampert, J B *et al*, 'Physical activity, physical fitness, and all-cause mortality: a prospective study of men and women', *Annals of Epidemiology* 1996; 6 : pp 452–7.

Shelton, Dr Herbert, M, *The Myth of Medicine*, Lodi, 1995.

To-Figueras, J *et al*, 'Glutathione S-transferase M1 GSTM1 and T1 GSTT1 polymorphisms and lung cancer risk among Northwestern Mediterraneans', *Carcinogenesis* 1997; 18[8]: pp 1529–33.

## If you do Nothing Else . . .

Guyton, Arthur C, *Textbook of Medical Physiology* (eighth edition), W B Saunders, 1991, pp 709–42.

*McCance & Widdowson's The Composition of Foods*, Milk Products and Eggs fourth Supplement, Royal Society of Chemistry, 1997.

Shelton, Dr Herbert, M, *Food Combining Made Easy*, Willow Publishing, 1982, pp 24–5.

Vander, Arthur J, *Human Physiology – The Mechanics of Function*, McGraw Hill, 1986, pp 459–503.

## Food Combining for Healthy Weight Loss

Author's personal correspondence with the Institute for Optimum Nutrition, dated 16 April 1992. Also a photocopy of research report on food combining from *Optimum Nutrition* newsletter, 1998; 11[3]: pp 12–13.

Cabot, S, 'A healthy liver and weight loss,' *Positive Health*, February 1999, pp 33–9.

Geiselman, P T and Novin, D, 'The role of carbohydrate in appetite, hunger and obesity', *Appetite*, 1982; 3 : pp 203–23.

Randolph, T G, 'Masked food allergy as a factor in the development and persistence of obesity', *Journal of Laboratory and Clinical Medicine*, 1947; 32 : p 1547.

Randolph, T G and Moss, R W, *Allergies – Your Hidden Enemy*, Thorsons, 1980.

Rodin, J, 'Comparative effects of fructose, aspartame, glucose and water preloads on calorie and macronutrient intake', *American Journal of Clinical Nutrition*, 1990; 51 : pp 428–35.

*Stay Young Longer*, Booklet by the editors of *Prevention Magazine*, 1996.

Toubro, S and Astrup, A, 'Randomised comparison of diets for maintaining obese subjects' weight after major weight loss: ad-lib, low-fat, high-carbohydrate diet versus fixed energy intake', *British Medical Journal*, 1997; 314 : pp 29–34.

Vogel, H C A, *The Nature Doctor*, Mainstream Publishing, 1989, pp 201–3.

'Weight – get yourself a healthy body', video produced by Iron Bridge Film and Television Ltd., 45 Muswell Road, London N10 2BS, telephone 020 8444 9574.

## Food Combining Detox: Better Breathing Techniques

Author's own interviews with practitioners.

'Your Healthy House', special report from *What Doctors Don't Tell You*, Wallace Press, 2000; 10[1]: pp 2–4

## The Importance of Exercise

'As weight goes up, so does breast cancer risk', *Tufts University Diet and Nutrition Letter*, 1996; 14[5]: pp 1–2.

The Arthritis Foundation website: www.arthritis.org

Dekkers, J C *et al*, 'The role of antioxidant vitamins and enzymes in the prevention of exercise-induced muscle damage', *Sports Medicine*, 1996; 21[3]: pp 213–38.

Kampert, J B *et al*, 'Physical activity, physical fitness, and all-cause mortality: a prospective study of men and women', *Annals of Epidemiology*, 1996; 6 : pp 452–7.

'Rx for arthritis sufferers: exercise', *Tufts University Diet and Nutrition Letter*, 1996; 14[5]: p 1

Weaver, C and Rajaram S, 'Exercise and iron status', *Journal of Nutrition*, 1992; 122 : pp 782–7.

## Easy Ways to Ease the Effects of Stress

Labott, S M and Martin, R B, 'The stress modulating effects of weeping and humour', *Journal of Human Stress*, 1987;13[4]: pp 159–64.

Schedlowski, M and Schmidt, R E, 'Stress and the immune system', extract translated from *Naturwissenschaften*, 1996;83[5]: pp 214–20.

Sheridan, J F *et al*, 'Psychoneuroimmunology: stress effects on pathogenesis and immunity during infection', *Clinical & Microbiological Review*, 1994; 7[2]: pp 200–12.

Sieder, W S *et al*, 'Modulation of human, natural killer cell activity by exposure the uncontrollable stress', *Stress, Brain, Behaviour and Immunity*, 1992; 9[2]: pp 141–59.

## Food Combining and Fluid Retention

'Eating less sodium means retaining more bone', report, Tufts *University Diet & Nutrition Letter*, 1996; 14[4]: pp 1–2.

Hanneman, R L, 'INTERSALT study: hypertension rise with age revisited', *British Medical Journal*, 1996; 312 : pp 1283–9.

Law, M R *et al*, 'Analysis of data from trials of salt reduction', *British Medical Journal*, 1991; 302 : pp 819–24.

'More salt suspicions', report, *The Food Magazine*, Jan March 1997, p15.

Notes taken from the DASH study (dietary, pattern and hypertension). 'Dietary approaches to stop hypertension', Department of Nutrition, University of Tennessee, Knoxville, 1997; 55[8]: pp 303–5.

Rocchini, A P *et al*, 'The effect of weight loss on the sensitivity of blood pressure to sodium in obese adolescents', *New England Journal of Medicine*, 1989; 321[9]: pp 580–5.

Ruppert, M, *et al*, 'Short-term dietary sodium restriction increases serum lipids, and insulin in salt-sensitive and salt-resistant normotensive adults', precis translation from German journal *Klin Wochenschr*, 1991; 69[25]: pp 51–7.

'Salt and blood pressure', nutrition feature, *The Food Magazine*, July/Sept 1995, p 15.

'The salt sellers', report, *The Food Magazine*, July/Sept 1991, pp 14–15.

Whelton, P K, *et al*, 'Sodium reduction and weight loss in the treatment of hypertension in older persons', *Journal of the American Medical Association*, 1998; 279 [11]: pp 839–46.

## Food Combing Detox: Long-term Protection – Reducing Your Exposure to Toxins

Blythman, Joanna, *The Food We Eat*, Michael Joseph, 1996.

Cox, Cat, *Chocolate Unwrapped: The Politics of Pleasure*, Women's Environmental Health Network, 1993.

Cox, Peter and Brussean, Peggy *Secret Ingredients*, Bantam Books, 1997.

Dibb, Sue, *What the Label Doesn't Tell You*, Thorsons, 1997.

Dinham, Barbara (compiler), *The Pesticide Hazard – A Global Health and Environmental Audit*, Zed Books, 1993.

'Dog flesh in animal feed', reported in *The Food Magazine*, July/Sept 1999, p 5.

Harvey, Graham, *The Killing of the Countryside*, Jonathan Cape, 1997.

Visioli, F *et al*, 'Low density lipoprotein oxidation is inhibited in vitro by olive oil constituents', *Arteriosclerosis*, 1995; 117 : pp 25–32.

'What the journals say', reported in *The food Magazine*, Oct/Dec 1991.

## Going into Detail

'Department of Health Dietary Reference Values for food energy and nutrients for the United Kingdom', reports of the Panel on Dietary Reference Values of the Committee on Medical Aspects of Food Policy (COMA), HMSO, 1991.

Grant, Doris and Joice, Jean, *Food Combining for Health*, Thorsons, 1984.

Guyton, Arthur C, *Textbook of Medical Physiology* (eighth edition), W B Saunders, 1991.

Hay, Dr William Howard, *Health via Food*, Harrap, 1934.

Hay, Dr William Howard, *A New Health Era*, 1934.

Marsden, Kathryn, *Food Combining in 30 Days*, Thorsons, 1984.

Marsden, Kathryn, *The Food Combining Diet*, Thorsons, 1993.

*McCance & Widdowson's The Composition of Foods* (fifth edition), Royal Society of Chemistry, 1991.

*McCance & Widdowson's The Composition of Foods* (fifth edition), Fruit and Nuts Supplement, Royal Society of Chemistry, 1992.

*McCance & Widdowson's The Composition of Foods* (fourth edition), Cereals and Cereal Products Supplement, Royal Society of Chemistry, 1988.

Shelton, Dr Herbert M, *Food Combining Made Easy*, Willow Publishing, 1951.

Vander, A J, Sherman, J H and Luciano D S, *Human Physiology: The Mechanisms of Human Function* (fourth edition), McGraw-Hill, 1986.

## Food Combining and Food Allergies

Bjarnason, I, Peters, T J and Levi, A J, 'Intestinal permeability: clinical correlates', *Digestive Diseases*, 1986; 4 : pp 83–92.

Bland, J, 'The food for one may be poison for another', *International Journal of Alternative and Complementary Medicine*, March 1995, pp 16–17.

Collins, A M *et al*, 'Bovine milk, including pasteurised milk, contains, antibodies directed against allergens of clinical importance to man', *Internal Archives of Allergy & Applied Immunology*, 1991; 96 : pp 362–7.

Crandall, M, 'Allergic predisposition in recurrent vulvovaginal candidiasis', *Journal of the Advancement of Medicine*, 1991; 4[1]: pp 21–38.

Grant, D, 'Allergies and the missing link', *Positive Health*, December 1998, pp 39–40.

Henzgen' M *et al*, 'Food hypersensitivity in patients with tree-pollen allergy and the influence of hyposensitization', *Allergologie* 1991; 14[3]: pp 90–4.

Randolph, T G and Moss, R W, *Allergies – Your Hidden Enemy*, Thorsons, 1980.

Sampson, H A *et al*, 'Spontaneous release of histamine from basophils and histamine-releasing factor in patients with atopic dermatitis and food hyper-sensitivity', *New England Journal of Medicine*, 1989; 321 : pp 228–32.

Walker-Smith, J A, 'Food sensitive enteropathies', *Clinics in Gastroenterology*, 1986; 15[1]: pp 55–69.

Young, E *et al*, 'A population study of food intolerance', *Lancet* 1994; 343 : pp 127–9.

# Postscript

My passion for food combining has, inevitably, attracted a bit of attention here and there. Over the years, I've been tagged food combining 'guru' and food combining 'evangelist'. I've also been called 'that food combining woman' by a journalist who couldn't remember my name, and 'food combining fanatic' by someone who was certain that food combining was a 'con'.

I accept that not everyone agrees that food combining is valuable, but I think it's sad and unfortunate that a few fault-finders feel it necessary to criticise food combining without learning about it first. This achieves nothing. 'One does not have to accept the dogmatic assertions of exspurts[sic], who know it all and know it all wrong,' said Dr Herbert Shelton, one of food combining's most diligent researchers. The half-a-dozen minor whinges that I've received in the past 16 years have all been of the unpleasant, sour-faced variety, from people who, when pressed, admitted that they've never actually tried food combining but just know that it definitely, absolutely, couldn't possibly work. Criticism is, of course, only ever constructive and fair if it emanates from a point of knowledge, not from one of ignorance.

I hope that, in the foreseeable future, funds will be made available so that researchers can carry out more detailed scientific study into food combining's many benefits. Acceptance of the system by orthodox medicine will surely come. It isn't weird or extreme. It isn't some new fad that has just been invented and never put properly to the test.

But change takes time.

Highly effective and talented practitioners of therapies such as chiropractic, acupuncture, herbalism and homoeopathy were once dismissed as practising quackery. They were then upgraded to 'fringe medicine', until grudging acceptance that they might know what they were talking about eventually promoted them to 'alternative'. Now that holistic and natural approaches have achieved such an enviable – and no longer ignorable – track record in restoring good health, conventional medics have had no choice but to accept them as complementary to the mainstream.

As the years pass, and more and more people discover better health as a result of food combining, perhaps it, too, will achieve the status it deserves.

Enjoy the blessings and the beauty of your life
Appreciate the gifts it has given you
They are far more significant than you think
Do something good every day for someone else
Sing
Smile
Laugh out loud
Eat your greens
File the compliments
Forget the insults
Make allowances for other people's bad moods
Don't be thoughtless with other people's affections
Protect yourself from people who are thoughtless with yours
Don't waste time being jealous or envious
Life is too short
Accept the ups and the downs of every day
Say thank you
Don't drop litter
Recycle
Go organic
Eat some fruit
Make time to stand and stare
Breathe more deeply
Treat wildlife and the countryside with respect
Drive a little slower and accept that delays often have good reason
The journey is the same
Be joyful
Life is precious

# Index